Intelligent Systems Reference Library

Volume 178

The aim of this series is to publish a Reference Library, including novel advances and developments in all aspects of Intelligent Systems in an easily accessible and well structured form. The series includes reference works, handbooks, compendia, textbooks, well-structured monographs, dictionaries, and encyclopedias. It contains well integrated knowledge and current information in the field of Intelligent Systems. The series covers the theory, applications, and design methods of Intelligent Systems. Virtually all disciplines such as engineering, computer science, avionics, business, e-commerce, environment, healthcare, physics and life science are included. The list of topics spans all the areas of modern intelligent systems such as: Ambient intelligence, Computational intelligence, Social intelligence, Computational neuroscience, Artificial life, Virtual society, Cognitive systems, DNA and immunity-based systems, e-Learning and teaching, Human-centred computing and Machine ethics, Intelligent control, Intelligent data analysis, Knowledge-based paradigms, Knowledge management, Intelligent agents, Intelligent decision making, Intelligent network security, Interactive entertainment, Learning paradigms, Recommender systems, Robotics and Mechatronics including human-machine teaming, Self-organizing and adaptive systems, Soft computing including Neural systems, Fuzzy systems, Evolutionary computing and the Fusion of these paradigms, Perception and Vision, Web intelligence and Multimedia.

** Indexing: The books of this series are submitted to ISI Web of Science, SCOPUS, DBLP and Springerlink.

More information about this series at http://www.springer.com/series/8578

Prasant Kumar Pattnaik ·
Suneeta Mohanty · Satarupa Mohanty
Editors

Smart Healthcare Analytics in IoT Enabled Environment

Springer

Editors
Prasant Kumar Pattnaik
School of Computer Engineering
KIIT Deemed to be University
Bhubaneswar, Odisha, India

Suneeta Mohanty
School of Computer Engineering
KIIT Deemed to be University
Bhubaneswar, Odisha, India

Satarupa Mohanty
School of Computer Engineering
KIIT Deemed to be University
Bhubaneswar, Odisha, India

ISSN 1868-4394 ISSN 1868-4408 (electronic)
Intelligent Systems Reference Library
ISBN 978-3-030-37553-9 ISBN 978-3-030-37551-5 (eBook)
https://doi.org/10.1007/978-3-030-37551-5

This Springer imprint is published by the registered company Springer Nature Switzerland AG
The registered company address is: Gewerbestrasse 11, 6330 Cham, Switzerland

Preface

The edited book aims to bring together leading researchers, academic scientists, and research scholars to put forward and share their experiences and research results on all aspects of wireless IoT and analytics for smart healthcare. It also provides a premier interdisciplinary platform for educators, practitioners, and researchers to present and discuss the most recent innovations, trends, and concerns as well as practical challenges encountered and solutions adopted in the fields of IoT and analytics for smart health care. The book is organized into fifteen chapters.

Chapter 1 presents an overview of smart healthcare analytics in IoT-enabled environment including its benefits, applications, and challenges.

Chapter 2 focuses on the use of mobile technologies in healthcare service and presents a selected list of emerging research areas. The review is an attempt to capture the most recent stage in the development of mobile communications and computing toward the domain of IoT in healthcare applications in recent years and identify the broad research challenges with the hope that it will aid researchers to identify the evolutionary path of the discipline and prepare their research program. This chapter describes the role of IoT in health care including from its current applications, some related projects, and the research issues in detail.

Chapter 3 discusses 5G in IoT. It also discussed some techniques, characteristics, and security challenges that may be faced by the fifth generation when it is used.

Chapter 4 presents a portable device (wearable gear) with its communication system which can be used to measure different health parameters and proper care of the child can be taken accordingly. This chapter brings an attempt and interest among the researchers to monitor the health of rural children in different "Anganwadi" centers.

Chapter 5 presents an approach to provide secured smart door knocker using IoT, that will check the details of the person who knocked the door, is authorized hospital visitor or not.

Chapter 6 presents an application of FCM-based segmentation method followed by an effective fusion rule to study and analyze the progression of Alzheimer's disease. Selection of salient features from each of the RGB plane of PET image and elimination of artifacts are done by applying fuzzy C-mean clustering approach.

Chapter 7 discusses the application and some of the case studies of machine learning in various medical fields like diagnosing diseases of brain and heart.

Chapter 8 focuses on the removal of salt and pepper noise from the contaminated Giemsa-stained blood smear image using probabilistic decision-based average trimmed filter (PDBATF). The experiments' outcomes are recorded and compared with recently reported algorithms. The proposed algorithm provides better accuracy level in terms of peak signal-to-noise ratio, image enhancement ratio, mean absolute error, and execution time.

Chapter 9 explains the importance of feature selection and feature creation related to biomedical data. It also discusses various methods of feature selection with its advantages and disadvantages for biomedical data. The experimental result of this chapter shows that the prediction accuracy of classifiers to be 100% in most of the cases. The accuracy of classifiers is much better with selected features and gives accurate results with less time and cost.

Chapter 10 presents a technique for real-time deep learning-based scene image detection and segmentation and neural text-to-speech (TTS) synthesis, to detect, classify, and segment images in real-time views and generate their corresponding speeches.

Chapter 11 focuses on a comparative study of different filter bank approaches in terms of classification accuracy using a binary classification BCI competition dataset which has obtained EEG signals from a single subject. Two fundamental types of filter banks have been used along with their non-overlapping and overlapping temporal sliding window-based techniques.

Chapter 12 states a new framework based on the denoising stack autoencoder and compressing sampling design. The method enables to solve an optimization problem without performing the product of large matrices; instead, it takes the advantage of the stacked and structure of compressing sampling providing better performance than traditional greedy pursuit CS methods. Compressing sensing (CS) has been considered for many real-time applications such as MRI, medical imaging, remote sensing, signal processing.

Chapter 13 presents an overview of big data framework for analytics of medical data. It discusses how does the proper selection of features and application of machine learning techniques can lead to a better understanding of diseases through experiments.

Chapter 14 presents an electroencephalography(EEG)-based approach for brain activity analysis on the multimodal face dataset to provide an understanding of the visual response invoked in the brain upon seeing images of faces (familiar, unfamiliar, and scrambled faces) and applying computational modeling for classification along with the removal/reduction of noise in the given channels.

Chapter 15 aims to present the state-of-the-art research relating to various IoT features, its architecture, security features, and different mechanisms to provide a secure working environment for an IoT system.

We are sincerely thankful to the Almighty to supporting and standing at all times with us, whether it is good or tough times and given ways to concede us. Starting from the call for chapters till the finalization of chapters, all the editors gave their contributions amicably, which is a positive sign of significant team works. The editors are sincerely thankful to all the members of Springer especially Prof. Lakhmi C. Jain for providing constructive inputs and allowing an opportunity to edit this important book. We are equally thankful to the reviewers who hails from different places in and around the globe shared their support and stand firm toward the quality chapter submission.

Bhubaneswar, India

Prasant Kumar Pattnaik
Suneeta Mohanty
Satarupa Mohanty

About This Book

Healthcare service is a multidisciplinary field that emphasizes on various factors like financial system, social factors, health technologies, and organizational structures that affect the health care of individuals, family, institutions, organizations, and populations. The goal of healthcare services includes patient safety, timeliness, effectiveness, efficiency, and equity. Health service research evaluates innovations in various health policies including medicare and medicaid coverage, discrepancy in utilization, and access of care. Smart health care comprises m-health, e-health, electronic resource management, smart and intelligent home services, and medical devices. The Internet of Things (IoT) is a system comprising of real-world things that interact and communicate with each other with the help of networking technologies. The wide range of potential applications of IoT includes healthcare services. IoT-enabled healthcare technologies are suitable for remote health monitoring including rehabilitation, assisted ambient living, etc. Healthcare analytics can be applied to the collected data from different areas to improve health care with minimum expenditure. This edited book is designed to address various aspects of smart health care to detect and analyze various diseases, the underlying methodologies, and their security concerns.

Key Features

1. Addresses the issues in healthcare services and requirements of analytics.
2. Addresses the complete functional framework workflow in IoT-enabled healthcare technologies.
3. Explores basic and high-level concepts, thus serving as a manual for those in the industry while also helping beginners to understand both basic and advanced aspects of IoT healthcare-related issues.
4. Based on the latest technologies, and covering the major challenges, issues, and advances in IoT healthcare.
5. Exploring intelligent healthcare and clinical decision support system through IoT ecosystem and its implications to the real world.
6. Explains concepts of location-aware protocols and decisive mobility in IoT health care for the betterment of the smarter humanity.
7. Intelligent data processing and wearable sensor technologies in IoT-enabled healthcare.
8. Exploring human–machine interface and its implications in patient-care system in IoT healthcare.
9. Exploring security and privacy issues and challenges related to data-intensive technologies in healthcare-based Internet of Things.

Contents

About the Editors

Prasant Kumar Pattnaik, Ph.D. (Computer Science), fellow IETE, senior member IEEE is a professor at the School of Computer Engineering, KIIT Deemed to be University, Bhubaneswar, India. He has more than a decade of teaching and research experience. He has published numbers of research papers in peer-reviewed international journals and conferences. He also published many edited book volumes in Springer and IGI Global Publication. His areas of interest include mobile computing, cloud computing, cyber security, intelligent systems, and brain–computer interface. He is one of the associate editors of *Journal of Intelligent and Fuzzy Systems*, IOS Press and Intelligent Systems Book Series Editor of CRC Press, Taylor Francis Group.

Suneeta Mohanty, Ph.D. (Computer Science) is working as an assistant professor at the School of Computer Engineering, KIIT Deemed to be University, Bhubaneswar, India. She has published several research papers in peer-reviewed international journals and conferences including IEEE and Springer as well as serves as an organizing chair (SCI-2018). She was appointed in many conferences as a session chair, reviewer, and track co-chair. Her research area includes cloud computing, big data, Internet of Things, and data analytics.

Satarupa Mohanty, Ph.D. (Computer Science) is working as an associate professor at the School of Computer Engineering, KIIT Deemed to be University, Bhubaneswar, India. She has published several research papers in peer-reviewed international journals and conferences. She was appointed in many conferences as a session chair, reviewer, and track co-chair. Her research area includes bioinformatics, big data, and Internet of Things.

Chapter 1
Smart Healthcare Analytics: An Overview

Suneeta Mohanty, Satarupa Mohanty and Prasant Kumar Pattnaik

Abstract The goal of healthcare services includes patient safety, timeliness, effectiveness, efficiency, and equity. Smart healthcare comprises of m-health, e-health, electronic resource management, smart and intelligent home services and medical devices. Internet of Things (IoT) enabled healthcare technologies are suitable for remote health monitoring with minimum expenditure. This chapter gives an overview including benefits, application, and challenges of smart healthcare analytics in IoT enabled environment.

Keywords Healthcare · Internet of Things (IoT) · Analytics · Security

1.1 Introduction

Healthcare is essentially defined as the improvement or maintenance of health and relevant facilities through the diagnosis, treatment and prevention of the disease, sickness, injury or mental disorders in people. Physicians and health professional provides healthcare services. The integral part of the healthcare industry comprises of Nursing, medicine, dentistry, optometry, pharmacy, physiotherapy and psychology. Access to healthcare depends on demography, socioeconomic conditions and health policies and may differ across nations, boundaries, communities and individuals. Healthcare systems are meant to address the health requirements of target populations. Healthcare is conventionally considered as an important factor for the well-being of people around the world. An impelling healthcare system can identify the irregular health conditions and make diagnoses from time to time. The swiftly aging populace and the related rise in chronic illness are playing a significant role

S. Mohanty (✉) · S. Mohanty · P. K. Pattnaik
School of Computer Engineering, KIIT Deemed to Be University, Bhubaneswar, India
e-mail: smohantyfcs@kiit.ac.in

S. Mohanty
e-mail: satarupafcs@kiit.ac.in

P. K. Pattnaik
e-mail: patnaikprasantfcs@kiit.ac.in

P. K. Pattnaik et al. (eds.), *Smart Healthcare Analytics in IoT Enabled Environment*,
Intelligent Systems Reference Library 178,
https://doi.org/10.1007/978-3-030-37551-5_1

in modern healthcare structures, and the demand for resources from hospital beds to expert medical personnel is increasing at an alarming rate. Evidently, a solution is needed to curtail the pressure on manual healthcare systems whilst continuing to implement high-quality care to unstable patients, by using all the technical advancement at our disposal. An efficient healthcare system can contribute to a significant part of a country's development, economy and industrialization.

1.1.1 Internet of Things (IoT)

In 1999, Kevin Ashton used the term Internet of Things (IoT) for the first time [1–6]. Internet of Things (IoT) is a system comprising of real world things that interact and communicate with each other with the help of networking technologies [7, 8]. The Internet of Things (IoT) can sense, assemble and transport the data without human intervention over network. IoT uses RFID technology, Sensor technology, Smart technology and Nanotechnology for tagging, sensing, thinking and shrinking of things respectively [9]. IoT architecture comprises of three layers: Physical layer, Network Layer and Application Layer [10]. The physical layer is responsible for the collection of data from things with the help of RFID, Bluetooth, 6LoWPAN technologies and convert them to digital setup. The network layer is responsible for transmission of data between physical layer and application layer securely in wired, wireless and satellite medium. The application layer represents the top most layer of IoT architecture and responsible for providing personalised user based application as per the requirements. In today's scenario, there exist many applications of IoT [11, 12] for industry [13] and healthcare [14].

1.1.2 IoT for Healthcare

Consolidation of IoT with healthcare has sharply increased across various specific IoT use-cases. IoT for healthcare is taking momentum to address the following issues:

- Making the healthcare accessible to remote area where people are deprived of good healthcare service due to several reasons.
- In case of emergency, patients information can be communicated to avoid delay in treatment.
- Reduction of manual patient's data entry by medical staff so that they can monitor the cases efficiently.

To make the IoT healthcare system well-organized, functional and successful, its ubiquitous influence needs to be considered. The IoT devices are required to be resistant to adverse environmental conditions. A particular use case in which IoT device is used by people living in remote and underdeveloped areas and getting involved in occupations like agriculture and construction activities. A damaged device might send inaccurate data. This adds limitations to the usage of such devices and keeping out of reach to such people. Certain other factors like humidity, moisture in the air, sweat and direct contact with water affect the connectivity and performance of IoT devices [15]. To solve this problem, hydrophobic nano-coating solutions can be used to maintain uptime and device reliability across the entire IoT domain. The full application of IoT in the area of healthcare lets medical centers function more competently and enables patients to obtain a better course of treatment. With the usage of a technology-based healthcare method, there are incomparable benefits which could improve the efficiency and quality of treatments as well as the health of the patients.

1.2 Benefits of Smart Healthcare

Health service research evaluates innovations in various health policies including medicare and medicaid coverage, discrepancy in utilization and access of care. Smart healthcare comprises of m-health, e-health, electronic resource management, smart and intelligent home services and medical devices. The Internet of Things (IoT) can sense, assemble and transport data without human intervention over the network. Thus, Internet of Things (IoT) enabled healthcare technologies are suitable for remote health monitoring.

1.2.1 Real-Time Reporting and Monitoring

Often, there have been situations where a patient falls extremely sick and by the time an ambulance is arranged and the patient to rushed to the hospital, the situation worsens. In case of medical emergency, real-time monitoring can save lives. Real-time monitoring can be achieved using IoT devices/Applications to collect and transfer health data like blood sugar and oxygen levels, blood pressure, ECG plots and weight to physician over Internet [16]. These collected data are stored in the cloud for further action by the authorised personnel regardless of their time and place. A study conducted via the Center of Connected Health Policy indicates that due to remote patient monitoring on heart failure patients reduced the readmission rate to 50%.

1.2.2 Affordability and End-to-End Connectivity

In IoT based healthcare system various connectivity protocols like Wi-Fi, Bluetooth, ZigBee etc. are used to automate the patient care workflow. Interoperability, data flow, machine-to-machine communication features of IoT enabled healthcare system provides revolutionary ways of treatment at lower cost. Smart healthcare system avoids unnecessary visits by utilizing quality resources and improves the recovery strategy thus bring down the cost.

1.2.3 Data Assortment and Analysis

To support the real-time application feature of IoT healthcare system, connected devices sends large amounts of data in a very short period. To store and manage such huge amount of data from multiple devices and to analyze the data in real-time, access to cloud is required. All these works will be done over cloud and the authorized personnel will get access to the reports with graphs. Thus, IoT healthcare system speed up decision-making with the help of these healthcare analytics irrespective of time and place. Real-time alerting, monitoring and tracking is possible using IoT which makes the medical treatment more efficient.

1.2.4 Remote Medical Assistance

In case of an emergency, a patient can contact a doctor situated at a distant location via a smart phone application only. With mobility solutions in healthcare, the doctor/physician can instantly check the vitals of the patient and identify the ailment. Besides, numerous healthcare delivery chains that are predicting the manufacture of machines which can deliver drugs on the basis of a patient's prescription and the data related to the aliment(s) available on the linked devices. This will act as an impetus to saving money and resources.

1.3 Challenges of Smart Healthcare

Technology has attracted more or less all industries inclusive of finance, business, healthcare, and others. Intending to revolutionize the treatment with a prior and proper diagnosis the healthcare industry is the right upfront to adopt the advancement in the technology. The IoT (Internet of Things) has considerably captured the healthcare industry in a comparably short period. For instance, due to the connected devices, there is the possibility of allowing older persons to concern the doctor safely in their place. It helps doctors to grant the benefit of having recourse with the respective specialists worldwide regarding the complex cases. However, every pro have its cons attached to it. Accordingly, any technological advancement comes up with its challenges which have to succeed with proper trafficking. Following are some challenges associated with its implication for the users of healthcare IoT devices.

1.3.1 Data Security and Privacy Threats

The privacy and security of storing and handling personal health information through connected devices is the fundamental concern for the regulatory of IoT facilities in healthcare. In real-time, IoT devices capture data and transmit those data through the connected environment. However, due to the lack of standardization of the protocols the security issues enter into the picture. Many healthcare industries have the illusion of storing their sensitive information in a secure and encrypted form, without any inside track over the security of data access point. This creates a remarkable threat which gradually increases with the introduction of new devices in the network. Additionally, there is the consequence of ambiguity come up concerning the data ownership regulation [17]. These components make the data immensely influenced or harmed by cybercriminals and hackers and ultimately endangering the Personal Health Information (PHI) of both doctor's as well as the patent's.

1.3.2 Multiple Devices and Protocols Integration

For the efficient deployment of IoT in the healthcare industry the principal obstacle is the integration of multiple heterogeneous devices. To collect the patient's data, most medical equipments have to be interconnected and have to be operated cooperatively [18]. For example, one individual suffering from diabetes can have heart disease as well. The point of concern is that the heterogeneous equipment has not followed a set of protocol standardization. This insufficiency homogeneity within the medical equipment scale down the purposeful deployment of IoT in healthcare.

1.3.3 Data Overload and Accuracy

The operational heterogeneity and unambiguousness in the communication standard and protocols cause to happen many complexities in the process of collection of data and its aggregation. IoT based medical equipments collect a flood of data and take advantage to derive the better solution deduce from the patient's report. Anyhow, extracting the insights from the tremendous data without data experts and refined analytics measure is quite challenging. Additionally, the growth of data makes it utmost critical for the physicians and medical specialists to identify the meaningful and actionable data and to reach to a flawless conclusion. Ultimately this result to the interference in the decision-making process and gives rise to poor quality result. On top of that, the concern is more problematic with the increase in the number of connected devices to the IoT [18].

1.3.4 Internet Disruptions

When checking the performance of medical IoT software, testing specialists deal with the load, network bandwidth, latency, and other metrics both for mobile and web applications. In case of crash under an unexpected load surge, it is unacceptable to have crashed in healthcare IoT. Especially for smart medical devices directly involved in patient care, such as a continuous patient monitoring system or a smart insulin pump it is completely unacceptable [19].

1.4 Applications of Smart Healthcare

The scope of large number of applications of IoT in healthcare instigate the individuals to avail the facility. The application of IoT in a medical centre provides a remote healthcare services as reducing tracking staff, patients and inventory, ensuring availability of critical hardware, reducing emergency room wait time and enhancing drug management and so on. Following sections addresses the various healthcare applications of remote monitoring of patient, elderly care, remote medication, telemedicine and providing consultancy through smart applications.

1.4.1 Glucose-Level Monitoring

The percentage of diabetic people is increasing day by day. Thus, monitoring their glucose level on a daily basis is highly required. IoT based healthcare has the capability of monitoring levels of glucose continuously in a non-invasive way. The patients can take help of the wearable sensors which has can able to track continuously the health parameters and can transfer the collected data to the healthcare providers [20]. The tracking device consists of a mobile phone, a blood glucose collector and an IoT-based medical procurement detector which can monitor the level of glucose.

1.4.2 Electrocardiogram (ECG) Monitoring

Electrocardiogram (ECG) monitoring is an essential requirement for heart patient. In this type of healthcare monitoring system, wireless transmitter and receiver are used to track heart rate and the basic rhythm, along with the identification of multifaceted arrhythmias, myocardial ischemia by recording the electrical activity of the heart [20].

1.4.3 *Blood Pressure Monitoring*

Blood Pressure (BP) monitoring can be done using wearable sensor device. The device should have a BP apparatus to record the BP and should have Internet based communication to transmit the data for analysis. Blipcare is an example of such device.

1.4.4 *Wearable Devices*

For the healthcare sector IoT has introduced a number of wearable devices like hearables, ingestible sensors, moodables and healthcare charting which has shaped a comfortable lives for patients. The hearables are new-age hearing tools that have entirely made over the lifestyle of the people who suffered from hearing issues and have entirely loosed the interaction with the outer world [21].

1.5 Conclusion

In the arena of Internet, there exists an array of alternative healthcare applications to provide smart healthcare. With the usage of a technology-based healthcare method, there are incomparable benefits which could improve the efficiency and quality of treatments as well as the health of the patients. Modern-day healthcare devices should analyze the collected data to find all possible solutions and should determine the optimal solution by taking into consideration different priorities and constraints of the applications.

References

1. Mingjun, W., Zhen, Y., Wei, Z., Xishang, D., Xiaofei, Y., Chenggang, S., et al.: A research on experimental system for Internet of Things major and application project. In: International Conference on System Science, Engineering Design and Manufacturing Informatization (ICSEM), pp. 261–263 (2012)
2. Rose, K., Eldridge, S., Chapin, L.: The Internet of Things (IoT): an overview—understanding the issues and challenges of a more connected world. In: Internet Society (2015)
3. Gubbi, J., Buyya, R., Marusic, S., Palaniswami, M.: Internet of Things (IoT): a vision, architectural elements, and future directions. Future Gener. Comput. Syst. **29**, 1645–1660 (2013)
4. Farooq, M., Waseem, M., Khairi, A., Mazhar, S.: A critical analysis on the security concerns of Internet of Things (IoT). Int. J. Comput. Appl. **111** (2015)
5. Rao, T.V.N., Saheb, S.K., Reddy, A.J.R.: Design of architecture for efficient integration of Internet of Things and cloud computing. Int. J. Adv. Res. Comput. Sci. **8** (2017)

6. Bandyopadhyay, D., Sen, J.: Internet of Things: applications and challenges in technology and standardization. Wireless Pers. Commun. **58**, 49–69 (2011)
7. Fan, Y.J., Yin, Y.H., Xu, L.D., Zeng, Y., Wu, F.: IoT-based smart rehabilitation system. IEEE Trans. Ind. Inform. **10**(2), 1568–1577 (2014)
8. Gershenfeld, N., Krikorian, R., Cohen, D.: The Internet of Things. Sci. Am. **291**(4), 76–81 (2004)
9. Bilal, M.: A review of Internet of Things architecture, technologies and analysis smartphone-based attacks against 3D printers. arXiv preprint arXiv:1708.04560 (2017)
10. Silva, B.N., Khan, M., Han, K.: Internet of Things: a comprehensive review of enabling technologies, architecture, and challenges. IETE Tech. Rev. 1–16 (2017)
11. Xu, L.D.: Enterprise systems: state-of-the-art and future trends. IEEE Trans. Ind. Inform. **7**(4), 630–640 (2011)
12. He, W., Xu, L.D.: Integration of distributed enterprise applications: a survey. IEEE Trans. Ind. Inform. **10**(1), 35–42 (2014)
13. Sauter, T., Lobashov, M.: How to access factory floor information using Internet technologies and gateways. IEEE Trans. Ind. Inform. **7**(4), 699–712 (2011)
14. Tarouco, L.M.R., Bertholdo, L.M., Granville, L.Z., Arbiza, L.M.R., Carbone, F., Marotta, M., et al.: Internet of Things in healthcare: interoperatibility and security issues. In: Proceedings of IEEE International Conference on Communications (ICC), pp. 6121–6125 (2012)
15. https://www.bresslergroup.com/blog/rugged-iot-considerations-for-electronic-components/
16. Gupta, P., Agrawal, D., Chhabra, J., Dhir, P.K.: IoT based smart healthcare kit. In: International Conference on Computational Techniques in Information and Communication Technologies (ICCTICT), IEEE, Mar 2016, pp. 237–242
17. Einab, K.A.M., Elmustafa, S.A.A.: Internet of Things applications, challenges and related future technologies. World Sci. News **67**(2), 126–148 (2017)
18. Laith, F., Rupak, K., Omprakash, K., Marcela, Q., Ali, A., Mohamed, A.: A concise review on Internet of Things (IoT)—problems, challenges and opportunities. In: 11th International Symposium on Communication Systems, Networks & Digital Signal Processing (CSNDSP) (2018)
19. Mayank, D., Jitendra, K., Rajesh, K.: Internet of Things and its challenges. In: International Conference on Green Computing and Internet of Things (ICGCIoT) (2015)
20. Vandana, S., Ravi, T.: A review paper on "IOT" & it's smart applications. Int. J. Sci. Eng. Technol. Res. (IJSETR) **5**(2), 472–476 (2016)
21. Upasana: Real World IoT Applications in Different Domains. https://www.edureka.co/blog/iot-applications/ (2019)

Chapter 2
Mobile Communications and Computing: A Broad Review with a Focus on Smart Healthcare

Debarshi Kumar Sanyal, Udit Narayana Kar and Monideepa Roy

Abstract Wireless networks are ubiquitous today. Cellular networks, wireless local area networks, and wireless personal area networks are among the most common ones. Simultaneously the proliferation of smartphones has led to new kinds of mobile applications. Notably, the healthcare industry has leveraged the benefits of mobile computing in several ways, including health monitoring and feedback, the swift transmission of diagnostic reports, and coordination with medical professionals. The progress notwithstanding, there are many research challenges in wireless networks and mobile computing that need to be addressed for wider deployment of the technology and better user experience. In this paper, we survey the state of the art in mobile communications and computing – with a special focus on the use of mobile technologies in healthcare service – and present a selected list of emerging research areas.

Keywords Mobile communications · Wireless networks · Survey · Standards · IoT · Healthcare

2.1 Introduction

Wireless communications has altered the world of interaction in an exceptional way, allowing people across continents to communicate in real-time. It was born in the 1890s with the pioneering works of Sir Jagadish Chandra Bose [13] and Marconi [47]. Radio communication systems were subsequently used in the Second World War. Although mobile transceivers for the public were available since the 1940s, widespread growth in mobile telephony began with the deployment of cellular net-

D. K. Sanyal
Indian Institute of Technology Kharagpur, Kharagpur, West Bengal 721302, India

U. N. Kar (✉) · M. Roy
School of Computer Engineering, Kalinga Institute of Industrial Technology (Deemed to be University), Bhubaneswar, Odisha 751024, India
e-mail: monideepafcs@kiit.ac.in

P. K. Pattnaik et al. (eds.), *Smart Healthcare Analytics in IoT Enabled Environment*, Intelligent Systems Reference Library 178,
https://doi.org/10.1007/978-3-030-37551-5_2

works in the early 1980s. It was followed by the use of fully digital systems from the early 1990s. *Cellular communications*– one of the most successful forms of wireless communications that divides a land area into cells and provides each with multiple frequencies and base stations – has evolved through several generations to provide integrated voice, video and data services at a high speed to mobile users. 3G/4G networks can transport high definition multimedia in addition to traditional voice transmission. Similarly, high bandwidth wireless local area networks are available for connecting laptops and tablets in offices and conferences. The ability to wirelessly connect using portable devices allows users to access information and software located at a different location and thus enables *mobile computing*. With the proliferation of sensors, tablets, and smartphones, it appears that most of the devices around us will soon be networked together. This envisioned connectivity among different devices – from embedded microprocessors to desktops – with each other and finally to the Internet will make computing possible everywhere and always. This is commonly hailed as ubiquitous or *pervasive computing*. It subsumes the field of mobile computing and plans for a completely connected ambiance of computing devices. Internet of Things (IoT) is all set to make it a reality [27]. Some recent surveys on mobile communications are [60] (published in 2012) and the papers included in the 2018 special issue [21] of the Elsevier journal *Computer Communications*. The latter papers retrospect how the field has matured over the last 40 years.

Contribution: This review is an attempt to capture the state of the art in mobile communications and computing, with an emphasis on IoT in healthcare applications, and what seems to lie in the foreseeable future. We identify the broad research challenges with the hope that it will aid researchers to identify the evolutionary path of the discipline and prepare their research program. Given the enormity of the subject, we only attempt an overview of the most active application-oriented topics (in particular, we do not discuss protocol details and open theoretical problems) and provide a carefully distilled bibliography of expository tutorials and recent comprehensive surveys of more focused topics. Although [60] discusses the landscape of wireless communications, their stress is more on radio technologies, while our view is more holistic. Unlike them, we also include a summary of the role of IoT in the healthcare sector. The rest of the chapter is organized as follows. In Sect. 2.2, we discuss the main network types classified by their spatial coverage. We outline the active research areas in mobile communications in Sect. 2.3. The main characteristics of mobile computing, or more specifically, smartphone computing, are described in Sect. 2.4, which is followed by a list of research areas in Sect. 2.5. The role of IoT in healthcare, including vignettes from its current applications, some related projects, and research issues are detailed in Sect. 2.6. We conclude in Sect. 2.7.

2.2 Mobile Communications

This section discusses the broad types of wireless networks in terms of their main technical features.

2.2.1 Common Mobile Wireless Networks

We discuss the main types of wireless networks categorized by their coverage area. The categories are shown in Table 2.1.

Wireless Wide Area Networks (WWAN) Cellular networks are the most common type of WWAN. Here a geographic area is divided into cells each with a base station and subscribers. Users in adjacent cells communicate using different frequencies while far-off cells can reuse the same frequencies. This is done to avoid interference caused by simultaneous transmissions in the same frequency.

The first generation (1G) cellular technologies (in the 1980s) used analog systems to carry voice. Introduction of digital cellular technology in the 1990s marked the second generation (2G) that provided both data (e.g., short message service) and voice, and allowed user mobility. The 3G or third generation (since ~ 2000) pioneered by standards like Universal Mobile Telecommunications Service (UMTS) and Code Division Multiple Access 2000 (CDMA2000) increased information transfer rates to 2 Mbps for walking users and 384 kbps for moving vehicles. The higher data rates allow streaming video, mobile television and Internet access from mobile devices. The 4G or fourth generation (~2010 onward) is built on revolutionary physical layer (PHY) techniques like MIMO-OFDM (expands to Multiple Input Multiple Output - Orthogonal Frequency Division Multiplexing) that uses *multiple antennas* at transmit and receive ends to increase data rate or reliability or both, and *orthogonal carriers* for interference reduction and better resilience to propagation loss [72]. It provides information rates of 100 Mbps to mobile users and up to 1 Gbps to indoor users. The role of MIMO in the dramatic growth of wireless communications cannot be

Table 2.1 Different categories of wireless networks

Wireless networks	Applications	Example standard
WWAN	Voice, data and multimedia transmission over long distance	LTE-A (for 4G)
WLAN	Extension or alternative to cabled LANs	IEEE 802.11 (Wi-Fi)
WMAN	Last-mile Internet connectivity to wireless users in large areas	IEEE 802.16 (WiMAX)
WPAN	Industrial and home automation	IEEE 802.15.4 (LR-WPAN)
WBAN	Health monitoring	IEEE 802.15.6

overemphasized. In case of an error-free wireless link with one antenna at the transmit side and one on the receive side, the capacity of the link, expressed in bits/sec/Hz is given by Shannon's formula $C = Q \log_2(1 + \chi)$ where χ is the ratio of signal power to noise power at receiver. This means, capacity increases only logarithmically with transmit power. Thus, to increase capacity, transmit power has to be increased significantly. Instead, if we use a $Q \times Q$ MIMO channel, i.e., Q parallel channels between the transmitter and receiver, and divide the transmit power equally among the channels, the capacity becomes $C = Q \log_2(1 + \frac{\chi}{Q})$ where we have assumed equal receiver noise. This is a multiplicative jump in capacity. Another feature of 4G is that it is supposed to be an all-IP network, i.e., it uses packet switching for both voice and data, unlike pre-4G technologies. Long-Term Evolution (LTE) and LTE-Advanced are well-known standards for 4G. The fifth generation (5G) mobile communications systems are currently being developed and expected to be standardized by 2020 [3]. It aims at 1000× improvement in aggregate data rates (i.e., the total amount of data the network can serve, characterized in bits/s per unit area) over 4G. It will provide 100 Mbps to 1 Gbps to users even in the worst network conditions. More active users per unit area and increased bandwidth can be afforded by transmitting in millimetre wave spectrum or visible light (indoor environment) and using massive MIMO (outdoor environment) [43]. Network architecture of 5G cellular networks are driven by the demand for high data rates. Given that the link efficiency has almost reached the Shannon limit, researchers are trying to increase the spectral efficiency by increasing the density of node deployment [12]. This ultra-dense network architecture has multiple tiers: macro-cells, pico-cells, and femto-cells. Femto-cells are more suited for indoor use and meant to reduce congestion and load at the macro-cell base station as shown in Fig. 2.1. The mobile terminal must be capable of analyzing and deciding with whom (out of the three kinds of cells) it should associate. 5G networks will also support a user-centric connectivity approach through direct device-to-device (D2D) communication in which devices in close geographic proximity will not use the radio access network but communicate directly with each other. This will lead to tremendously high data rates and very low end-to-end delays. Development of full-duplex transceivers will also lead to a magnification of data rates [39].

Wireless Metropolitan Networks (WMAN) WMAN provides connectivity to large areas like an entire campus or an entire town. IEEE 802.16 (also called WiMAX) is a standard for the physical and medium access control (MAC) layers that provide WMAN scale communications [4]. It explicitly supports Quality of Service (QoS) by defining different scheduling policies for different traffic classes like constant bit rate traffic, real-time traffic, best effort traffic, etc. [10, 20]. Mobile devices connect to a WiMAX base station to achieve Internet connectivity. Explicit support for terminal mobility in WiMAX led to the development of IEEE 802.16m or mobile WiMAX standard. However, the markets adoption of LTE has been significantly greater than that of WiMAX for 4G communications.

Wireless Local Area Networks (WLAN) Predating the WMANs for wireless data connectivity is the WLAN. Reduced costs have made it immensely popular in offices, academic campuses, electronic campuses, houses, hotels, airports, and remote areas.

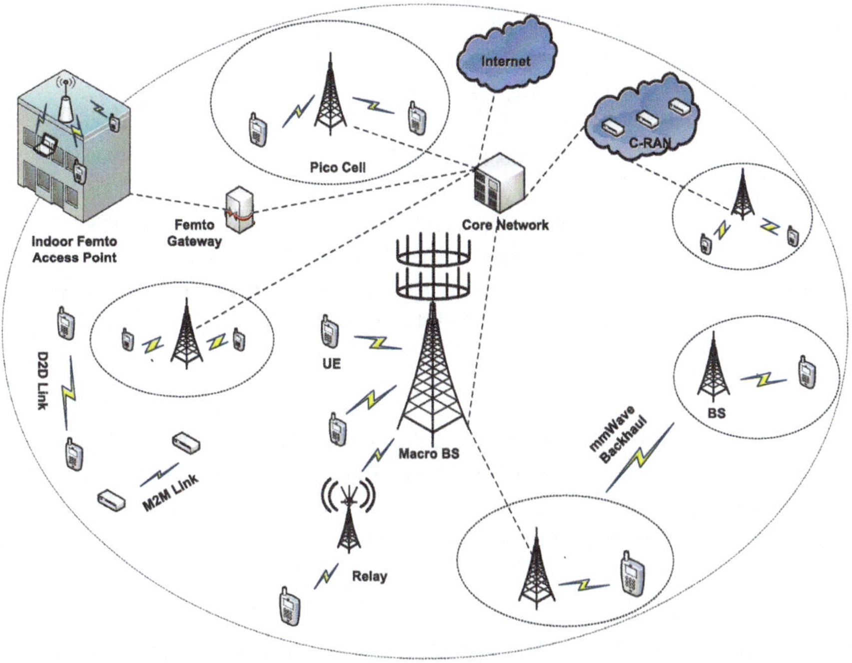

Fig. 2.1 Architecture of 5G network

The IEEE approved 802.11 standard (also called Wi-Fi) for WLANs operates in the license-free 2.4 and 5 GHz ISM band [30]. An IEEE 802.11 style WLAN is based on a cellular architecture; each cell (called a basic service set or BSS) is a set of fixed or mobile devices running the 802.11 protocol. The network architecture may be infrastructure-based where nodes communicate only via a distinguished station called an access point (AP), or ad hoc where nodes communicate directly with each other. We found from an analysis of contemporary and upcoming standards as given in Table 2.2 that the evolution is primarily driven by (1) throughput requirements (e.g., 802.11n, ac, ax), (2) ease of network use (e.g., 802.11y, 802.11aq), (3) QoS requirements (e.g., 802.11e, 802.11ae), and (4) spectrum expansion (e.g., 802.11ad, af, ah). High data rates are achieved in IEEE 802.11n with MIMO while multiuser-MIMO (where access point uses many antennas to simultaneously serve multiple downlink user devices, each equipped with only one or two antennas), advanced modulation and coding schemes and channel bonding raise the rate even higher in IEEE 802.11ac.

Wireless Personal Area Networks (WPAN) In 2003, the IEEE 802.15.4 standard was approved that is particularly suitable for ad hoc wireless networks of resource-constrained sensor devices. More specifically, IEEE 802.15.4 specifies the PHY and MAC layers for *low rate wireless personal area networks (LR-WPAN)*. It offers data rates between 20 and 250 kbps and incurs extremely low power consumption [68].

Table 2.2 Selected IEEE WLAN standards

Standard	Main features	Status
IEEE 802.11	Up to 2 Mbps in 2.4 GHz	Approved 1997
IEEE 802.11a	Up to 54 Mbps in 5 GHz	Approved 1999
IEEE 802.11b	Up to 11 Mbps in 2.4 GHz	Approved 1999
IEEE 802.11e	Support for QoS at MAC layer	Approved 2005
IEEE 802.11n	Up to 600 Mbps in 2.4 and 5 GHz	Approved 2009
IEEE 802.11ac	At least 1 Gbps in 2.4 and 5 GHz	Approved 2013
IEEE 802.11ax	High average throughput per user in high density deployments in 2.4 and 5 GHz	Under development (Expected 2019)

The ZigBee consortium has standardized the higher layers of 802.15.4. WSNs built with IEEE 802.15.4/ZigBee and RFIDs are expected to form the key building blocks of IoT. Bluetooth is another WPAN technology used for connecting small devices in very close proximity ($\sim$10m) but with data rates as high as 2 Mbps. For both IEEE 802.15.4 and Bluetooth, single-hop star topologies and multi-hop topologies are defined and both operate in license-free 2.4 GHz ISM band.

Wireless Body Area Networks (WBAN) An extreme case of short-range ad hoc wireless network is a WBAN that uses low-power wearable sensors for reliable real-time health monitoring. WBAN systems may use radio waves, ultrasonic waves or diffusion-based molecular communications.

2.3 Research Areas in Mobile Communications

We tried to understand research trends by analyzing publication counts related to the above communication systems from the Scopus[1] bibliographic database. We used queries like

```
TITLE-ABS-KEY ( "wireless local area network" OR "wireless lan"
OR "wlan" OR "wifi" OR "wi-fi" OR "802.11" ) AND SUBJAREA ( comp
OR engi ) AND PUBYEAR > 1996 AND PUBYEAR < 2002
```

Parts of the query strings are shown in Table 2.3. Results were retrieved on 5-October-2018. The corresponding plot in Fig. 2.2 reveals that the WLAN research community is extremely active (owing to widespread use of WLAN and the large number of IEEE standards on them) and surpasses other groups in productivity except from 2017 onwards when most of the focus has shifted to 5G. There is also continuing interest in WPAN and WBAN due to their ubiquity in sensor networks and IoT.

[1] https://www.scopus.com/.

Table 2.3 Query strings used to search title, abstract, keywords and subject area in Scopus to generate Fig. 2.2

WWAN	WLAN	WMAN	WPAN	WBAN
TITLE-ABS-KEY ("cellular wireless network" OR "wireless cellular network" OR "wireless wide area network" OR "wwan" OR "cellular network" OR "5G") AND SUBJAREA (comp OR engi)	TITLE-ABS-KEY ("wireless lan" OR "wireless local area network" OR "wifi" OR "802.11") AND SUBJAREA (comp OR engi)	TITLE-ABS-KEY ("wireless metropolitan area network" OR "wman" OR "wimax" OR "802.16") AND SUBJAREA (comp OR engi)	TITLE-ABS-KEY ("wireless personal area network" OR "wpan" OR "bluetooth" OR "zigbee" OR "802.15.4") AND SUBJAREA (comp OR engi)	TITLE-ABS-KEY ("wireless body area network" OR "wban" OR "802.15.6") AND SUBJAREA (comp OR engi)

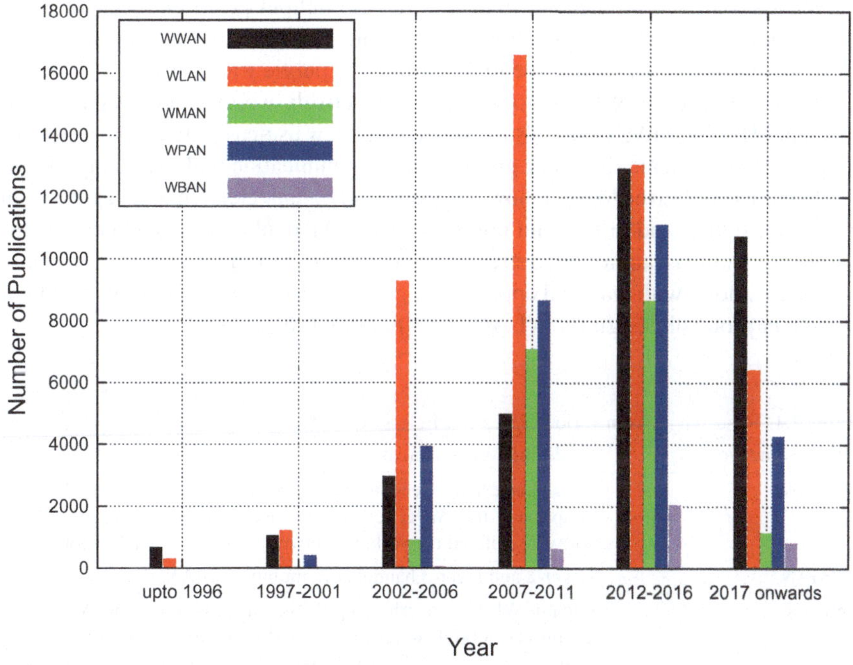

Fig. 2.2 Research trends in mobile communications

2.3.1 Network-Specific Research Directions

We summarize some of the most engaging current research topics for each of these networks below and in Table 2.4.

1. WWAN: The major challenges (especially in 5G) pertain to the overwhelming customer base which is being tackled with hierarchy of cells, massive MIMO (where the pilot contamination problem is critical), mmWave (which is unused but has poor propagation characteristics and generally work only for line-of-sight communication) and D2D communication (where it is often challenging to decide whether a mobile should use D2D mode or cellular mode given multiple optimization criteria) [36]. Software-defined networking is sometimes advanced as a means to simplify dynamic resource allocation. These areas individually and in combination bubble with numerous research challenges [31, 37].
2. WMN: Handover remains an important issue [59] although overall research interest is waning due to lack of business thrust.
3. WLAN: The requirement of high average throughput per user, QoS for high-definition multimedia applications and presence of dense overlapping cells (e.g., in stadiums, campuses, residential apartments, public transport, etc.) drive the research agenda in WLAN. Researchers are actively working on designing efficient PHY and MAC protocols for WLANs for new use-cases. Example problems include how clients should be grouped for communication with AP in uplink and downlink multiuser-MIMO, how to dynamically adapt clear channel assessment (CCA) signals and/or transmit powers in dense AP deployments and how to efficiently multicast audio/video streams [9]. IEEE 802.11ax addresses some of these issues. Along with classical approaches, game theory is expected to play a major role in protocol design for WLAN [19, 48, 50, 63–67].

Table 2.4 Research areas in various types of wireless networks

Wireless network type	Emerging research areas
WWAN	Ultra-dense heterogeneous networks, adoption of massive MIMO, adoption of mmWave, device-to-device communication, software-defined networking, network function virtualization
WMAN	Layer-2 and layer-3 handover in mobile WiMAX
WLAN	Gigabit WLANs, overlapping BSSs, transmission in mmWave, adoption of uplink and downlink multiuser-MIMO, dynamic channel bonding, QoS for multimedia applications
WPAN	Co-existence issues (with other wireless networks in the same frequency band), object identification/naming systems in IoT, forming robust, autonomous networks, standardization aspects of IoT
WBAN	Channel modelling (in-body and off-body channels), standardization, development of energy-efficient protocols, co-existence issues

4. Bluetooth and ZigBee: These devices exist in the same 2.4 GHz ISM band as most IEEE 802.11 WLANs and hence suffer from high co-channel interference. The situation is serious since Bluetooth and ZigBee devices operate at far lower transmit power than WLAN devices. Hence co-existence issues should be investigated in detail by the WPAN community.
5. WBAN: Developing suitable models for both in-body and off-body channels, designing energy-efficient protocols, and standardizing the protocols are contemporary research topics [18]. Sensors are used in IoT where many issues like identification of all *smart* objects, forming robust, autonomous networks and standardization of different technologies and interfaces attract significant research attention. A survey with research directions in IoT appears in [27]. Most of these standards are also being explored for implementation of smart grid applications [24].
6. Mobile Ad hoc Network (MANET): In spite of several hundred research papers published in the field of MANETs in the last two decades, general-purpose MANETs shown in Fig. 2.3 did not really take off as a commercial success.

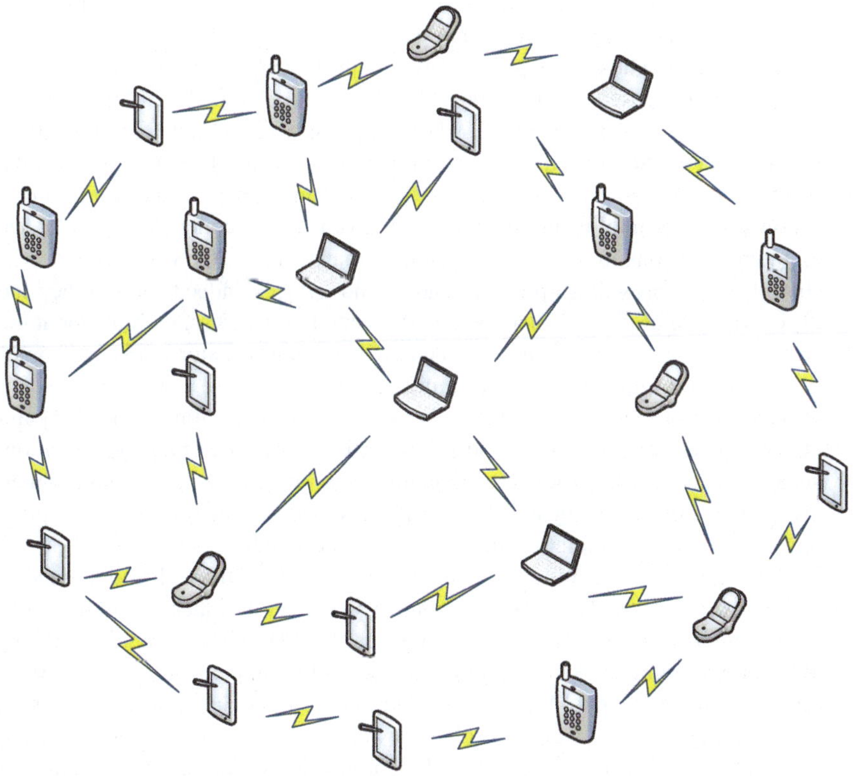

Fig. 2.3 Mobile ad hoc network made of laptops, smartphones, and personal digital assistants

Instead, specialized networks built on the same principles but adapted to specific applications became popular. Conti and Giordano [22] attribute the success of the MANET specializations to five factors: application-oriented development, complexity reduction, focused research, use of realistic simulation models and development of real network testbeds with the users involvement. In the coming days, increasing efforts will go into standardizing various features of MANETs in the specific contexts of WSN, vehicular ad hoc networks, and delay tolerant networks. Considerable research has been done and is in progress on connectivity, routing, medium access control [35] and security protocols of MANET [7, 74].

2.3.2 Generic Research Directions

We now identify a set of generic research topics cutting across network types. The five contemporary research directions we mention below need more attention for improved performance and wider deployment of wireless networks. Progress in these fields will be extremely useful for most of the network types we surveyed.

1. Cognitive Systems: The explosive rate of increase in the customer base of cellular networks and the scarcity of available spectrum are motivating researchers to develop cognitive radios [29] that can coexist with legacy/primary spectrum holders and share the licensed spectrum provided they induce limited or no interference at primary receivers. For example, when the primary user is not communicating, its spectrum could be used by the cognitive radios. It must, though, release the spectrum as soon as the primary user returns. Cognitive radio is a powerful innovation since it is intelligent enough to perceive network conditions to influence its future decisions in aspects like resource management, QoS, security, access control, etc. for providing optimized end-to-end services. Indeed, interference due to co-existence of multiple networks in the same frequency (e.g., think about the crowded unlicensed ISM band) is gradually becoming a major issue, and cognitive techniques might be useful to mitigate them. Cognitive radio networks are also envisioned to use the abundant TV white spaces opportunistically [15] and improve spectrum utilization in the TV transmission band. Introducing cognition, adaptation and learning into network elements is, however, a non-trivial problem involving technical and legal intricacies [70]. No wonder they continue to remain largely confined to simulators and experimental testbeds.
2. Security and Privacy: Wireless channels are, by definition, shared broadcast medium. Hence it makes eavesdropping easy. A host of attacks including jamming, denial-of-service, spoofing, etc. are possible [81]. Cryptographic solutions like a public or private key cryptosystem are hard to implement if no infrastructure is available (as in a MANET) since keys need to be distributed by a trusted source. Extremely lightweight mechanisms need to be devised and embedded in various layers of the protocol stack [54]. Wireless networks are usually deployed in unprotected areas making physical vulnerability another major concern. The

emergence of RFIDs and contact less credit cards has exposed new security threats like relay attack, mafia attack and terrorist attack which must be appropriately addressed [40]. Security and standardized security protocols for WBAN are also a very important research area.

3. Quality of Service (QoS): Wireless networks operate in error-prone conditions. The topology itself is highly volatile. Hence best effort service is the typical service model for data communications. Differentiating high and low priority traffic in terms of bit rate and resource reservation is quite challenging. But QoS support is needed in many applications. In cellular networks, increasing customer base threatens QoS of telephonic calls and can cause congestion and call drops. QoS is pivotal for reliable message delivery in VANETs [62]. Similarly, it may be needed in different sensor networks, especially those used for industrial automation where reliability and real-time response must be simultaneously achieved [78]. Research in QoS provisioning (e.g., one approach is software-defined networking that enables flexible allocation of network resources) is an absolute must if wireless networks are planned to be deployed for heterogeneous applications and multiple business verticals [10, 11, 23, 55].
4. Energy Efficiency: Consider the case of MANETs, especially WSNs. Most routing protocols bootstrap for new destinations by flooding that consumes enormous bandwidth and power. Energy depletion of nodes may partition the network and disconnect distant nodes. Clever methods are needed to couple routing with energy management techniques [58]. Nodes should be selected for routing in such a way that the network is not disconnected. Wireless interfaces also consume a lot of energy. So the transceiver is normally switched off when no transmission or reception occurs. Although it is relatively easy to coordinate the sleep schedules in infrastructure networks, it is a hard problem in highly mobile ad hoc networks. Energy harvesting, that is, extracting energy from the ambient sources like magnetic fields, mechanical vibrations, wind, etc., is also being investigated by researchers [28, 76]. Massive MIMO towers and cloud servers will also require proper power management and cooling systems. Thus energy-efficient design is needed in network deployment, transmission scheme, and resource management.
5. Research Methodology: There are different methodologies to analyze the problems in wireless networks. In general, one encounters optimization problems that are often non-convex and require different advanced techniques for solving. One often also needs lightweight sub-optimal algorithms rather than involved optimal solutions. Some very general frameworks that have recently gained prominence include network utility maximization [52], game theory [6] and matching theory [26]. Researchers usually validate their proposed ideas in a simulator or a testbed. Several simulators for wireless networks are available including ns-2,[2] ns-3,[3] OMNeT++[4] and TOSSIM[5] [53]. Though widely used, there lurk important open

[2]https://www.isi.edu/nsnam/ns/.

[3]https://www.nsnam.org/.

[4]https://omnetpp.org/.

[5]http://networksimulationtools.com/tossim/.

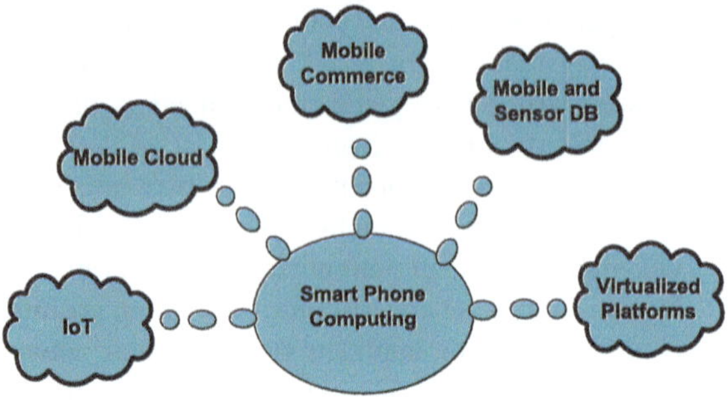

Fig. 2.4 Characteristics of smartphone computing

issues regarding the models (e.g., interference models, mobility models) used by these simulators. Hence researchers are increasingly turning to testbeds for protocol evaluation. Designing and deploying open testbeds will be crucial to reliable validation of complex network protocols required in next-generation systems. In fact, [22] remarks that a reason for the failure of general-purpose MANETs in transitioning from lab to market is the lack of credible simulations and experiments. More interaction between academic researchers and professional engineers, and diffusing research output into real systems and standards are needed [69].

2.4 Mobile Computing

The wide availability of mobile devices has catapulted the adaptation of many traditional applications from static to the mobile environment and the development of many new ones. We feel the emerging mobile computing ecosystem can be roughly captured by calling it *smartphone computing that uses virtualized platforms and likely to use mobile and sensor databases to perform run various mobile apps frequently for sensor-based tasks and mobile commerce, occasionally using mobile cloud and communicating with other IoT devices*. We now elaborate the above italicized terms (also shown in Fig. 2.4).

1. Smartphone Computing: Todays smartphones are equipped with powerful CPUs and adequate memory along with a number of sensors. Thanks to Global Positioning System (GPS) and apps like Life360,[6] mobile devices are aware of their geographic locations and can learn about others' locations. This allows common location- or context-aware information services (like a list of hotels near the user, etc.), as well as online interaction with acquaintances present nearby. The intersection of mobile networks with online social networks (like Facebook[7] and MySpace[8]) is often called *mobile social networking* [38]. The presence of sensors

[6]https://www.life360.com/.

[7]https://www.facebook.com/.

[8]https://myspace.com/.

in smartphones spurred the development of several indoor localization apps that are useful in large uncharted buildings. Smartphones are encouraging another new computing paradigm, *crowdsensing* [17, 44]. For illustration consider this: one can collect information about the physical world (e.g. road traffic condition in a city) using sensors in their smartphones and share them with other smartphone users using cellular or Wi-Fi connections; such crowdsourced collection and processing of data can be beneficial where other reliable data sources are not available. One can build local maps on traffic congestion or a profile of local hospitality services using crowd-sourced data if no commercial help desks are available in the proximity. This is also called *participatory sensing* although one might question the quality of collected information and whether the privacy of participants is protected. Guarantee of privacy protection and other incentives might be needed to motivate users to participate at all. Soon smartphones will also be capable of using machine learning algorithms to construct higher-level concepts from the raw signals recorded by its multi-modal sensors [56]. As smartphone sensing becomes more ubiquitous, information about the physical world will be more liberally available. However, there is a usability requirement: one must have easy ways to query databases of sensed data. Given the plethora of heterogeneous sensors, efforts are needed to define *interoperability standards*. Many researchers and consortiums suggested XML as a means of encoding sensor descriptions, sensor deployments and sensor measurements in the context of WSNs [2]. Defining sharing policies for smartphone readings is an open issue. The sensor databases should be ideally accessible via the Web, thus constituting a worldwide sensor web. One also needs search engines to seek information from the sensor web and regular feeds to run automated monitoring services. Although sensor web and sensor search engines initially proposed in the context of WSNs did not become a business reality, smartphones and IoT might catapult them back into focus.

2. Virtualized Application Platform: Mobile applications need a trusted execution environment to run due to the high probability of malware infections in a mobile network. A simple method to achieve this is application *virtualization*. Here an application is compiled to bytecodes of a software-defined virtual machine which may be then translated to native code (as in Android runtime[6]) and stored. Later the native code is executed by the runtime. Hence the application does not directly interface with the operating system. This controls memory accesses at runtime and guarantees security to a large extent. Virtualization also plays a pivotal role in resource sharing in cloud computing.
3. Mobile and Sensor Databases: Databases for mobile devices need to conform to the low processing power and restricted memory of the device. SQLite[9] and Oracle Database Lite[10] are examples of databases for mobile devices. Oracle Database Lite can also be used to connect and synchronize with a remote enterprise Oracle database. ACID (Atomicity, Consistency, Isolation, and Durability) properties are

[9]https://www.sqlite.org/index.html.

[10]https://www.oracle.com/technetwork/es/database/database-lite/overview/index.html.

usually weakened for transactions in mobile scenarios. Databases for WSNs are more specialized. In fact, such a network may be viewed as a distributed database that collects measurements from the physical world, indexes them and allows queries on them, under power constraints of the nodes, inherent unreliability of routes, and unpredictable delays in data arrival to the sink node. Long-running, continuous queries are common. An example WSN query could be "For the next 2 hours, retrieve the temperature in each town of Bhubaneswar every 15 min". It augments traditional Structured Query Language (SQL) with new clauses to express aspects like duration for the query should run and the frequency at which sensors should take readings. Similarly, there are notions of probabilistic queries that ask for measurements with a certain probability of correctness since uncertainty (noise) is an intrinsic component of sensor readings. Some queries where a maximum (`MAX`) or an average (`AVG`) reading is desired are usually implemented using in-network aggregation. Here, instead of processing the query completely at an external server by collecting together all sensor readings, each node in the query-response propagation path computes a running value (e.g., a partial maximum or a partial average as the case may be) using its own measurement and the inputs it receives from its neighbors, and propagates them to the next hop. This incrementally generates the final report without propagating all the raw readings to the sink. TinyDB from Berkeley is an example sensor database management system [45]. With the proliferation of sensors in smartphones and IoT, sensor databases might emerge as commonplace applications in the near future.

4. Mobile Commerce: Commerce using mobile devices has become popular and is a major leap from offline transactions [73]. Mobile financial transactions (e.g., money transfer, banking, brokerage, auctions, etc.), mobile advertising (e.g., sending custom made advertisements according to users physical location), and mobile shopping (e.g., searching, selecting and ordering products from a mobile terminal) are commonplace. But for many developing countries, more emphasis is needed to address fundamental issues like low network bandwidth that may introduce unacceptable delays or disconnections during transactions.
5. Mobile Cloud Computing: One rapidly upcoming field is cloud computing. Stated very simply, it is a model for providing dynamic on-demand access to a shared pool of configurable resources like servers, storage applications, etc. The end-users can use these resources for computational and storage purposes, thus reducing the cost of procuring them at their end and instead, paying on a usage-basis. Hence it is an attractive business paradigm for the IT houses. The most common cloud service models are cloud Software as a Service (SaaS), cloud Infrastructure as a Service (IaaS), and cloud and cloud Platform as a Service (PaaS) shown in Fig. 2.5. The amalgamation of mobile computing and cloud computing is termed as mobile cloud computing (MCC) [77]. Immediate means to leverage the benefits of cloud computing in the mobile environment are offloading computing power and data storage requirements from mobile devices into resource-rich computers and data centers in the cloud, and delegating computation-heavy baseband signal processing at each cell in a cellular network to more powerful machines in the cloud.

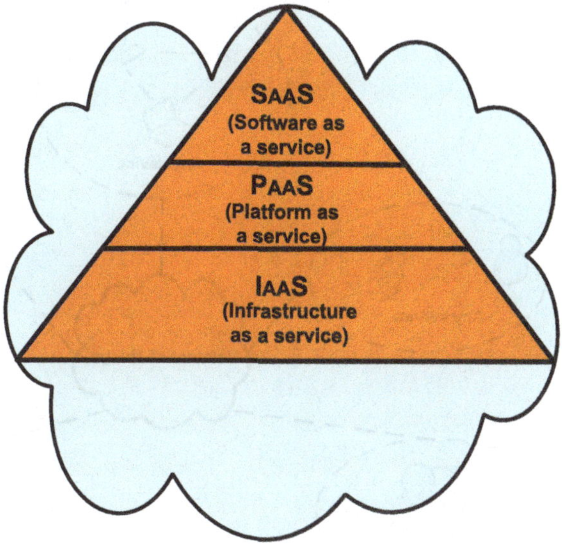

Fig. 2.5 Mobile cloud computing stack

6. IoT: It is an intelligent ambience with interconnected *smart* objects. To leverage the power of IoT, innovative applications that can auto-adapt to various contexts must be developed. These services could be made available via the Internet to the end-users. They should communicate with each other through standard interfaces so that higher-level services can be composed shown in Fig. 2.6. In this respect, service-oriented architectures (SOA) may be adopted and suitably optimized [5]. The adoption of IPv6 is essential for the realization of IoT. With IPv4, there are not sufficient addresses to register all connected devices. IPv6 expands the address space and thus makes it possible to build the IoT network [32]. IoT is also likely to generate humongous amounts of data called big data that multiply fast, has a surprising variety, and is usually noisy (e.g., not all data sources are trusted, the right data is usually surrounded by unimportant data, etc.) [1]. *Machine learning* techniques (in particular, deep learning) are used to analyze these data at scale [46]. IoT also demands an adequate emphasis on privacy protection as the data encode everyday activities of individuals. Recently, IoT has found immense applications in a smart city, healthcare, and agriculture.

2.5 Research Areas in Mobile Computing

We consider the followings as some of the most important research topics in contemporary mobile computing. They are graphically highlighted in Fig. 2.7.

1. Security and Privacy: The rise of m-commerce, mobile social networks, and IoT has catapulted flow of huge amounts of data that can be used by business houses to

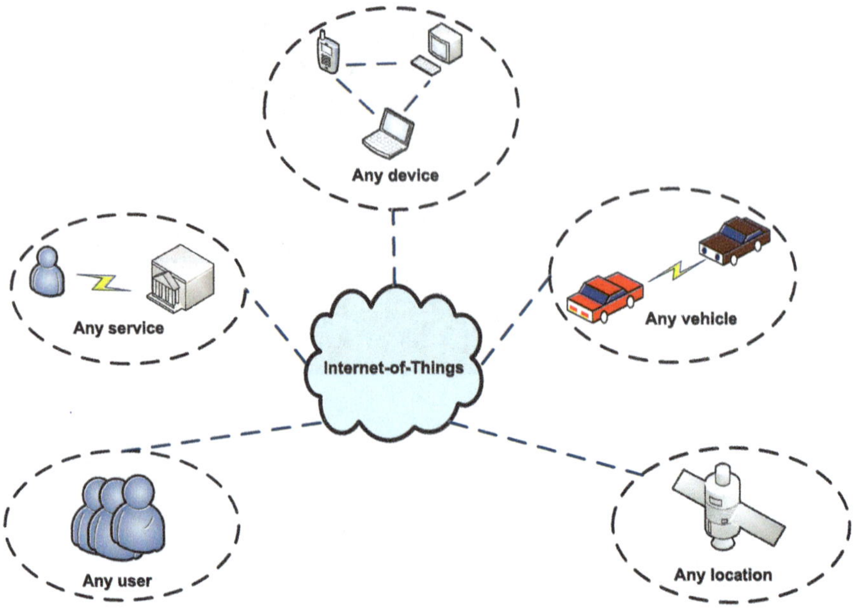

Fig. 2.6 IoT aims to connect any user with any device at any location at any time

Fig. 2.7 Some important research areas in mobile computing

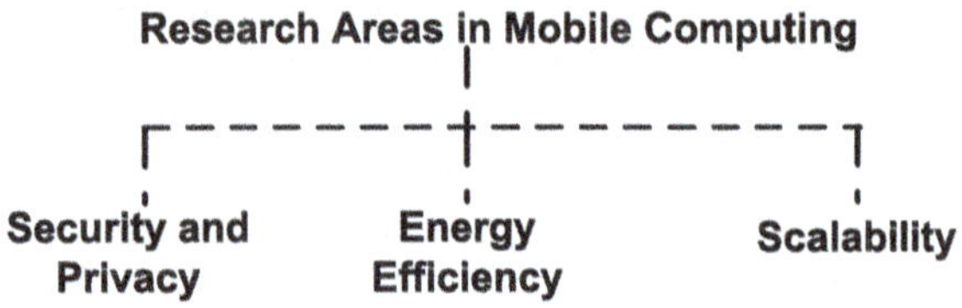

identify and target the right customers. It can also be used by the scientific community to understand human behavior, health issues, and environmental conditions. Mobile users can also benefit from the easy availability of information. But it also makes personally identifying information liberally available to interested parties. Today most search engines and online shops contain accurate data about the location, preferences, and purchase habits of its customers. More research is needed to ensure that personal data are secure and privacy breaches are avoided [71, 79]. In particular, it is important to understand the impact of demographic factors – age, literacy, gender – in m-commerce users and apprise the users of the risks.

2. Energy Efficiency: In a smartphone, agglomeration of technologies, especially to support multimedia services, leads to heavy power consumption and short battery life. Hence both applications and operating systems should cooperatively perform efficient energy management. For example, the video bit rate may be reduced if bandwidth and battery power are low. Similarly, sensors in smartphones might trade accuracy for energy savings. One might also offload computation (e.g.,

think about image search, speech recognition, sensor data processing or complex mathematical calculations) to more resourceful devices in the cloud or to nearby Wi-Fi access points [42]. Researchers need to develop software frameworks with the above intelligence embedded so that application developers can transparently build energy-efficient mobile apps

3. Scalability: As mobile networks grow, researchers must carefully consider these two dimensions: *interfacing technology* and *efficient data processing*. Easy software interfacing (e.g., through SOA) is needed so that applications running on one device can communicate with those on another device if needed by end-users. Moreover, the heterogeneity in devices owned by companies and end-users should also be exploited for collaborative computing. The other important research goal is to find means (e.g., query languages) to process and query the big data generated by IoT and use the mined information to make automated decisions. IoT will sometimes work with human users in the loop; so, applications must be able to accept and process feedback reliably and in real-time [51].

2.6 IoT in Smart Healthcare

IoT represents the interconnection among devices used in everyday life. We can say, IoT is a framework where various devices like sensors, wireless transmitters, local processors, software, and central management stations are interconnected to each other. Hence, collecting and sharing information becomes easier. IoT in healthcare management system has huge benefits. It can be extremely beneficial to people who do not have immediate access to medical facilities. With the help of IoT, various wearable medical devices can be connected to an online network. This simplifies the exchange of patient information, long term observation, and availing medicines quickly. IoT in healthcare ecosystem is an efficient and cost effective solution [33]. Notwithstanding the benefits of IoT in healthcare management, there are some undesirable aspects that sometimes limit its adoption. Medical wearable devices have restricted capabilities; there are issues in accuracy of recorded data. With so many devices connected together, the issue of interoperability is also crucial [75]. Due to the high cost of medical wearable devices, patients and hospitals are sometimes reluctant to use IoT.

2.6.1 IoT-Based Healthcare Applications

IoT-based healthcare applications help in taking care of kids, women, senior citizens, and a wide diversity of patients in a well-organized manner. We have shown a basic IoT-based healthcare system in Fig. 2.8. Various types of sensors are attached to the human body. Every sensor attached to the body has its own specific role. They collect health related data on a regular and timely basis. All real-time data collected by the

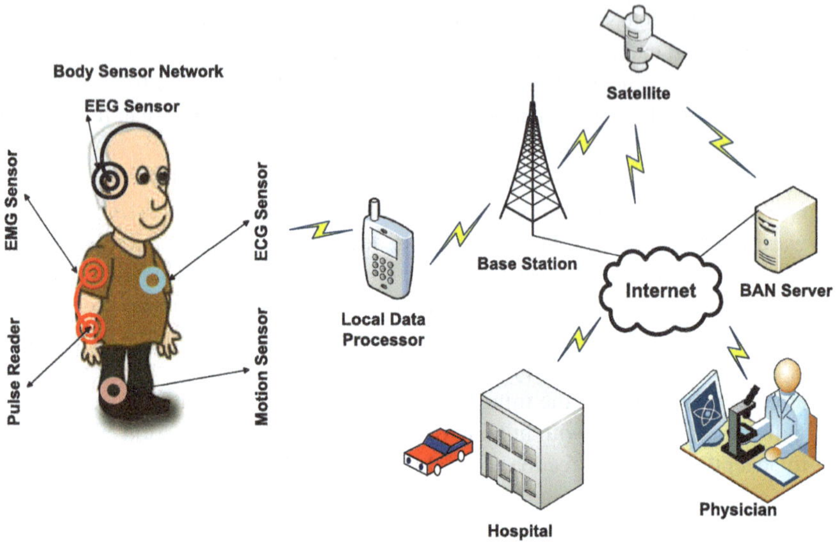

Fig. 2.8 IoT-based healthcare system. The person *on the left* carries several health wearables including EEG (electroencephalogram) sensor, ECG (electrocardiogram) sensor and EMG (electromyogram) sensor

sensors are processed by a local processor. In case of any serious issues identified, the patient can be given immediate medical care. Accurate data collection and transmission to hub, permanent storage, continuous medical observation, minimal risk in terms of data loss, and minimal power consumption are some of the key features of IoT-based healthcare applications. Some specific IoT-based healthcare applications are as follows.

1. Monitoring Senior Citizens: Ultrasound techniques available in the hospital can be used to track the daily activities of a person. It can also be deployed as a personal home care system so that monitoring the daily and recent activity of aging family members is easier. A wearable sensor device can be just like a wristwatch connected to the human body. The sensor collects data and sends it to the ultrasound receiver. The collected data can be further communicated to the home care gateway through a WLAN. The data is monitored and analyzed at the gateway. If any critical condition is detected, the data can be broadcast with the help of WWAN. It can help the patient to avail immediate medical help [57].
2. IoT-Based Heart Rate Monitoring: Electrocardiogram (ECG) is used to monitor cardiac functions. IoT-based heart monitoring system has been used for detection of ventricular tachycardia, bradycardia, arterial fibrillation and myocardial infraction [8]. An ECG-based monitoring device consists of a wearable ECG sensor and wireless receiving processor. Cardiac data is collected by the sensor in real-time. The wireless receiver receives the data and generates an alarm if any anomaly is detected.

3. Monitoring of Glucose Level: The demand for self-monitoring of diabetics patients is increasing gradually. For self-monitoring, an optoelectronic sensor has been integrated into m-Health system [34]. In this m-IoT concept, sensors connected to the human body transmit the glucose level data to the hospital using IPv6 connectivity.
4. Continuous Blood Pressure Monitoring: Keep in Touch (KIT) technology has been developed for collecting and forwarding necessary health-related data from patients using mobile phones [24]. The KIT system includes a smart card (that identifies the patient) and a Near Field Communication (NFC)-enabled mobile phone along with the medical equipment (like blood pressure meter) to read health data (like blood pressure) from the patient. Once the blood pressure is measured by the meter, the patient touches the phone with her smart card and then touches the meter. The data is immediately transferred to the mobile phone using NFC. It can then be sent to a secure remote server to which a physician has access. The server sends periodic alerts to the physician to monitor the data. It also forwards the feedback to the patient.

2.6.2 Representative Research Projects on IoT-Based Healthcare

In today's scenario, technicians in hospitals are not very adept in capturing data in real-time. This is due to limited time, low accuracy and low attention. Therefore, automation through IoT can be a great alternative. Reliance on IoT in the healthcare domain is increasing day by day. The philosophy *right care to the right person at the right time* can be achieved if IoT is properly implemented and adopted in healthcare. We mention below two representative academic research projects on IoT-based healthcare.

1. Remote Healthcare by Information Technology Research Academy (ITRA): This is one of the biggest research projects initiated by ITRA. Regular analysis and collection of healthcare data through sensors, storing, and accessing the data from sensor-based cloud infrastructure and maintaining QoS are some of its primary objectives. As a part of the project, a JSON (JavaScript Object Notation) tree-based healthcare framework for remote areas has been developed. The framework allows a patient to send request for the medical assistance through a mobile device. Thereafter, immediate assistance is provided to the patient based upon the location and the nature of the disease. The JSON tree framework helps in matching user information with the information stored in the cloud. Once matched, additional information is retrieved dynamically, and quick assistance is provided to the patient [25].
2. E-Skin for Motion Monitoring: Recently researchers at Indian Institute of Technology Hyderabad (IITH) developed an E-skin. It mimics human skin. The designed E-skin is attached to the human neck, elbow, and hand. It can analyze

the touch sensation and monitor the corresponding body movements. The sensed data is transmitted to a smartphone through a Bluetooth integrated with the E-skin. Hence, it enables smartphone assisted personal healthcare monitoring [61].

Whenever there is a problem like congestion in the communication network, data transmission and reception for IoT-based healthcare systems may be affected. In such a scenario, D2D communications standardized by Third Generation Partnership Project (3GPP Release 12) can play a big role [36]. Not only in terms of transmission speed but also in terms of computational offloading it can sometimes be a viable alternative [49].

2.6.3 IoT in Healthcare: Open Research Issues

Even though IoT provides a great platform in terms of healthcare perspectives, there are some big challenges as elucidated below. They need to be investigated thoroughly.

1. Infrastructure: The wearable medical devices not only monitor the patient continuously but also collect a huge amount of data. This is where big data comes into the picture. It is necessary to have a large storage for this gigantic volume of health data. Similarly, the IoT healthcare network, applications, and databases need to be highly scalable [33].
2. Restriction on Computation: The devices used in IoT for healthcare have very low memory, low processing speed, and low energy consumption. Hence, compute-heavy tasks are difficult to execute. Researchers should focus on reducing resource consumption [16].
3. Standardization: IoT-based healthcare technologies are yet to be standardized. This is why interoperability issues still persist. To make a great technology like IoT in health acceptable and adaptable on a large scale, a dedicated group must focus on standardizing it [33].
4. Power Consumption: There are so many wearable healthcare devices available nowadays. These devices require very low power. They can sleep at any point in time. In power-saving mode, they do not gather or transmit any data. This can sometimes prove detrimental. Hence, researchers must focus on developing a protocol that trades off power saving properly with the collection of data [14].
5. Uncertainty: The use of IoT-based healthcare devices is increasing enormously. These health wearables collect massive amount of health-related data and are likely to prove pivotal in critical decision making in future healthcare systems. In this context, Knowles et al. [41] raise the issue of *uncertainty* which they define as "a lack of understanding about the reliability of a particular input, output, or function of a system that could affect its trustworthiness". Unless both patients and doctors understand the reliability of a system, it is unlikely that they will trust or even engage with it. But again, it is difficult to communicate the technical nuances of a system to a lay consumer. Also, being aware of the limitations of the

system may not necessarily increase trust. In summary, the area is replete with conflicting issues and requires more research.

6. Security: Healthcare wearables deal with the most personal and private data of individuals. IoT-based wearables connected to the Internet might be targeted by hackers. Security threats like denial-of-service, eavesdropping, data tampering, and unauthorized access can be crafted by attackers to manipulate health data and interfere with a medical diagnosis. Hence, the basic security factors – confidentiality, integrity, and availability – should be scrutinized properly [33, 80].
7. Cost: Cost is one of the major challenges for IoT in healthcare. Health wearables available today are too costly. To make the devices widely available to a large population, researchers and vendors should focus on the cost minimization.

2.7 Conclusion

The advancements in mobile and ubiquitous computing have removed the information and communication boundaries of the world. The emergence of IoT promises to take healthcare to many more people in the remotest of regions. But it is also true that there are many accompanying problems. Constrained bandwidth and data rates reduce user satisfaction in many developing countries; frequent and unexpected disconnections cripple mobile computing in critical applications. User privacy in online social networks and other online platforms is a monstrous issue in modern times. Power consumption in large data centers and base stations is a contributor to global warming. No doubt, fault tolerance, service availability, service differentiation, security and privacy, and greener technologies remain challenging research topics.

References

1. Ahmed, E., Yaqoob, I., Gani, A., Imran, M., Guizani, M.: Internet-of-things-based smart environments: state of the art, taxonomy, and open research challenges. IEEE Wirel. Commun. **23**(5), 10–16 (2016)
2. Al Nuaimi, K., Al Nuaimi, M., Mohamed, N., Jawhar, I., Shuaib, K.: Web-based wireless sensor networks: a survey of architectures and applications. In: Proceedings of the 6th International Conference on Ubiquitous Information Management and Communication, pages 113:1–113:9. ACM (2012)
3. Andrews, J.G., Buzzi, S., Choi, W., Hanly, S.V., Lozano, A., Soong, A.C.K., Charlie Zhang, J.: What will 5G be? IEEE J. Sel. Areas Commun. **32**(6), 1065–1082 (2014)
4. Andrews, J.G., Ghosh, A., Muhamed, R.: Fundamentals of WiMAX: Understanding Broadband Wireless Networking. Pearson Education (2007)
5. Atzori, L., Iera, A., Morabito, G.: The internet of things: a survey. Comput. Netw. **54**(15), 2787–2805 (2010)
6. Bacci, G., Lasaulce, S., Saad, W., Sanguinetti, L.: Game theory for networks: a tutorial on game-theoretic tools for emerging signal processing applications. IEEE Sig. Process. Mag. **33**(1), 94–119 (2016)

7. Banik, A., Sanyal, D.K.: WoLiVe: wormhole detection through link verification in wireless networks with error-prone channel. In: Proceedings of IEEE India Council International Conference (INDICON), pp. 1–6. IEEE (2015)
8. Bayasi, N., Tekeste, T., Saleh, H., Mohammad, B., Khandoker, A., Ismail, M.: Low-power ECG-based processor for predicting ventricular arrhythmia. IEEE Trans. Very Large Scale Integr. (VLSI) Syst. **24**(5), 1962–1974 (2016)
9. Bellalta, B., Bononi, L., Bruno, R., Kassler, A.: Next generation IEEE 802.11 wireless local area networks: current status, future directions and open challenges. Comput. Commun. **75**, 1–25 (2016)
10. Bhakta, I., Chakraborty, S., Mitra, B., Sanyal, D.K., Chattopadhyay, S., Chattopadhyay, M.: A diffserv architecture for QoS-aware routing for delay-sensitive and best-effort services in IEEE 802.16 mesh networks. J. Comput. Netw. Commun. **2011**, 1–13 (2011)
11. Bhakta, I., Majumdar, K., Bhattacharjee, A.K., Das, A., Sanyal, D.K., Chattopadhyay, M., Chattopadhyay, S.: Incorporating QoS awareness in routing metrics for wireless mesh networks. In: Proceedings of the World Congress on Engineering, vol. 1 (2010)
12. Bhushan, N., Li, J., Malladi, D., Gilmore, R., Brenner, D., Damnjanovic, A., Sukhavasi, R., Patel, C., Geirhofer, S.: Network densification: the dominant theme for wireless evolution into 5G. IEEE Commun. Mag. **52**(2), 82–89 (2014)
13. Bondyopadhyay, P.K.: Under the glare of a thousand suns-the pioneering works of Sir J C Bose. Proc. IEEE **86**(1), 218–224 (1998)
14. Borgia, E.: The internet of things vision: key features, applications and open issues. Comput. Commun. **54**, 1–31 (2014)
15. Brown, T.X., Pietrosemoli, E., Zennaro, M., Bagula, A., Mauwa, H., Nleya, S.M.: A survey of TV white space measurements. In: Proceedings of the International Conference on e-Infrastructure and e-Services for Developing Countries, pp. 164–172. Springer, Berlin (2014)
16. Bui, N., Zorzi, M.: Health care applications: a solution based on the internet of things. In: Proceedings of the 4th International Symposium on Applied Sciences in Biomedical and Communication Technologies, p. 131. ACM (2011)
17. Calabrese, F., Ferrari, L., Blondel, V.D.: Urban sensing using mobile phone network data: a survey of research. ACM Comput. Surv. **47**(2), 25:1–25:20 (2015)
18. Cavallari, R., Martelli, F., Rosini, R., Buratti, C., Verdone, R.: A survey on wireless body area networks: technologies and design challenges. IEEE Commun. Surv. Tutorials **16**(3), 1635–1657 (2014)
19. Chakraborty, S., Dash, D., Sanyal, D.K., Chattopadhyay, S., Chattopadhyay, M.: Game-theoretic wireless CSMA MAC protocols: measurements from an indoor testbed. In: Proceedings of the IEEE International Conference on Computer Communications (INFOCOM), pp. 1063–1064. IEEE (2016)
20. Chakraborty, S., Sanyal, D.K., Chakraborty, A., Ghosh, A., Chattopadhyay, S., Chattopadhyay, M.: Tuning holdoff exponents for performance optimization in IEEE 802.16 mesh distributed coordinated scheduler. In: Proceedings of the 2nd International Conference on Computer and Automation Engineering (ICCAE), vol. 1, pp. 256–260. IEEE (2010)
21. Conti, M., Dressler, F.: Editorial. Comput. Commun. **131**, 1. COMCOM 40 years (2018)
22. Conti, M., Giordano, S.: Mobile ad hoc networking: Milestones, challenges, and new research directions. IEEE Commun. Mag. **52**(1), 85–96 (2014)
23. Dipti, D., Sanyal, D.K.: Steiner system-based topology-transparent priority scheduling for wireless ad hoc networks. Internet Technol. Lett. **2**(3), e102 (2019)
24. Dohr, A., Modre-Opsrian, R., Drobics, M., Hayn, D., Schreier, G.: The internet of things for ambient assisted living. In: Proceedings of the 7th International Conference on Information Technology: New Generations, pp. 804–809. IEEE (2010)
25. Giri, S., Datta, S., Roy, M.: A json based healthcare framework for remote areas and emergency situations. In: Proceedings of the 7th International Conference on Advances in Computing, Communication and Informatics (ICACCI), pp. 1320–1327. IEEE (2018)
26. Gu, Y., Saad, W., Bennis, M., Debbah, M., Han, Z.: Matching theory for future wireless networks: fundamentals and applications. IEEE Commun. Mag. **53**(5), 52–59 (2015)

27. Gubbi, J., Buyya, R., Marusic, S., Palaniswami, M.: Internet of Things (IoT): a vision, architectural elements, and future directions. Future Gener. Comput. Syst. **29**(7), 1645–1660 (2013)
28. Han, T., Ansari, N.: Powering mobile networks with green energy. IEEE Wirel. Commun. **21**(1), 90–96 (2014)
29. Haykin, S., et al.: Cognitive radio: brain-empowered wireless communications. IEEE J. Sel. Areas Commun. **23**(2), 201–220 (2005)
30. Hiertz, G.R., Denteneer, D., Stibor, L., Zang, Y., Costa, X.P., Walke, B.: The IEEE 802.11 universe. IEEE Commun. Mag. **48**(1), 62–70 (2010)
31. Hossain, E., Hasan, M.: 5G cellular: key enabling technologies and research challenges. IEEE Instrum. Measur. Mag. **18**(3), 11–21 (2015)
32. HQSOFTWARE. The history of iot: a comprehensive timeline of major events, infographic. https://hqsoftwarelab.com/about-us/blog/the-history-of-iot-a-comprehensive-timeline-of-major-events-infographic July 2018. Accessed on 05 Dec 2018
33. Islam, S.M.R., Kwak, D., Kabir, M.H., Hossain, M., Kwak, K.: The Internet of Things for health care: A comprehensive survey. IEEE Access **3**, 678–708 (2015)
34. Istepanian, R.S.H., Hu, S., Philip, N.Y., Sungoor, A.: The potential of Internet of m-health Things "m-IoT" for non-invasive glucose level sensing. In: Proceedings of the Annual International Conference of the IEEE Engineering in Medicine and Biology Society, pp. 5264–5266 (2011)
35. Kar, U.N., Dash, D., Sanyal, D.K., Guha, D., Chattopadhyay, S.: A survey of topology-transparent scheduling schemes in multi-hop packet radio networks. IEEE Commun. Surv. Tutorials **19**(4), 2026–2049 (2017)
36. Kar, U.N., Sanyal, D.K.: An overview of device-to-device communication in cellular networks. ICT Express **4**(4), 203–208 (2017)
37. Kar, U.N., Sanyal, D.K.: A sneak peek into 5G communications. Resonance **23**(5), 555–572 (2018)
38. Kayastha, N., Niyato, D., Wang, P., Hossain, E.: Applications, architectures, and protocol design issues for mobile social networks: a survey. Proc. IEEE **99**(12), 2130–2158 (2011)
39. Kim, D., Lee, H., Hong, D.: A survey of in-band full-duplex transmission: from the perspective of PHY and MAC layers. IEEE Commun. Surv. Tutorials **17**(4), 2017–2046 (2015)
40. Kitsos, P.: Security in RFID and Sensor Networks. Auerbach Publications (2016)
41. Knowles, B., Smith-Renner, A., Poursabzi-Sangdeh, F., Lu, D., Alabi, H.: Uncertainty in current and future health wearables. Commun. ACM **61**(12), 62–67 (2018)
42. Kumar, K., Liu, J., Lu, Y.-H., Bhargava, B.: A survey of computation offloading for mobile systems. Mobile Netw. Appl. **18**(1), 129–140 (2013)
43. Larsson, E.G., Edfors, O., Tufvesson, F., T.L. Marzetta. Massive MIMO for next generation wireless systems. IEEE Commun. Mag., **52**(2), 186–195 (2014)
44. Ma, H., Zhao, D., Yuan, P.: Opportunities in mobile crowd sensing. IEEE Commun. Mag. **52**(8), 29–35 (2014)
45. Madden, S.R., Franklin, M.J., Hellerstein, J.M., Hong, W.: TinyDB: an acquisitional query processing system for sensor networks. ACM Trans. Database Syst. **30**(1), 122–173 (2005)
46. Mahdavinejad, M.S., Rezvan, M., Barekatain, M., Adibi, P., Barnaghi, P., Sheth, A.P.: Machine learning for internet of things data analysis: a survey. Digit. Commun. Netw. **4**(3), 161–175 (2018)
47. Marconi, G.: Improvements in transmitting electrical impulses and signals, and in apparatus therefor. British patent No. 12039, 2nd June, 1896
48. Mitra, B., Sanyal, D.K., Chattopadhyay, M., Chattopadhyay, S.: A novel QoS differentiation framework for IEEE 802.11 WLANs: a game-theoretic approach using an optimal channel access scheme. In: Das, V.V., Thankachan, N. (eds.), Computational Intelligence and Information Technology, volume 250 of Communications in Computer and Information Science, pp. 500–502. Springer (2011)
49. Mittal, D., Kar, U.N., Sanyal, D.K.: A novel matching theory-based framework for computation offloading in device-to-device communication. In: Proceedings of the 14th IEEE India Council International Conference (INDICON), pp. 1–6. IEEE (2017)

50. Mukherjee, S., Dey, S., Mukherjee, R., Chattopadhyay, M., Chattopadhyay, S., Sanyal, D.K.: Addressing forwarders dilemma: a game-theoretic approach to induce cooperation in a multi-hop wireless network. In: Das, V.V., Stephen, J. (eds.), Advances in Communication, Network, and Computing, vol. 108. Lecture Notes of the Institute for Computer Sciences, Social Informatics and Telecommunications Engineering, pp. 93–98. Springer (2012)
51. Nunes, D.S., Zhang, P., Silva, J.S.: A survey on human-in-the-loop applications towards an internet of all. IEEE Commun. Surv. Tutorials **17**(2), 944–965 (2015)
52. Palomar, D.P., Chiang, M.: A tutorial on decomposition methods for network utility maximization. IEEE J. Sel. Areas Commun. **24**(8), 1439–1451 (2006)
53. Pan, J., Jain, R.: A survey of network simulation tools: current status and future developments. Washington University in St. Louis, Technical report, Department of Computer Science and Engineering (2008)
54. Pathan, A.-S.K.: Security of Self-organizing Networks: MANET, WSN. WMN. CRC Press, VANET (2016)
55. Pavlou, G., Psaras, I.: The troubled journey of QoS: from ATM to content networking, edge-computing and distributed internet governance. Comput. Commun. **131**, 8–12 (2018)
56. Pejovic, V., Musolesi, M.: Anticipatory mobile computing: a survey of the state of the art and research challenges. ACM Comput. Surv. **47**(3), 47:1–47:29 (2015)
57. Ram, S.: Internet-of-Things (IoT) advances home healthcare for seniors. Embedded Intel®. Extension Media (2016)
58. Rault, T., Bouabdallah, A., Challal, Y.: Energy efficiency in wireless sensor networks: a top-down survey. Comput. Netw. **67**, 104–122 (2014)
59. Ray, S.K., Pawlikowski, K., Sirisena, H.: Handover in mobile WiMAX networks: the state of art and research issues. IEEE Commun. Surv. Tutorials **12**(3), 376–399 (2010)
60. Raychaudhuri, D., Mandayam, N.B.: Frontiers of wireless and mobile communications. Proc. IEEE **100**(4), 824–840 (2012)
61. Sahatiya, P., Badhulika, S.: Eraser-based eco-friendly fabrication of a skin-like large-area matrix of flexible carbon nanotube strain and pressure sensors. Nanotechnology **28**(9), 095501 (2017)
62. Saini, M., Alelaiwi, A., Saddik, A.E.: How close are we to realizing a pragmatic VANET solution? a meta-survey. ACM Comput. Surv. **48**(2), 29:1–29:40 (2015)
63. Sanyal, D.K., Chakraborty, S., Chattopadhyay, M., Chattopadhyay, S.: Congestion games in wireless channels with multipacket reception capability. In: Das, V.V., Vijaykumar, R (eds.), Information and Communication Technologies, volume 101 of Communications in Computer and Information Science, pp. 201–205. Springer (2010)
64. Sanyal, D.K., Chattopadhyay, M., Chattopadhyay, S.: Improved performance with novel utility functions in a game-theoretic model of medium access control in wireless networks. In: Proceedings of the IEEE Region 10 Conference (TENCON), pp. 1–6. IEEE (2008)
65. Sanyal, D.K., Chattopadhyay, M., Chattopadhyay, S.: Performance improvement of wireless MAC using non-cooperative games. In: Ao, S.-I., Gelman, L., (eds.), Advances in Electrical Engineering and Computational Science, volume 39 of Lecture Notes in Electrical Engineering, pp. 207–218. Springer (2009)
66. Sanyal, D.K., Chattopadhyay, M., Chattopadhyay, S.: Non-cooperative games in wireless collision channels. In: Bauer, J.P. (ed.) Computer Science Research and Technology, volume 3, pp. 113–135. Nova Science Publishers, Inc. (2011)
67. Sanyal, D.K., Chattopadhyay, M., Chattopadhyay, S.: Recovering a game model from an optimal channel access scheme for WLANs. Telecommun. Syst. **52**(2), 475–483 (2013)
68. Schiller, J.H.: Mobile Communications. Pearson Education (2003)
69. Schulzrinne, H.: Networking research–a reflection in the middle years. Comput. Commun. **31**, 2–7 (2018)
70. Sharma, S.K., Bogale, T.E., Chatzinotas, S., Ottersten, B., Le Bao, L., Wang, X.: Cognitive radio techniques under practical imperfections: a survey. IEEE Commun. Surv. Tutorials **17**(4), 1858–1884 (2015)

71. Sicari, S., Rizzardi, A., Grieco, L.A., Coen-Porisini, A.: Security, privacy and trust in internet of things: the road ahead. Comput. Netw. **76**, 146–164 (2015)
72. Stuber, G.L., Barry, J.R., Mclaughlin, S.W., Li, Y., Ingram, M.A., Pratt, T.G.: Broadband MIMO-OFDM wireless communications. Proc. IEEE **92**(2), 271–294 (2004)
73. Turban, E., King, D., Lee, J.K., Liang, T.-P., Turban, D.C.: Mobile commerce and ubiquitous computing. In: Electronic Commerce: A Managerial and Social Networks Perspective, pp. 257–308. Springer Texts in Business and Economics. Springer (2015)
74. Tziakouris, G., Bahsoon, R., Babar, M.A.: A survey on self-adaptive security for large-scale open environments. ACM Comput. Surv. **51**(5), 100:1–100:42 (2018)
75. Walker, J., Pan, E., Johnston, D., Adler-Milstein, J., Bates, D.W., Middleton, B.: The value of health care information exchange and interoperability. Health Aff. **24**(Suppl1), W5–10 (2005)
76. Wang, X., Vasilakos, A.V., Chen, M., Liu, L., Kwon, T.T.: A survey of green mobile networks: opportunities and challenges. Mobile Netw. Appl. **17**(1), 4–20 (2012)
77. Wang, Y., Chen, R., Wang, D.-C.: A survey of mobile cloud computing applications: perspectives and challenges. Wirel. Pers. Commun. **80**(4), 1607–1623 (2015)
78. Willig, A.: Recent and emerging topics in wireless industrial communications: a selection. IEEE Trans. Ind. Inform. **4**(2), 102–124 (2008)
79. Zhang, R., Chen, J.Q., Lee, C.J.: Mobile commerce and consumer privacy concerns. J. Comput. Inform. Syst. **53**(4), 31–38 (2013)
80. Zia, T., Zomaya, A.: Security issues in wireless sensor networks. In: Proceedings of International Conference on Systems and Networks Communications (ICSNC), pp. 40 (2006)
81. Zou, Y., Zhu, J., Wang, X., Hanzo, L.: A survey on wireless security: technical challenges, recent advances, and future trends. Proc. IEEE **104**(9), 1728–1765 (2016)

Chapter 3
A State of the Art: Future Possibility of 5G with IoT and Other Challenges

Mohammed Abdulhakim Al-Absi, Ahmed Abdulhakim Al-Absi, Mangal Sain and Hoon Jae Lee

Abstract With the high demand for faster speeds and the greater volume of information exchange, 4G will be unable to meet these requirements. 5G, it is an extension after 4G. South Korea, Japan, and Europe are all investing in considerable resources to develop 5G networks. The fifth generation is expected to include a significant increase in bandwidth with high-frequency carriers, high density in connection stations and a large number of antennas in each communication device. The first relatively large deployments took place in April 2019. In South Korea, SK Telecom claimed 38,000 base stations, KT Corporation 30,000 and LG U Plus 18,000. 85% are located in six major cities. They use a spectrum of 3.5 GHz and speeds tested range from 193 to 430 Mbit/s. 5G network speed and accessibility are more powerful, and will jump from the mobile Internet to really connect all things, so that urban life, including transportation, security, education, tourism, and other aspects, become more intelligent, artificially intelligent, automatic driving, remote surgery, smart cities will be popularized, All things connected, because of 5G. In this article, we will discuss 5G in IoT, reasons why we don't yet have 5G, address some of these techniques, characteristics and a security challenge that may face the fifth generation when it is used.

Keywords IoT · 2G · 3G · 4G · 5G challenges · IoT challenges

3.1 Introduction

To put it simply, the Internet of Things technology is a network technology that connects items to the Internet and exchanges information and communication to realize

M. A. Al-Absi · M. Sain (✉) · H. J. Lee (✉)
Division of Information and Communication Engineering, Dongseo University, 47 Jurye-ro, Sasang-gu, Busan 47011, Republic of Korea
e-mail: hjlee@dongseo.ac.kr

A. A. Al-Absi
Department of Smart Computing, Kyungdong University, 46 4-gil, Bongpo, Gosung, Gangwon-do 24764, Republic of Korea
e-mail: absiahmed@kduniv.ac.kr

P. K. Pattnaik et al. (eds.), *Smart Healthcare Analytics in IoT Enabled Environment*, Intelligent Systems Reference Library 178,
https://doi.org/10.1007/978-3-030-37551-5_3

intelligent identification, location, tracking, monitoring and management functions. There is no doubt that IoT technology is based on and based on Internet technology. The completion of information exchange and communication processes is based on Internet technology. However, the core of IoT technology is not just "Internet". It is focused on creating a new network architecture connected by intelligent objects. With the massive deployment of 5G base stations and the widespread use of 5G mobile phones, the economic advantages of IoT applications under 5G networks will be fully highlighted.

- In the 5G environment, the IoT device can directly connect to the 5G mobile phone and transmit the sensing layer data through the 5G base stations, so that the dependence of the IoT application on the network layer in the three ubiquitous structural layers will be greatly reduced. Therefore, the use of network layer devices such as switches and routers can be effectively reduced, thereby saving a large amount of equipment purchase "installation" and "maintenance" upgrade costs;
- IoT applications in the context of 5G networks can be directly implemented through IoT products, enabling intelligent upgrades without extensive renovation and destruction of buildings, which can save a lot of IoT application costs and promote smart home products. Popularity.

The relationship between 5G and the internet of things is very close. Rather than developing 5G to meet the needs of human daily communication, it should be said that the development of 5G is for the internet of things. However, from the perspective of different information interaction objects, the future 5G applications will cover three types of scenarios: enhanced mobile broadband (eMBB), massive machine type communication (mMTC) and ultra-reliable low-time. Yan (uRLLC). The eMBB scenario refers to the further improvement of the performance of the user experience based on the existing mobile broadband service scenario, and mainly pursues the ultimate communication experience between people. mMTC and uRLLC are the application scenarios of the Internet of Things, but their respective focuses are different: mMTC is mainly the information interaction between people and things, and uRLLC mainly reflects the communication requirements between objects and objects.

mMTC will be developed in the frequency band below 6 GHz and applied to large-scale Internet of Things. The more visible development is NB-IoT. In the past, Wi-Fi, Zigbee, Bluetooth, etc., are relatively small-scale technologies for home use. The backhaul (Backhaul) is mainly based on LTE. Recently, the technical standards such as NB-IoT and LoRa covered by a large range have been released. It is expected to make the development of the Internet of Things more extensive.

5G represents the fifth generation of mobile technology, a new revolution in the mobile phone market, which has transformed the use of mobile phones into extremely high bandwidths. Users have never experienced this high-value technology, including all kinds of advanced features, and in the near future the 5G technology will be the most powerful and demanding [1, 2].

When it comes to two-way wireless communication, you can't help but mention Motorola. If AT&T was the king of wired communications, Motorola was the pioneer of mobile communications.

Initially, wireless communication technology was mainly used in the national aerospace and defense industry, with military color, as well as Motorola's development.

Founded in 1928 [3], Motorola signed a contract with the US Department of the Army to develop wireless communication tools during World War II. In 1941, Motorola developed the first cross-generation product SCR-300, which is still the most classic image of American communications giants in the movie.

Although the SCR-300 weighs 16 kg and even needs a dedicated carrier, or is installed on vehicles and airplanes, the SCR-300 uses FM technology to make the call distance reach an unprecedented 12.9 km, enough for the artillery. The observers contacted the artillery positions and also allowed the ground forces to communicate with Army Aviation [4].

Due to the poor quality and confidentiality of the 1G analog communications and the unstable signal, people began to develop new mobile communication technologies. In the late 1980s, with the maturity of the application of large-scale integrated circuits, microprocessors and digital signals, mobile operators at that time gradually turned to digital communication technology, and mobile communication entered the 2G era.

Since the communication industry is a national strategic industry, the competition between communication standards is a comprehensive struggle between countries and alliances. Once lost, one party must continue to pay high patent fees to the other alliance, and it is easier for the other party to grasp the industry.

The name GSM is the abbreviation of the Mobile Expert Group (French: Groupe Spécial Mobile), and the meaning of this abbreviation was later changed to "Global System for Mobile communications" to promote GSM to the world.

The core technology of GSM is Time Division Multiple Access (TDMA), which is characterized by distributing one channel equally to eight talkers, one person can speak at a time, and each person uses 1/8 of the channel time in turn.

The drawback of GSM is its limited capacity [5]. When the user is overloaded, more base stations must be established. However, the advantages of GSM are also outstanding: easy to deploy, and the use of a new digital signal encoding to replace the original analog signal; also supports international roaming, providing a SIM card to allow users to still store personal data when replacing the phone; can send 160 words in length SMS. It can be said that the technology and application of mobile communication have made amazing progress in the 2G period.

Qualcomm's CDMA technology is superior to the European Union's GSM TDMA technology in terms of capacity and call quality. However, GSM was deployed one step earlier and quickly launched the world in a short period of time. As a result, CDMA was only a small thunderstorm at the time, and Qualcomm was once in crisis [6].

Before the 1100000000010 development of CDMA, South Korean operators, mobile phones and other communications equipment manufacturing industry is quite weak. In November 1990, Qualcomm and the Institute of Electronics and Communications (ETRI) signed a CDMA technology transfer agreement [7].

South Korea did not move closer to Europe supporting GSM, and chose CDMA as the 2G standard, mainly for low-cost patent concessions. Although it assumed certain risks, it eventually obtained corresponding returns.

Through the development of CDMA, Korea's mobile communication penetration rate has rapidly increased. In just five years, the number of mobile communication users has reached 1 million, and SK Telecom has become the world's largest CDMA operator. Communications equipment manufacturers have sprung up, and Samsung has become the world's first CDMA mobile phone exporter.

CDMA not only promoted the development of the Korean communications industry, but also promoted the development of the entire Korean economy. So many people said: "Korean people saved Qualcomm", Qualcomm has since become a global multinational company.

South Korea's success model proved the possibility of commercial CDMA commercialization for the first time to the world, and also enabled some US operators and equipment vendors to resume confidence in CDMA technology [8].

With the development of smart phones, mobile traffic demand has increased, and W-CDMA has evolved 3.5G High-Speed Downlink Packet Access (HSDPA) and 3.75G High-Speed Uplink Packet Access (HSUPA), but the CDMA technology framework has not changed. The 1x EV-DO evolved from Qualcomm CDMA was accepted as one of the 3G technical standards in 2001. In 2003, the IEEE introduced Orthogonal Frequency Division Multiplexing (OFDM) and introduced an improved version of 802.11b, 802.11g to increase the transmission speed from the original 11 to 54 Mbps [9–11].

Nowadays, the Wi-Fi we use is mainly 802.11n, compatible with 802.11a, 802.11b, 802.11g, and adopts MIMO technology, which improves the transmission speed and distance, and the speed can reach 600 Mbps.

OFDM + MIMO technology solves multipath interference, improves spectrum efficiency, and greatly increases system throughput and transmission distance. The combination of these two technologies has made Wi-Fi a great success.

As the map continues to expand, IT giants are beginning to set off a big pie in the cellular mobile communications market, 4G.

The Wi-Fi standard is IEEE 802.11, and the standard for IT giants to enter the telecommunications industry is 802.16, called WiMax.

In 2005, Intel and Nokia and Motorola jointly announced the development of the 802.16 standard for interoperability testing of mobile terminal devices and network devices.

The 4G is associated with what is known today as the long-term development of networks (LTE). The evolution of long time is an important technical revolution. This changes the structure of cellular communication and this is a breakdown of the layers between devices. Users use equipment and are provided with service provider (for example, the Internet). Users who increased their efficiency and capacity in an unprecedented manner as they developed RISC Multicore processors and the development of ground stations. The eNB is broken down to separate it from the ground stations Second and third generations. Many tasks and services remain to be addressed and performed in land stations for the fourth generation and disposed of station control stations.

Many countries are experiencing the installation and operation of 4G LTE networks, known as "long-range development" for broadband wireless technology, and with the high demand for faster speeds and greater data exchange, 4G will be unable to meet these requirements. This is why the development of a fifth generation of cellular communication networks has begun to take place to cope with the steady increase in services expected to include the fifth generation mobile increase, including high frequency bandwidth with high frequency carriers, high density of communication stations and a large number of antennas. The fifth generation most provides service to users anywhere, anytime and with any available technology. The fifth generation should also be able to connect between different types of users whether human-human or human-machine or machine-machine. The transition from one generation to another in cellular communication has always meant a radical change in the technology used with the incompatibility between the new generation and the previous one. However, the fifth generation must be seamlessly compatible with the previous generation and with the local telecommunications networks operating. In this article we will address some of these technologies, their characteristics and the challenges that the fifth generation may face when using them.

3.2 Fifth Generation (5G)

The biggest change in the fifth generation is to achieve communication between people and people to communicate between people, things and things, to achieve interdependence of all things and promote social development.

In terms of speed: from 4G 100 Mbps, the speed can reach 5G to 10 Gbps, or 100 times faster than 4G, it is easy to watch 3D movies or 4 and 8 K movies.

Power and power consumption: For applications like Internet of Things (IoT) and smart homes, the 5G networks will be able to accommodate more device connections while maintaining low-power endurance.

Low latency: industrial factories must have 4.0 smart, automotive networks, telemedicine and other applications latency is very low. Low latency and Internet connections means that broadband can provide a variety of services, requiring more flexible networks and distribution, requiring NFV/SDN software/cloud transformation and IT networking to achieve network fragmentation.

Virtualization has opened an open source platform, allowing more third parties and partners to participate, inspiring more innovation and value to the mature communications network that has been operating for many years. 5G is business model transformation and ecosystem integration.

As defined in NGMN, 5G is a comprehensive ecosystem that will create a fully mobile and connected society.

5G mainly includes three aspects: environment, customer and business model. It provides a consistent service experience that creates value for customers and partners through current and new usage situations and sustainable business models.

The birth of 5G will change our lives and our society and promote a new information revolution. It's coming, let's wait and see.

3.3 10 Things that Have 5G Networks Than 4G

In June 2018, South Korea auctioned 280 MHz of spectrum in the 3420–3700 MHz range on a national basis for 5G use, raising a total of ~USD 2, 89 billion from the sale of three licenses. Figure 3.1 shows the current countries that have the high band spectrum licensed for mobile use. We can see, only three countries (Italy, South Korea, and US) assigned Millimetre-wave (mm-wave) spectrum for 5G [12].

Began with the spring of 2019 another spring advancing a revolution in the world of communications; but in various areas, the spring of the fifth generation networks 5G, a number of phones that support the technology, in conjunction with the support of a number of telecommunications companies in some countries. These include the Galaxy S10 5G from Samsung and the OnePlus 7 Pro 5G.

Today we show you 10 things that are characterized by the fifth generation 5G networks for the fourth generation 4G:

- Broadcast video at 8 K resolution: With the high speed of a advancing technology, you can transfer the same amount of data faster, while you can transfer more data,

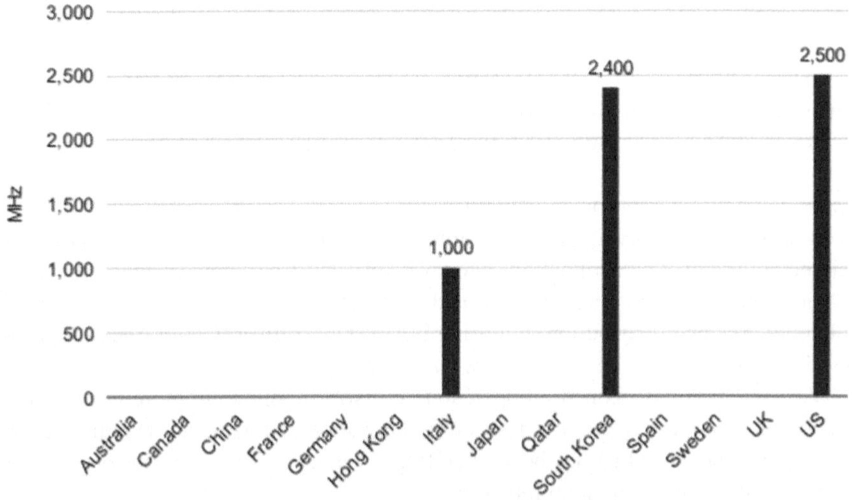

Fig. 3.1 Current awarded countries with high-band mobile spectrum

the time needed to broadcast 4 K without delay on 4G networks is enough to broadcast 8 K on 5G networks.
- Massive depths of downloads at a glance: The ability of 5G networks to transmit video at 8 K without delay naturally means that they can also download 8 K video more quickly than 4G networks. The same applies to different data types, including games, data, and applications.
- Support live streaming of games without delay as if stored on the device: Playing online with mobile devices is relatively slow because of its reliance on the speed of the Internet. The slower game has suffered some delay, but with the tremendous speeches offered by the 5G VG networks, it will not happen. Stored on your device.
- Broadcast VR games, speaking of gaming, virtual reality games will be the fastest and most accurate: Thanks to the availability of 5G networks of a much higher speed compared to 4G networks. This is not only the broadcast of the games, but the events and conferences that are broadcast via virtual reality technology will be better.
- Broadcast events with virtual reality technology: One of the new technologies, still rare, is the virtual reality event, including: sporting events. However, because of the low penetration of virtual reality glasses and the current low speed, it takes some time, but 5G networks are expected to accelerate Spread.
- Increasing the direct broadcast of events and events: It's not about smart phones, but live TV is going to be better than before. With current transmission technologies, companies are constrained at low speeds and are restricted by large-scale equipment, such as transmission trucks.
- Holographic calls: The current 4G networks provide video calling, but with 5G V5, it is possible to make stereo calls, which Vodafone has already done.
- Improve enhanced reality techniques: Enhanced reality technology is emerging technology in recent years, yet it is still in the early stages, so the 5G VG networks may change the future of this technology. With high speeds, a reality-enhancing experience can be provided with the best image.
- Spread auto-driving: 5G networks may play an important role in self-driving vehicles, which must be able to share data with other vehicles and smart roads to operate effectively, requiring high Internet speeds, which is a 5G network.
- Houses and cities smarter: One of the most important areas waiting for the deployment of 5G networks is IoT, which includes Internet-connected devices, which will make homes and cities smarter, including the ability to monitor pollution, traffic, pedestrian traffic, power consumption, and that, instantaneously.

3.4 5G NR (New Radio) and How It Works

5G NR (New Radio) is a new standard in 5G wireless technology that offers a faster, more efficient and scalable network. The 5G NR technology allows you to connect many objects at low latency [13] and light speed.

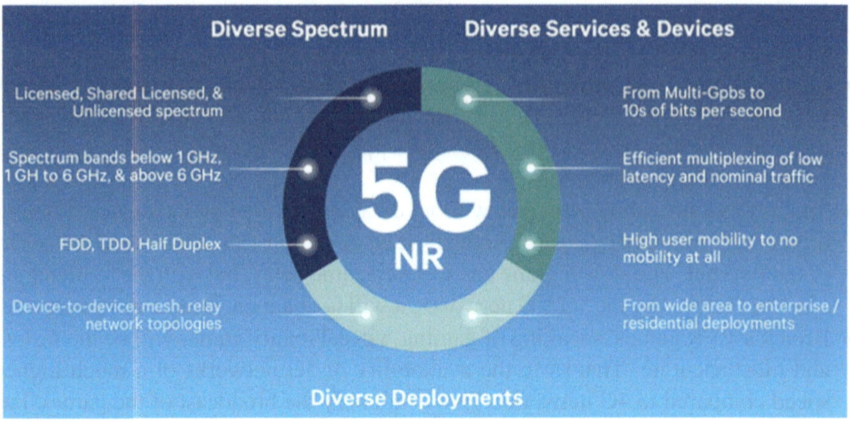

Fig. 3.2 5G NR (New Radio) [14]

Since the introduction of 3G mobile networks, we have been able to send and receive data over mobile networks. The current 4G technology offers faster data rates than previous generations, but is limited by the bandwidth, scalability and number of users in a single cell.

The 5G NR (Fig. 3.2) is designed to effectively expand the network in the next 10–15 years. Subsequent improvements do not affect your current network and can improve performance.

3.5 Spectrum in 5G

In addition to basic LTE capabilities, another important aspect to consider in the future is the spectrum that will be used to deploy these new technologies and the availability of new frequency bands. A quick scan of the proposed frequency bands reveals that the new TDD spectrum is universally available in the range of 3–6 GHz (LTE 6 GHz or less) for LTE Advanced Pro and 5G NR Phase 1. For the fifth generation phase 2, the plan is to use mmWave with high bandwidth frequency.

Figure 3.3 shows the new frequency of 5G NR. There are two frequency bands that play an important role in NR 5G. For the 3–6 GHz band, there is generally a large general range in areas from 3.3 to 3.8, 3.8 to 4.2 and 4.4 to 4.9 to GHz. This range depends on TDD or Scatter Spectrum and typically uses a larger bandwidth than the previous 4G. This is especially important in planning user equipment using 4G LTE receivers and 5G wireless transmission. In addition to bands licensed in the 3–6 GHz band, additional unlicensed bands are used to reduce available bandwidth.

Another aspect of innovative 5G NR is the MMWave spectrum. The mmWave range has a wider reach range and can be used in many areas that provide a multi-GHz spectrum. Industry agreement on the MMWave spectrum usage model for fixed

Region	New F_{LOW}	New F_{HIGH}	Existing F_{LOW}	Existing F_{HIGH}	Existing Band	BW	Total BW
Korea	3400	3700				300	300
EU			2570	2620	38	50	450
	3400	3800	3400	3800	42+43	400	
Japan			2496	2690	41	194	1494
	3600	4200	3400	3600	42	800	
	4400	4900				500	
U.S.			2496	2690	41	194	344
			3550	3700	48	150	
China			2300	2400	40	100	790
			2555	2655	41B	100	
	3300	3600	3400	3600	42	300	
	4400	4500				100	
	4800	4990				190	

Region	F_{HIGH}	Band	BW	Total BW
Korea	26.50	29.50	3.00	3.00
EU	24.25	27.35	3.10	7.70
	31.80	33.40	1.60	
	40.50	43.50	3.00	
Japan	27.50	29.50	2.00	2.00
U.S.	27.50	28.35	0.85	10.85
	37.00	38.60	1.60	
	38.60	40.00	1.40	
	64.00	71.00	7.00	

Fig. 3.3 Candidate spectrum for 5G NR [15]

wireless applications. Implementation of the MMWave technology on mobile devices will be a very technical challenge in the near future.

The 5G technology provides high capacity, low latency (very low transmission time), using mmWave spectrum and sub 6 GHz.

3.6 Direct Device-to-Device (D2D) Communication

This means direct communication between devices where there is no user movement of the aircraft across all network infrastructure, as shown in Fig. 3.4. Under normal circumstances, the network reduces the interference caused by controlling the use of radio resources directly. The goal is to expand the scope, provide unloading of the backlink, provide backup connections, and increase the use of spectrum and capacity in each region.

Moving Networks Infrastructure Used to extend a large group that is potentially part of a shared device. Figure 3.1 shows a mobile network node or a set of nodes that can constitute a "mobile network" and communicate with its environment (i.e. fixed or other mobile nodes within or outside the mobile entity).

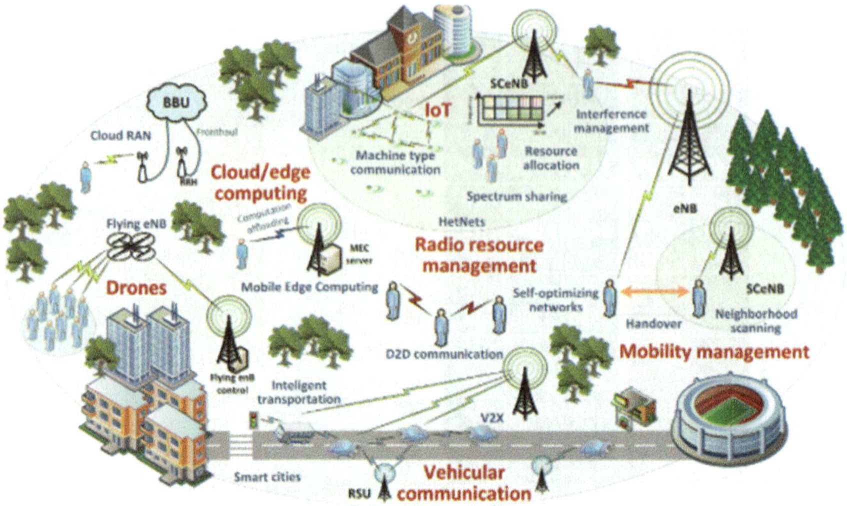

Fig. 3.4 Device-to-device communication in cellular networks (D2D) [16]

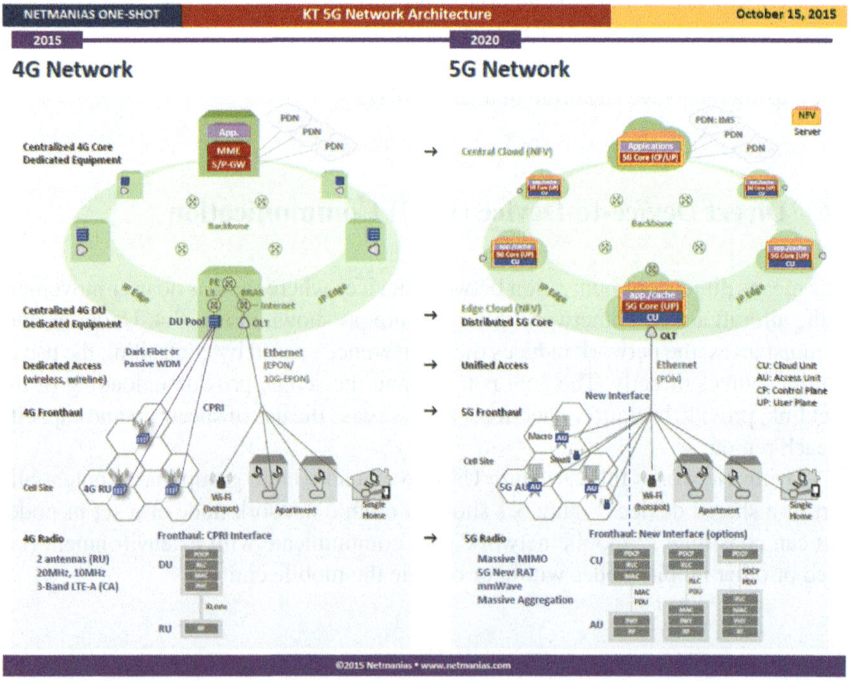

Fig. 3.5 4G network to 5G network evolution [17]

3.7 Nodes and Antenna Transmission

As shown in Fig. 3.5, Multi-input, Massive-MIMO provides very high data rates and spectral efficiency, improved correlation reliability, coverage and/or energy efficiency.

Advanced node coordination is expected to improve spectral efficiency, user productivity, and improve users in harmful wireless environments. METIS is currently looking at three broad research trends related to coordination between nodes. The first is to improve classic adaptation techniques. Network intensification, reliability, and support for mobile networks can be a key component of wireless architecture, unlike conventional wireless networks where relay connections and multi-hop connections are multi-hop connections as an addition. Intensive research addresses the issues of network integration using relays and wireless backhaul technology deployed in the infrastructure. In particular, METIS believes that wireless network encryption, cached helper relays, and detailed interference flow processing are promising research trends and can achieve wireless relays to obtain effective connectivity in the wireless band.

3.8 Application Scenario

In 2015, the ITU defined the 5G vision in Recommendation ITU-R M.2083-0 [18], and identified three major application scenarios supported by 5G in the Recommendation, including enhanced mobile broadband, referred to as eMBB, massive machine type communications (MMTC) and ultra-reliable and low latency communications (URLLC) [18]. Figure 3.6 shows the potential use scenarios of future IMT2020.

Specifically, the characteristics of each of the three types of scenarios are mainly [19]:

(1) Enhanced Mobile Broadband. This type of scenario primarily addresses the human-centric potential requirements of providing a 100 Mbps user experience rate, such as 3D/Ultra HD video, Virtual Reality (VR)/Augmented Reality (AR), etc.
(2) Large-scale machine type communication. This kind of scenario mainly deals with the communication problem of large-scale intelligent devices, and requires the connection service of supporting millions of low-power Internet-connected device terminals such as various wearable devices.
(3) Ultra-reliable and low-latency communication. This type of scenario deals with special application scenarios that require extremely high reliability and extreme delay. It requires ultra-high transmission reliability while ensuring a delay of less than 1 ms. Such as assisted driving, automatic driving, industrial automation and remote mechanical control.

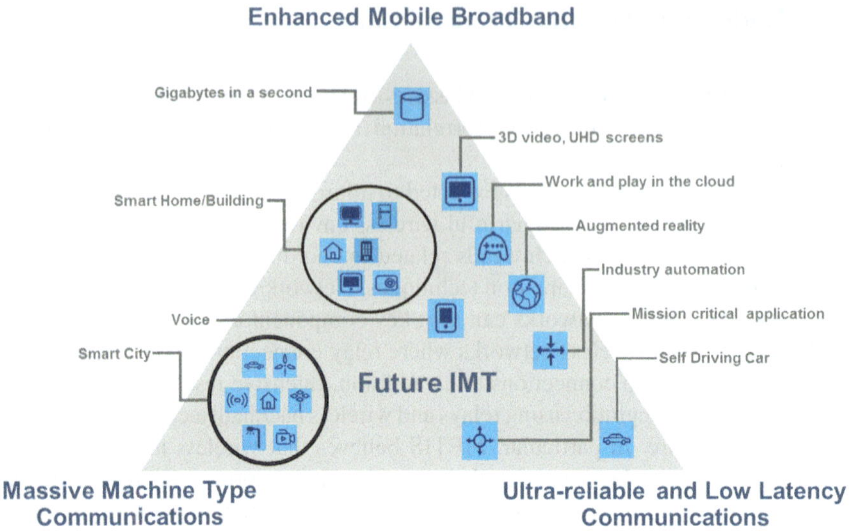

Fig. 3.6 Scenarios of IMT for 2020 and beyond [18]

3.9 Requirements for 5G Mobile Communications

On the fifth generation of wireless communication to achieve three basic requirements is the speed of information transfer and reduce the delay time and finally reduce the energy consumed and cost. Achieving these demands depends on the quality of the targeted application; there are applications that require very high data transfer speeds but are not affected by the delay in transferring such data, such as downloading videos recorded over the network. While applications do not require high-speed but highly sensitive data transfer delays, such as safety applications and remote control applications.

1. Information Flow Rate

The need to send a lot of digital information via mobile wireless communication is now much larger in our world than the voice communications that the older generation is designed to communicate with. The rate of data flow or the speed of information is therefore critical to the success of any new technology. There are several definitions of the speed of information:

- The speed of the total data or the amount of data on the space means the speed of the data that can be provided by the network on the unit of the geographical area of the networked unit. Bits/s per unit area and its measurement unit. The increase required in this parameter is likely to multiply by 1111 times compared to the fourth generation.
- The maximum data transfer speed is measured by the number of pulses sent per second, which is the best possible access to the data transmission speed (bps) per the best conditions, which is usually theoretically and commercially significant

and the probability of reaching it is very small. The maximum possible data speed determines the actual network status of any cell in terms of the number of callers and how the network manages its available resources.

2. Delay Time

The fourth generation of mobile communications has a total delay time of 41 and this is considered ms for information when moving from sender to receiver is less than acceptable for many applications. However, future applications such as instantaneous feeds over the network, virtual reality applications, and remote control in industrial and household equipment over the network may require delay time of up to 0. Therefore, researchers and developers working to reach the fifth generation need ms to look for new technologies and algorithms that you can achieve this goal.

3. Energy and Cost

If the fifth generation of mobile wireless communication has to achieve more than 100 times as much as the rate of transmission of information, this requires reducing the energy consumed and the cost paid per pulse the same proportion. Since the millimeter frequency is the expected bandwidth of the fifth generation, which is much higher than the frequencies currently used in the third and fourth generation, the cost of bandwidth in the milli-metric field must be ten times lower. Also, to achieve very high intensity of the stations, the area of each cell will decrease significantly, which means reducing the cost of stations and reduce the energy consumed from the points of contact in both directions.

3.10 5G Security and Challenges

1. Wireless Device Challenges

Wireless devices mainly include baseband digital processing units and analog devices such as ADC/DAC/inverter and RF front-end.

5G in pursuit of higher throughput and lower air interface user plane delay, using shorter scheduling cycles and faster HARQ feedback, requires higher baseband processing capability for 5G systems and terminals, thus enabling digital baseband processing chip processing Bring more challenges.

The 5G supports higher frequency bands, wider carrier bandwidth, and more channels. It also places higher demands on analog devices, including ADC/DAC, power amplifier, and filter. To support a wider carrier bandwidth (such as 1 GHz), the ADC/DAC needs to support higher sampling rates. Power amplifiers are designed to support high-band frequencies above 4 GHz and higher power amplifier efficiencies, requiring GaN materials. The number of channels on the base station side increases sharply, resulting in a corresponding increase in the number of filters. It is necessary to further reduce the filter volume and weight in the engineering, such as the use of ceramic filters or miniaturized metal cavity design.

In short, the main challenge of analog devices is the lack of industrial scale. The output power/efficiency, volume, cost, power consumption of new power amplifier devices and the filtering performance of new filters are still not meeting the commercial requirements of 5G scale, especially RF components and In terms of terminal integration RF front-end, although it has certain R&D and production capacity, it needs to be further improved in terms of industry scale, yield, stability and cost performance. As for the future millimeter wave band, whether it is an active device or a passive device, the performance requirements are higher, and the industry needs to make greater efforts.

2. Terminal Technology Challenges

Compared with 4G terminals, in the face of diversified scenarios, 5G terminals will evolve along the trend of morphological diversification and technical performance differentiation. In the early 5G, the terminal product form was dominated by mobile phones in the eMBB scenario, and the terminal plans of other scenarios (such as URLLC and mMTC) will gradually become clear as the standards and industries mature.

The 5G multi-band large-bandwidth access and high-performance indicators pose new challenges for antennas and radios for terminal implementation. From the perspective of network performance, in the future 5G mobile phone, the 2T4R can be used as the basic scheme of the transceiver in the sub 6 GHz (below 6 GHz) frequency band. An increase in the number of antennas will cause terminal space and antenna efficiency problems, and the antenna design needs to be optimized. The RF front-end devices in the sub-6 GHz band need to be optimized for hardware and algorithms according to new 5G requirements (such as high frequency band, large bandwidth, new waveform, high transmit power, low power consumption, etc.) to further promote the development of the RF front-end industrial chain in this band.

3. Network Architecture Flexibility Challenges

5G carries a wide variety of services, with different service characteristics and different network requirements. Business Needs Diversity brings new challenges to 5G network planning and design, including network design, architecture, resources, routing and many other aspects of customized design challenges. 5G network will realize network virtualization and cloud deployment based on NFV/SDN and cloud native technology. Currently, the container technology standard is not yet clear and the industry development is not yet mature. The 5G network is designed based on the service architecture. Through the network function modularization, control and forwarding separation and other enabling technologies, the network can be rapidly deployed according to different service requirements, dynamic expansion and reduction, and network slice lifecycle management, including end-to-end Flexible construction of end network slices, flexible scheduling of service routes, flexible allocation of network resources, and end-to-end service provisioning across domains, platforms, vendors, and even carriers (roaming), etc., all for 5G network operations and Management brings new challenges.

4. Access Security

Access control plays a very important role in 5G security, and plays a role in protecting spectrum resources and communication resources. It is also a prerequisite for providing 5G services for devices. It is different from 4G homogeneous network access control (that is, through unified hardware). The USIM card is used to implement network access authentication. The 5G support for heterogeneous access technologies and heterogeneous devices makes 5G access control a huge challenge. Specifically, 5G issues to be solved are:

a. User/Device Certification

- A unified authentication framework spanning the underlying heterogeneous multi-layer radio access network: from different network systems (5G, 4G, 3G, Wi-Fi), different access technologies, different types of sites (macro/small/microcell) Parallel/simultaneous access will become the norm. Therefore, a unified authentication framework is required to implement flexible and efficient two-way authentication for various application scenarios, and a unified key system is established;
- Frequent access to mass terminal equipment: The vertical industry supported by 5G will use a large number of IoT devices. Unlike traditional terminals, the total number of IoT devices is large, computing power is low, and there is a sudden network connection. Into the feature. Therefore, it is necessary to develop a more efficient access authentication mechanism for IoT devices.

b. Anti-denial of Service Attacks

- The purpose of denial-of-service (DoS) attacks is to make network resources exhausted and unable to provide normal services. In 5G, hackers use massive IoT devices to initiate distributed networks. Denial of service attacks will cause more harm to the network than traditional terminals. Limiting or blocking excessive requests for resources can avoid DoS attacks to a certain extent; on the other hand, minimize the number of requests for network resources. Consumption will also be a measure to mitigate DoS attacks. How to avoid DoS attacks will also become an important research content for the future of 5G networks.

3.11 Promising Technologies for the 5G

The main purpose of proposed or proposed technologies for the fifth generation of wireless communications with a diverse architecture is to increase the capacity of the communication system with the total use of the components and resources of this system in terms of available bandwidth, energy consumption and user requirements and expectations. According to the Shannon theory of the capacity of the communication channels, the total capacity of the structure similar to the above will be

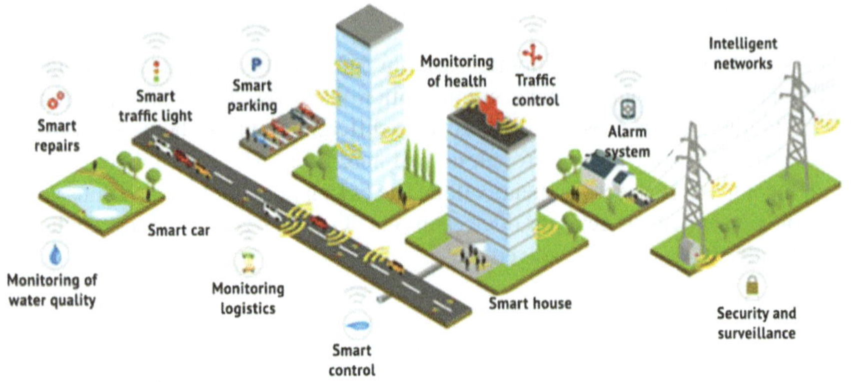

Fig. 3.7 Structure of the fifth generation of mobile communications [20]

standard, equal to the total capacity of the available channels with the total available capacities of all the techniques used. The capacity available for each channel is directly proportional to the channel bandwidth allocated to the channel and is logarithmically proportional to the required signal strength to the electrical noise. Taking into account the use of dense antennas, the amplitude of this technique is proportional to the number of antennas used in high-dispersion and low-correlation radio channels between electromagnetic waves transmitted on different antennas. Here are some techniques that may be the way to leap into the capacity of mobile communication systems (Fig. 3.7).

3.12 Geographical Condensation of Transmitting Stations and Networks

The direct and proven way to increase the capacity of mobile communications networks is to minimize the area covered by each station and add new stations to cover the remaining space by reusing the spectrum. This method has been proven to be efficient by the continuous development of mobile communications generations where the single cell in the older generation covers areas estimated at hundreds of square kilometers and in subsequent generations the size of the area has now decreased to a fraction of the square kilometer in urban areas. The intensification of stations covering geographical areas was accompanied by a steady increase in capacity and the number of subscribers in mobile networks. In the fifth generation, the target distance may be between two adjacent stations to less than 11 m. Intensification of stations requires the use of techniques to control the signal level relative to the interference effect of nearby stations involved in wireless resources. The process of minimizing coverage is enhanced by the transition to millimeter waves where the propagation of electromagnetic waves is confined to a small area around the station. Other technologies, such as Wi-Fi and other networks, can be used in so-called different networks (Heterogeneous Networks HetNet), where these networks load the burden of dealing with users within their range rather than the main network for mobile communications. There are many difficulties that will face the process of intensifying stations to reach the level (Picocell) and Wolfo cell as well as connectivity with various networks, including how to maintain the continuity of users to the network (Handoff) as they move through the cells and mini-networks between various. Also, the cost of installing and maintaining a large number of mini-stations, as well as how to connect the user and transfer his data between the main network and the various networks.

3.13 Multiple Dense Antennas

By adding a number of antennas at both transmitter and receiver, another dimension can be added to the communication system, thus increasing the system efficiency and increasing the available capacity. Multiple antennas are used in a number of systems, such as Wi-Fi, WiMAX and 4G mobile communications. By placing a number of antennas at both ends of the communication system, the communication channel is transformed into a matrix of values that depends on many factors, such as the distance between multiple antenna elements at each end and the mutual and geo-polarization of the communication channel.

When the communication channel matrix elements are independent of each other and there is no significant correlation between them, the channel turns into a similar set of multiple parallel channels, thus doubling the amount of information transmitted to the channel without using new frequencies or additional time slots. In the case of multiple antenna systems for one user, the number of antennas that can be used is limited to the size of the transmitter. In the case of a number of ground station operators, the system can deal with the antennas in each connection as a multi-antenna system geographically distributed according to the location of the callers and not grouped into one device. This gives greater efficiency in terms of ensuring the independence of electromagnetic signals in each antenna as a result of their geographical distance from each other. This is what has been called a multi-antenna system across a number of users (Multiuser MIMO). When the fourth generation of mobile communications began, multi-antenna technology was available; therefore, it was used to significantly increase communication speeds compared to 3G, using 4 to 2 antennas in the mobile device and up to 0 antennas in base stations. The number of antennas in stations is increased exponentially so that the number is much greater than the number of callers at any moment. This process will significantly increase the efficiency of spectrum usage and make the multi-component communication channel easier to filter out the changing channel response due to a large number of signal (Spatial Diversity) diversity. Intensive antennas create semi-perpendicular channels between the ground station and the callers Thereby reducing the overlap between them.

3.14 Millimeter Waves

Most mobile communications are carried out across a frequency spectrum ranging from several hundred MHz to several GHz with wavelengths ranging from several centimeters to about one meter, where this area is filled in crowded areas such as markets and festivals; new frequencies are needed to cover the continuous demand for speed Connect and increase the number of users. There is a trend to consider the use of the highest frequencies in the radio frequency spectrum in frequency bands from 30 to 300 GH which are equivalent to wavelengths between 1 to 10 mm, which are called Millimeter waves. Within this frequency range there is room around frequency 60 GH that is particularly important as a non-standard area, which means that users and operators do not need authorization from the regulatory authorities to use these frequencies. With the development of electronic circuits operating in this area and gradually lowering their prices, this has given a strong impetus to considering the use of the 60 GH frequency band by mobile communications. There are several points you need to look for before using the millimeter waves. First, the propagation of the millimeter waves. As the signal loss increases with the increase in the frequency of the signal, these waves are expected to suffer from a short coverage distance. On the other hand, this is an advantage since interference with nearby cells will be significantly reduced. Second, the millimeter waves suffer an increase in the loss due to blocking of some impediments and the weakness of the diffraction phenomenon, which gives the electromagnetic waves the ability to reach points blocked from the source of transmission. As a result of micrometer wave shortness, a simple movement at the transmitter or receiver location would mean a significant change in the angles of the receiving signals and the frequency change from Doppler would be doubled due to the high wave frequency of the millimeter. In general, the development of mathematical models for the propagation of radio waves at millimeter frequencies will be a major requirement for the design of any system at these frequencies. Third: the difficulty of designing antennas at these frequencies, which will be small. This means that there is less space available to receive millimeter signals. This difficulty can be compensated by using a matrix of antennas to increase signal strength. Here, another difficulty is how to control the multiple antennas so that their signals are harmoniously grouped to strengthen the signal. The use of the antenna matrix will make the millimeter signal propagate in a specific direction as a precise line, as happens to the light when it is spread from a central light source, which means the need for a system that searches in all directions to connect the station with the users around it. One of the problems with the use of millimeter waves is the absorption of air and rain for millimeter waves in an impressive way, as loss due to the absorption of oxygen to the wave at 60 GH ~ 15 dB/km [21].

3.15 Optical Communication

Visual optical communication is the use of visible light for wireless communication rather than infrared light waves. It is known that the capacitance increases by increasing the carrier frequency of the data. The amplitude will be a percentage of the carrier frequency. In optical communications frequencies are located in the range of 1012 cycles per second and for the magnitude of these figures the light is usually measured in wavelength by millimeters or nanometers. Visible wavelengths range from 400 to 800 nm. Optical fiber optic communication can provide up to 20 Tpulse/s communication speeds. It is therefore used as a way to connect large communication networks across continents and countries by passing optical fiber cables under the ocean and connecting high speed points within cities as applications require connectivity of various banks and control centers. It suffers from a major weakness: fiber optic cables must be reached for all network access points. Differently, wireless optical communications have high communication speeds. Recent research has shown their ability to transmit up to 3.5 Gpulse/s and flexibility in communication without the need for direct connection to optical fiber, but they are short-lived and susceptible to climatic conditions. The goal of integrating wireless optical communications with the mobile communications network as the fifth generation is to enable the user to overcome the obstacle of possible pulse speed at the current network access point. Optical visual communications will be naturally confined to indoor and short distances, which means no interference with wireless telecommunications networks operating in adjacent rooms. The wireless optical network consists of a cheap light emitting diode where the information is included for the purpose of transmitting and two photosensitive to reception. Data embedding is done by changing the signal intensity. Because the signal strength always takes a positive value, it means that the techniques used in wireless transmission of electromagnetic waves are not used in terms of coding and detection methods. Therefore, special processors for optical signals must be designed.

3.16 Comparison of 1G to 5G Mobile Technology

In 1979, Japan Telephone and Telegraph Corp. (NTT) established Japan's first-generation mobile communications network. In the early 1980s it gained popularity in the United States, Finland, the United Kingdom and Europe. This system uses analog signals and due to technical limitations it has many disadvantages [2, 22–24].

Most popular 1G system in the eighties

- Nordic Mobile Phone System (NMTS)
- European Total Access Communication System (ETACS)
- Advanced Mobile Phone System (AMPS)
- Total Access Communication System (TACS).

Key features (technology) of 1G system

- Bandwidth: 10 MHz (666 duplex channels with bandwidth of 30 kHz)
- Modulation: Frequency Modulation (FM)
- Mode of service: Voice only
- Frequency 800 and 900 MHz
- Technology: Analogue switching
- Access technique: Frequency Division Multiple Access (FDMA).

Disadvantages of 1G system

- Poor voice quality due to interference
- Large sized mobile phones (not convenient to carry)
- Limited number of users and cell coverage
- Poor battery life
- Less security (calls could be decoded using an FM demodulator)
- Roaming was not possible between similar systems.

2G—Second generation communication system GSM

The second-generation mobile communications system introduced a new digital wireless transmission technology, also called the Global Mobile Telecommunications System (GSM). GSM technology has become a fundamental standard for wireless standards development. This standard can support data rates of up to 14.4 kbps (maximum), enough to support SMS and email services.
Code Division Multi Access (CDMA) was developed by Qualcomm and implemented in the mid-1990s. In terms of spectrum efficiency, number of users and data rate, CDMA contains more features than GSM.

Key features of 2G system

- Digital system (switching)
- Encrypted voice transmission
- Low data rate
- Less features on mobile devices
- SMS services is possible
- Enhanced security
- First internet at lower data rate
- Limited mobility
- Limited number of users and hardware capability
- Roaming is possible
- Disadvantages of 2G system.

2.5G and 2.75G system

GPRS service has been successfully deployed to support high data rates. The GPRS data transfer rate is 171 kbps (maximum).
EDGE—Enhanced GSM Evolution data has also been developed to increase GSM data rate. EDGE can support up to 473.6 kbps (maximum).
Another popular CDMA2000 technology has been introduced to support the high data rate of CDMA networks. This technology can provide data rates of up to 384 kbps (maximum).

3G—Third generation communication system

3G mobile communications started with the introduction of UMTS, a global terrestrial/mobile communications system. UMTS boasts a data transfer rate of 384 kbps and is the first to support video calls on mobile devices.
Since the launch of 3G mobile communications systems, smartphones have gained popularity around the world. We have developed specific applications for smartphones for multimedia chat, games, video calls, email, healthcare and social media.

Key features of 3G system

- Video calling
- Mobile app support
- Location tracking and maps
- High quality 3D games
- Enhanced security, more number of users and coverage
- Multimedia message support
- Better web browsing
- Higher data rate
- TV streaming.

3.5G to 3.75 systems

Two technical improvements have been introduced in the network to increase data transfer rate for existing 3G networks. HSDPA—High-speed downlink and HSUPA access—High-speed access to uplink packages developed and deployed in 3G networks. 3.5G networks can support data rates of up to 2 Mbps.
System 3.75 is an improved version of a 3G network that uses HSPA + high-speed packet access. Later, the system will evolve into a more powerful 3.9G system called LTE.

Disadvantages of 3G systems

- Higher bandwidth requirements to support higher data rate
- Costly mobile devices
- Costly infrastructure, equipment's and implementation
- Compatibility with older generation 2G system and frequency bands
- Expensive spectrum licenses.

4G—Fourth generation communication system

The 4G system is an improved version of the 3G network developed by IEEE to provide higher data rates and handle more advanced multimedia services. LTE and LTE have developed wireless technology for 4G systems. In addition, compatibility with earlier versions makes it easy to deploy and upgrade advanced LTE and LTE networks.
LTE systems can transmit voice and data at the same time, greatly improving data rates. All services, including voice services, can be transferred over IP packets. The complex modulation scheme and the carrier range are used to multiply the uplink/downlink capacity.
Wireless transmission technologies such as WiMAX have been introduced in 4G systems to improve data rates and network performance.

Key features of 4G system

- Reduced latency for mission critical applications
- Voice over LTE network VoLTE (use IP packets for voice)
- Enhanced security and mobility
- High definition video streaming and gaming
- Much higher data rate up to 1 Gbps.

Disadvantages of 4G system

- High end mobile devices compatible with 4G technology required, which is costly
- Costly spectrum (most countries, frequency bands are is too expensive)
- Wide deployment and upgrade is time consuming
- Expensive hardware and infrastructure.

Kevin and Francesco [25] presented a various 4G download speeds seen throughout the day in different countries around the world. For example, Korean analyses showed that 4G downloads are the fastest in 77 countries. However, the average download speed in Korea is 47.1 Mbps, which is not constant throughout the day. Depending on the number of hours, the average speed may increase to 55.7 Mbps or drop to 40.8 Mbps. Although the speeds of Korea and Singapore vary greatly from time to time according to measurements, Korea and Singapore are always the only two countries with average user frequencies of 40 Mbps.

5G—Fifth generation communication system

5G uses the latest technology to provide its customers with a high-speed Internet and multimedia experience. The current LTE network will be transformed into a distinct 5G network in the future. To achieve higher data rates, 5G uses a millimeter wave and an unlicensed spectrum for data transfer.
Complex modulation techniques have been developed to support the massive data rate for Internet of things.
The cloud-based network architecture extends the functions and capabilities of analysis for industrial, independent, health care and safety applications [26].

Key features of 5G technology

- Total cost deduction for data
- Higher security and reliable network
- Forward compatibility network offers further enhancements in future
- Low latency in milliseconds (significant for mission critical applications)
- Uses technologies like small cells, beam forming to improve efficiency
- Cloud based infrastructure offers power efficiency, easy maintenance and upgrade of hardware
- Ultra-fast mobile internet up to 10 Gbps.

Table 3.1 presents the comparative study of 1G to 5G Mobile Technology.

3.17 Reasons Why You Don't yet Have 5G

5G is slowly entering the cities of Korea, United States and other parts of the world, but it appears once it provides an exciting way to improve everyday life.

Although the 5G has already reached a small community among most of the world's major cities, it does not happen simultaneously due to a series of problems.

Several reasons are the time required to implement devices for the next generation wireless network, the need for regulatory approval, the lack of coverage for the 5G battery, and the cost of building the network.

Table 3.1 Comparison of 1G to 5G Mobile Technology [1, 27–31]

Generation	1G (1970–1980s)	2G (1990–2000)	2.5G to 2.75G (2001–2004)	3G (2004–2005)	3.5G (2006–2010)	4G (2010 onwards)	5G (expecting at the end of 2019)
Speed	14.4 kbps	9.6/14.4 kbps	171.3 kbps 20–40 kbps	3.1 Mbps 500–700 kbps	14.4–3 Mbps	100–300 Mbps. 3–5 Mbps 100 Mbps (Wi-Fi)	1–10 Gbps
Technology	AMPS, NMT, TACS	TDMA, CDMA	GPRS	CDMA2000(1xRTT, EVDO) UMTS and EDGE	HSPA	WiMax, LTE and Wi-Fi	LTE advanced schemes, OMA and NOMA [2, 21–29]
Key features	Voice only service, limited coverage, expensive	Voice and data service	Web mobile internet, voice and data service, low speed streaming service and email service, more coverage, more affordable	Voice, data and access to the internet (email, audio and video), first mobile broadband, people begin using their phones as computers	All the services from 3G network with enhance speed and more mobility	Voice, data, high-speed access to the internet on smartphones, tablets, laptops, true mobile broadband; unlimited plans; devices used as hotspots, streaming, new applications, online gaming	Super-fast mobile internet, low latency network for mission critical applications, Internet of Things security and surveillance, HD multimedia streaming, autonomous driving smart healthcare applications

(continued)

Table 3.1 (continued)

Generation	1G (1970–1980s)	2G (1990–2000)	2.5G to 2.75G (2001–2004)	3G (2004–2005)	3.5G (2006–2010)	4G (2010 onwards)	5G (expecting at the end of 2019)
Time to download 2-h movie	N/A	N/A	N/A	10–26 h	1 h	6 min	3–4 s
Primary service	Analog phone calls	Digital phone calls and messaging	Digital phone calls and messaging	Phone calls, messaging, data	Phone calls, messaging, data	All-IP service (including voice messages)	High speed, high capacity and provide large broadcasting of data in Gbps
Weakness	Poor spectral efficiency, major security issue	Limited data rates, difficult to support demand for internet and email	Limited data rates, difficult to support demand for internet and email	Real performance fail to match type, failure of WAP for internet access	Real performance fail to match type, failure of WAP for internet access	Battery use is more, required complicated and expensive hardware	N/A?

3.17.1 5G Networks Are Limited in Range

If you can access the 5G network quickly in all regions of the world, you can access the network through 5G phones and hot spots. However, the type of signal sent by the 5G mobile tower significantly limits its range based on the range of equipment.

Many 5G networks operate at high radio frequencies called millimeters, but can transmit large amounts of data within a limited range (less than one square mile in general) (for example, for high-speed video streams at speeds). Data transmitted over these types of 5G networks is easily blocked for common things like trees and buildings.

With a limited range of 5G, users can access less than 5G of a single cell tower. This means that in order to serve more customers, you should set up a lot of small antennas. Otherwise, only a few local devices can enter the network.

However, placing hundreds of thousands of small cells across the country is not a quick task, and providers have other related problems such as local regulations.

3.17.2 Some Cities Aren't on Board

Without widespread deployment of 5G devices and related equipment (antennas, towers, wires etc.), the 5G can reach its maximum potential. Unfortunately, some regulators in the city did not have enough ambitions to work with telecom companies to install the fifth-generation devices, and the programs they approved proved to be obstacles.

City regulations may be one of the biggest obstacles to the 5G rapid release. Some examples include area designation policies, long licensing procedures, unreasonable fees, and even aesthetic problems that arise with the installation of 5G devices on street lighting and telephone poles.

Most importantly, some people worry about how safe, because a secure 5G network is a new type of network that operates at a frequency different from the old network like 4G or 3G to you.

It is difficult to issue 5G on time if the relevant jurisdiction does not have an appropriate admission. In fact, fifth generation networks may appear randomly at an early stage, until fifth-generation companies are properly installed to install fifth-generation towers in small communities and even large cities.

3.17.3 Testing Is Crucial

As with all development techniques, the exact test is complete before the actual 5G start. For example, a company that launched a new mobile phone does not offer customers until it operates as advertised and can provide the best buyer experience. This applies to 5G networks as well.

Currently, most mobile operators around the world are testing 5G. Some run internal 5G tests and other external tests, and some companies test 5G moving vehicles and other vehicles through fixed wireless access points.

If you plan to launch business products tested by 5G companies, then you need a thorough test. It has no quick processing.

3.17.4 Spectrum Needs to Be Purchased

Parts of the 5G radio spectrum are available free of charge, but also require permission from a network operator of an regulatory agency such as the US FCC. However, before the carrier pays part of the spectrum, the international organization needs to agree on which part of the spectrum can be used for mobile communications. These steps seem simple, but it can take years to complete. According to the GSMA, "even after the redistribution of a certain set of portable devices, there are still operations that allow current spectrum users (such as broadcasters or defense programs) to exclude them from management functions".

3.17.5 It's Expensive to Roll Out 5G

Another factor behind the launch of the fifth generation is that it is not cheap to create a new mobile network. There are several ways to start a 5G network, some of which are described above.

In fact, telecom companies are expected to invest up to $ 270.5 billion in 5G infrastructure by 2025.

Mobile phone operators need to pay all the following charges before launching the 5G

- Spectrum license
- Physical hardware used to deploy 5G
- Hire a technician to install the necessary hardware
- Network testing and retesting
- Regulatory bodies require installation costs.

3.18 IoT Healthcare System Architecture

Healthcare in IoT applications has turned it into a faster, smarter, and more accurate way. Figure 3.8 shows the different IoT Healthcare architecture.

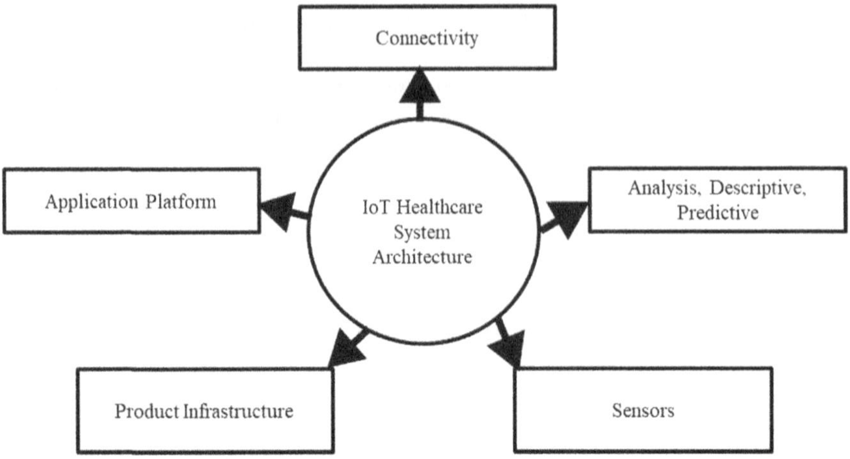

Fig. 3.8 Healthcare System Architecture

- Application Platform: The IoT system accesses all the details of a healthcare professional on all patient monitoring devices.
- Sensors: The IoT in medical field has different sensor devices, such as hermometer, blood pressure, sphygmomanometer, pulse oximetry that can read the patient's current condition.
- Product infrastructure: Displays and reads sensor signals on a dedicated device.
- Analysis: The medical system can analyze sensor and related data to obtain patient health standards and raise patient health based on analysis data.
- Connectivity: The IoT systems improve the connection of devices (using WiFi, Bluetooth, etc.) devices or sensors from the microcontroller to the server and vice versa to read data.

3.18.1 IoT Challenges in Healthcare

Data security and privacy, Integration: Multiple devices and protocols, data overload, accuracy and cost are the most healthcare challenges. The application of IoT technology raises many concerns about the privacy and security of personal data. Many devices provide information to the cloud in a secure manner, but they are still vulnerable to hackers.

In addition to theft and misuse of personal data, IoT devices can also be used for damage. In short, the Internet of Things in health care can be a life threat if not properly protected. One fictional example is the 2012 TV series Homeland Security. It features a pacemaker that causes a heart attack in the patient. Later, former US Vice President Dick Cheney called for disabling wireless pacemaker capabilities. In 2016, Johnson & Johnson warned that network-connected insulin pumps were weak and that patients might receive unauthorized insulin injections. These are just a few of the medical attacks that caused the Internet of Things.

In response to these risks, the US Food and Drug Administration (FDA) has issued a number of comprehensive safety guidelines for the establishment of connected medical devices, and regulators do not use connected devices for patients. There is a possibility for further monitoring. At the end of 2018, the FDA and the Department of Homeland Security signed a memorandum of understanding to implement a new framework for cyber security for medical devices established by two agencies. In addition, the FDA also released product sales to manufacturers of connected medical devices in 2018. The previous manual draft was updated to ensure overall safety of the medical device during the design and development phase.

3.19 Conclusion

The Internet of Things will be the main driving force for the development of 5G. The industry believes that 5G is designed for the Internet of Everything. By 2021, there will be 28 billion mobile devices connected, of which 16 billion will be IoT devices. In the next decade, the service targets in the Internet of Things will be extended to users in various industries, and the number of M2M terminals will increase dramatically, and applications will be ubiquitous. From the perspective of requirements, the Internet of Things first satisfies the need for identification and information reading of objects, followed by the transmission and sharing of such information through the network, followed by system management and information data brought by the growth of networked objects. Analysis, and finally change the business model of the enterprise and the lifestyle of people to achieve the Internet of Everything. The future IoT market will change towards segmentation, differentiation and customization. The future growth is likely to exceed expectations. If the number of IoT connections will reach 50 billion by 2020, then this is only a starting point. The number of IoT connections in the future will be nearly 10 trillion.

The future 5G will be widely used in all aspects of life. At present, 4G communication technology cannot meet the scene, such as autonomous vehicles, drone flight, 5G VR/AR, mobile medical, remote operation of complex automation equipment, etc. will be 5G to show their talents. In the automatic driving scenario, assuming that the car is driven at a speed of 120 km/h, if the car is delayed by 1 m in 4G communications, this distance is enough to cause an accident, but in the case of 5G communications, the car only travels a few cm times. In terms of AR/VR, the current experience is still relatively poor. With the advent of 5G, its high bandwidth and low latency characteristics will help high-end VR devices get rid of the shackles of data transmission lines. The edge computing technology introduced by 5G combines the characteristics of high bandwidth. Not only improve the rendering quality of the content, but also greatly reduce the hardware cost of the display.

5G network speed and accessibility are more powerful, and will jump from the mobile Internet to really connect all things, so that urban life, including transportation, security, education, tourism and other aspects, become more intelligent, artificially intelligent, automatic driving, remote surgery, smart cities will be popularized, All things connected, because of 5G. 5G not only brings changes in Internet speed, but also changes in thinking and business models.

Acknowledgements This work was supported by Institute for Information and Communications Technology Promotion (IITP) grant funded by the Korea government (MSIT) (No. 2018-0-00245), And it was also supported by the Basic Science Research Program through the National Research Foundation of Korea (NRF) funded by the Ministry of Education, Science, and Technology (grant number: NRF2016R1D1A1B01011908).

References

1. Vora, L.J.: Evolution of mobile generation technology: 1G to 5G and review of upcoming wireless technology 5G. Int. J. Mod. Trends Eng. Res. (IJMTER) **2**(10), 281–290 (2015)
2. Gawas, A.U.: An overview on evolution of mobile wireless communication networks: 1G-6G. JRITCC **3**(5) (2015)
3. In the United States District Court for the Northern District of Illinois Eastern Division, Case No. 1:17-cv-(1973). https://www.courthousenews.com/wp-content/uploads/2017/03/Motorola2.pdf
4. Marshall, G.C.: Radio Set SCR-300-A. War Department Technical Manual TM 11-243, Feb 1945. http://www.radiomanual.info/schemi/Surplus_NATO/SCR-300A_serv_user_TM11-242_1945.pdf
5. Nura, M.S.: Coverage and capacity improvement in GSM network. Int. J. Novel Res. Electr. Mech. Eng. **2**(3), 57–62 (2018)
6. Laishram, P.: A comparative study of three TDMA digital cellular mobile systems (GSM, IS-136 NA-TDMA and PDC) based on radio aspect. Int. J. Adv. Comput. Sci. Appl. **4**(6), 139–143 (2013)
7. InnChan, L.: Successful Innovation of the Korean Mobile Communications Industry and SK Telecom's Role, June 2007, pp. 1–33
8. Heedong, Y., Youngjin, Y., Kalle, L., Joong-Ho, A.: Diffusion of broadband mobile services in Korea: the role of standards and its impact on diffusion of complex technology system. In: Workshop on Ubiquitous Computing Environment, Cleveland, 24–26 Oct 2003
9. Andrews, J.G., et al.: What will 5G be? IEEE J. Sel. Areas Commun. **32**(6), 1065–1082 (2014)
10. Schaich, F., Wild, T.: Waveform contenders for 5G—OFDM vs. FBMC vs. UFMC. In: 6th International Symposium on Communications, Control and Signal Processing (ISCCSP), Athens (2014)
11. Chen, Y., Schaich, F., Wild, T.: Multiple access and waveforms for 5G: IDMA and universal filtered multi-carrier. In: 2014 IEEE 79th Vehicular Technology Conference (VTC Spring), Seoul, South Korea, pp. 1–5 (2014)
12. David, A., Janette, S., Chris, N.: Global race to 5G-update. REF2015448-103, analysis mason, final report CTIA, Apr 2019. https://api.ctia.org/wp-content/uploads/2019/03/Global-Race-to-5G-Update.pdf
13. Haider, Th., Salim, A., Abdul, H.M., Ahmed, S.A., Faisal, T.A.: Analysis of the efficient energy prediction for 5G wireless communication technologies. Int. J. Emerg. Technol. Learn. (iJET) **14**(8), 23–37 (2019)
14. What is 5G NR (New Radio) and how it works. https://www.rfpage.com/what-is-5g-nr-new-radio-and-how-it-works/
15. Preparing for 5G New Radio networks and devices. https://www.mpdigest.com/2017/06/23/preparing-for-5g-new-radio-networks-and-devices/

16. 5G mobile research lab. http://5gmobile.fel.cvut.cz/activities/
17. LG U+ 5G white paper, LG U+ Telecom (2015)
18. ITU-R: IMT vision—framework and overall objectives of the future development of IMT for 2020 and beyond. Recommendation ITU-R M.2083-0. http://www.itu.int/rec/R-REC-M.2083 (2015)
19. 3GPP: Evolved Universal Terrestrial Radio Access (EUTRA); physical layer procedures for control (Release 15). TS 38.213, Dec 2017
20. Mathematicians model 5G mobile communication of the future. https://phys.org/news/2017-10-mathematicians-5g-mobile-future.html
21. Surajo, M., Abdulmalik, S.Y., Isiyaku, Ya.: Design of 5G mobile millimeter wave antenna. ATBU, J. Sci. Technol. Educ. (JOSTE) **7**(2), 178–185 (2019)
22. Mukhopadhyay, S., Agarwal, V., Sharma, S., Gupta, V.: A study on wireless communication networks based on different generations. Int. J. Curr. Trends Eng. Res. (IJCTER) **2**(5), 300–304 (2016). e-ISSN 2455–1392
23. Yadav, S., et al.: Review paper on development of mobile wireless technologies (1G to 5G). Int. J. Comput. Sci. Mob. Comput. **7**(5), 94–100 (2018)
24. Pachauri, A.K., Singh, O.: 5G technology—redefining wireless communication in upcoming years. Int. J. Comput. Sci. Manage. Res. **1**(1) (2012)
25. Kevin, F., Francesco, R.I.F.: How 5G will solve the congestion problems of today's 4G networks. OPENSiGNAL, Feb 2019. https://www.opensignal.com/sites/opensignal-com/files/data/reports/global/data-2019-02/the_5g_opportunity_report_february_2019.pdf
26. Gupta, A., Jha, R.K.: A survey of 5G network: architecture and emerging technologies. IEEE Access (2015)
27. Evolution of wireless technologies 1G to 5G in mobile communication, 28 May 2018. https://www.rfpage.com/evolution-of-wireless-technologies-1g-to-5g-in-mobile-communication/
28. Agiwal, M., Roy, A., Saxena, N.: Next generation 5G wireless networks: a comprehensive survey. IEEE Commun. Surv. Tutor. (2015)
29. A survey on key technology trends for 5G networks-slideshare. https://www.slideshare.net
30. 5G technology—evolution of technology towards 2020. www.engineersgarbage.com
31. 5G technology. www.electronicshub.org

Chapter 4
Design Model of Smart "Anganwadi Center" for Health Monitoring

Sasmita Parida, Suvendu Chandan Nayak, Prasant Kumar Pattnaik, Shams Aijaz Siddique, Sneha Keshri and Piyush Priyadarshi

Abstract We live in an Era where the technology has taken over all the sphere of our daily life, but still, the World Bank estimates that India is one of the highest-ranking countries in the world for the number of children suffering from malnutrition. It is mostly seen in rural areas. Some of the infants die due to hunger, malnutrition and related disease. We know doctors in rural areas visits at most twice a month but it is not sufficient for proper health care therefore somehow if we narrow-down he gap of regular checkups then proper health care could be seen in rural areas also. In this paper, we make a portable device (wearable gear) which can be used to measure different health parameters and proper care of child can be done accordingly. The chapter brings an attempt and interest among the researchers to monitor the health of rural child in different "Anganwadi centers". We have implemented the working model and study its different performance parameters.

Keywords Helath care · Monitoring · IoT · Rural development · Anganwadi center

4.1 Introduction

Being healthy should be the main priority of the individual. HealthCare is the basic right of each and every person but due to the lack of proper guidance, infrastructure, non-access to essential medicines and basic medical facilities more than 60% population of India faces the major health issues. In India maximum percentage of the

S. Parida (✉) · S. C. Nayak
IT, CTIS, iNurture Education Solutions Private Limited, Bangalore, India

P. K. Pattnaik
School of Computer Engineering, KIIT University, Bhubaneswar, India

S. A. Siddique
Cognizant Technology Solutions, Kolkata, India

S. Keshri
Robert Bosch Engineering and Business Solutions, Hyderabad, India

P. Priyadarshi
Infosys Technologies Limited, Bangalore, India

P. K. Pattnaik et al. (eds.), *Smart Healthcare Analytics in IoT Enabled Environment*, Intelligent Systems Reference Library 178,
https://doi.org/10.1007/978-3-030-37551-5_4

population live in rural areas. Rural health care is the most difficult and challenging issue for the Department of Health ministry in India.

In recent years, we have seen the rapid increase in technology and transformation towards the digital life [1]. Today playing with the technology is the new interest for everyone [2, 3]. If we combine these two important terms we can have a better life. Focussing on the health issue of rural children, it is seen that they suffer from various disease and due to an absence of proper guidance, medicinal facilities, monitoring system etc. they have to suffer a lot. The government has started various schemes for decreasing health issue among children but due to lack of proper guidance, it turns into failure.

"Anganwadi" a child care center was started by the government of India as part of Integrated Child Development Services program but due to improper monitoring of the health of children, they are facing serious issues. If the child is suffering from disease and taking medicine in proper time is necessary for him/her but due to the absence of daily visit of a doctor at Anganwadi center, his/her health is not monitored properly. So if we implement e-health care in these "Anganwadi Center" we can have better outcomes.

Nowadays Internet of Things (IoT) acts as a backbone of smart India. Due to the various technology improvements in the area of the wireless sensor network, the presence of small and low power consumption processor, various electronic devices like wearable sensors, actuators makes the existence of IoT in reality. IoT is a paradigm in which each and every object are observed, controlled, addressable by means of Internet and these smart object can communicate among themselves [4]. The wide dispersal of IoT has demonstrated its potential to create a significant effect in the everyday lives of people. IoT can be implemented on several domains, one such application areas that can gain maximum profit is e-health care which can be characterized as health care practices monitored by smart electronic gadgets that can incorporate electronic medicinal records, electronic remedies, remote checking. In e-health care scenario, sensors like temperature sensors, body sensors, blood pressure sensors, heartbeat sensor etc. are used for regular monitoring and these devices are easily available [5].

In this chapter, we present the design model to make the Anganwadi centers smarter for child health monitoring in rural areas. The aim of the work is to provide a better health service to rural child through the Anganwadi center. The work presents 6 sections; Sect. 4.2 presents the related study to make a smart health monitoring system. The IoT platform and its significance is presented in Sect. 4.3. The proposed working model, different modules and flow-chart is discussed in Sect. 4.4. Section 4.5 demonstrates the implementation and the result discussion. Finally, the conclusion is presented in Sect. 4.6.

4.2 Related Work

Health monitoring has been rapidly increased nowadays and has integrated monitoring, treatment, and diagnosis of patients [1]. Thus it improves patient's life and helps them track their health data in continuous manner. Among the various applications provided by the Internet of Things (IoT), nowadays best and connected health care are necessary one. Various wireless and networked sensors, either worn by the human or embedded in our living environments collect the wealthy data which indicates our physical and mental state [6]. The captured data are integrated, aggregated and mined in such a way that it creates a positive impact on health care landscape.

Nowadays, various e-health technologies are present in the industry. Many of them are simplified and implemented in daily life to monitor routines for athletes or to monitor the health condition of those people who need continuous monitoring like elderly and physical disabled people. Various sensors like body sensors are integrated to watches in combination with mobile applications and other personal devices, which provides method for real-time data monitoring facility to improve the health care of patients. These devices provides various information like measure of temperature of human body, heartbeats per minute, blood pressure, any bone damage and other vital signs [7].

The measurement of temperature is essential as if the temperature is either too high or too low during a specific time then patient might need emergency service [8]. Similarly heartbeat rate monitoring is also important. If the rate is too high or too low during a specific period of time or it changes drastically, the patient might need to be in emergency situation [9]. Patient's blood pressure is also an important signal that can be continuously monitored. Patient having low blood pressure may faint whereas they may suffer from chest pains, headaches and other symptoms if they have high blood pressure. Furthermore information about the position of patient (standing or sitting, left, right, prone and supine) can be measured by using an accelerometer is important measurement for elders.

All the above mentioned body signs can be continuously measured so that these data can be used to provide urgent medical care to patients especially to those people who belongs to risk zone and requires continuous monitoring and attention. This information can be used to describe complex situation, doctors can make use of all this data to improve their diagnosis. The existences of various types of sensors are noteworthy and a software platform is needed for integrating these devices to make large amount of data. This platform provides a high level interface that helps the end-users to make use of them.

4.3 IoT Platform

A high degree of heterogeneous combination of software and hardware are responsible for characterization of IoT environments. Several devices are integrated with different capabilities and functionalities and using different network protocol for running these devices. Aim of creating a value added IoT applications by combining the resources from Internet, it is essential to have high-level models which can provide abstractions over physical devices and it also provide interoperability and several levels of transparency [2].

IoT is a scalable and standardized approach in which we integrated several devices to make it "smart objects" in Web which leads to creation of multi level of interaction process. In initial stage called as lower stage/level we simply integrate several heterogeneous physical devices with each other. In intermediate stage, data available from the devices are sending to Internet. At higher level, a standardized programming model is present which provides the facilities of assembling and transforming information from all the present sensing devices. At this level, abstraction is provided so that user can easily interact with these devices without having any specific knowledge about these physical devices [4].

An IoT middleware is an item organize among application and basic (communication, processing and sensing) structure that offers regulated plans to get to data and services gave by smart objects through a high-level interface. The requirement of IoT Platform are due to presence of several functional elements which provides functionalities like a scalable interoperability, management of large amounts of data, an efficient dynamic support, an efficient device discovery, context-awareness capabilities, issue related to security and privacy, and also provide provision of a high-level interface.

IoT platform is supported by cloud computing. Cloud computing is a new era of Internet Technology where the resources are rented the user as per requirements using "pay per use" model [10, 11]. As the IoT uses multiple types of sensors, it requires more physical storage space which is not cost effective. So, the better option is to use cloud database for storage of sensor data. However, to access and computing these data a mobile cloud model is better option for the IoT applications.

4.4 Proposed Work

In our proposed system we have monitored health parameters of children in rural areas and our sole objective was to keep parents aware about the health of their wards with minimum or no cost on daily basis. This system consist of a Beaglebone black which is the main controlling device, DS18S20 Temperature Sensor, REES52 pulse sensor amped, regulated power supply as hardware units. In our proposed system all the sensors are attached to the Beaglebone black, that will measure the health related parameters and the received data from each sensor will be collected into the centralized database. In software part different components used are Python, PHP, SQL, HTML, HTTP PROTOCOL, REST API, MYSQLDB, SQLITE3, WEB SERVER and website. The proposed designed model is shown in Fig. 4.1.

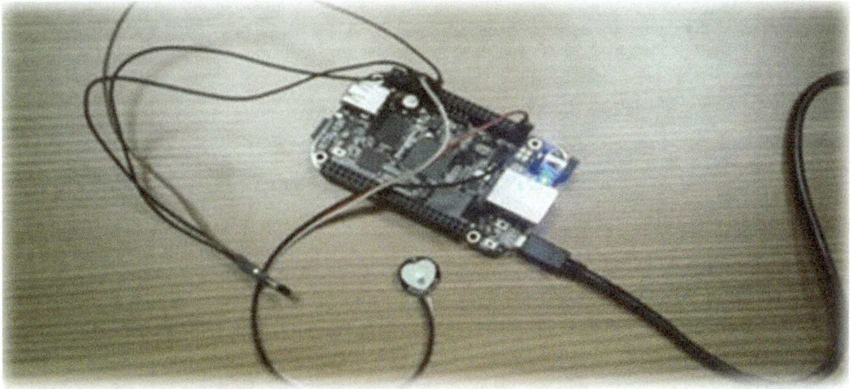

Fig. 4.1 Proposed system

4.4.1 Working Principle

First we have to set up our device. All the sensors should be plugged in the correct pin of the Beaglebone black and the device is now powered ON. After successful configuration the device is ready to be used. Before using the device, user has to register in the website so that they will become valid users to use the device. In the website there is a register button, user has to click there and a form will be open. The form contains different fields like First Name, Last Name, Blood Group, Father's Name, Mother's Name, Phone Number, Pin code, Address etc. After filling up the details they have to submit the form. Once the Form is successfully submitted that user will become the registered user and a user_id and password will be generated and a table will be created for the particular user.

When the device is powered ON then first the user will be authenticated. The authentication is done from the SQLite database present in the device. On successful authentication the valid user is now required to hold temperature sensor first for few seconds so that correct data can be recorded. After that, the user is required to hold the pulse rate sensor for few seconds. After the data has been recorded, it is now pushed to the central server in the corresponding user table and concurrently the web server will be updated. Along with this, a message will be send to the registered mobile number which will contain information about the recorded data (e.g. temperature = 36 °C, Heart rate = 74 bpm). For each child in the Anganwadi every day the health parameters will be recorded. And if anybody wants to know the detailed information about the health condition of a child then they can get that after logging into the website with proper credential. On weekly basis the information's about the health of children will be send to the proper authority and doctors and they can access those dataset after successful authentication (Figs. 4.2 and 4.3).

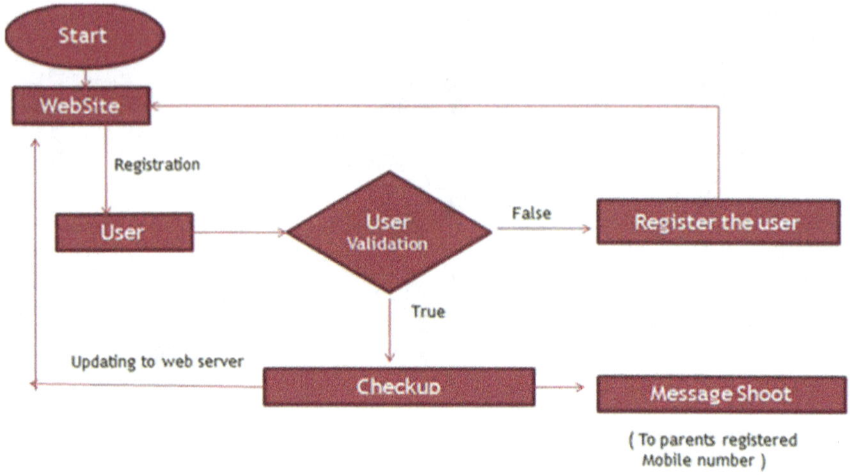

Fig. 4.2 Proposed flow-chart for registration

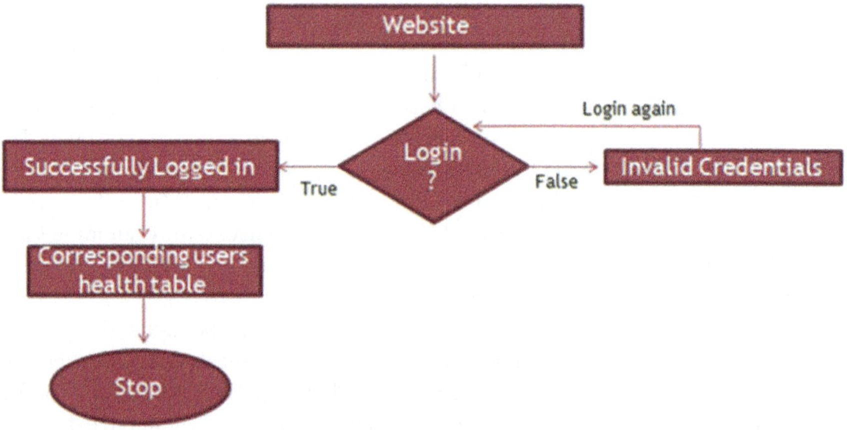

Fig. 4.3 Proposed flow-chart for web login

4.4.2 Hardware Required

4.4.2.1 Beaglebone Black

The Beaglebone black is a low-power development platform which is approximately 86 × 53 mm in size and has all the basic functionalities of a basic computer as shown in Fig. 4.4. It includes AM335x 1 GHz ARM Cortex-A8 processor, The board is provided with built-in storage and memory which includes 512 MB DDR3 RAM, 2x 46 pin headers for connection of different sensors, 4 GB 8-bit eMMC on board

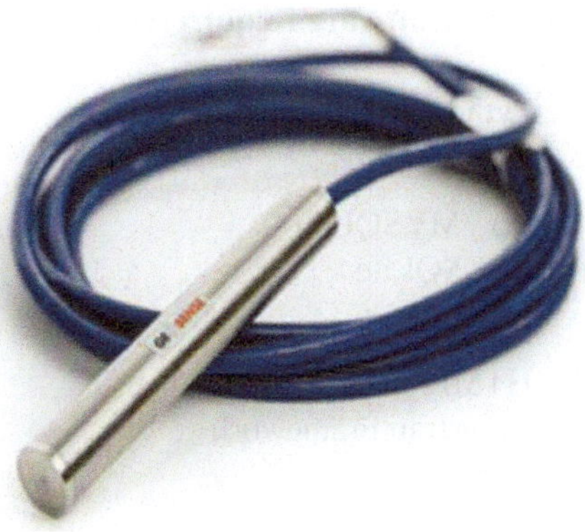

Fig. 4.4 Basic components of proposed model (Beaglebone black, DS18S20 Temperature Sensor and REES52 pulse sensor amped)

flash storage, SGX530 PowerVR GPU for accelerated 2D and 3D rendering, NEON floating-point accelerator, 2x PRU 32-bit microcontroller. Video out is provided through separate HDMI connections, 1x standard A host port, 1x mini B device port, 2.1 mm × 5.5 mm 5 V jacks, 4x UART, 8x PWM. The processor can run Linux, Debian, Android, Ubuntu, Cloud9 IDE, Minix, RISC OS, Symbian and FreeBSD. This is the main controlling device in our proposed system.

4.4.2.2 DS18S20 Temperature Sensor

DS18S20 is a 1-wired digital thermometer which gives measurement of 9-bit Celsius temperature and incorporates alert capacity with client programmable trigger focuses. The DS18S20 Temperature Sensor has only one data line for establishing communication with the central processor. It operates at the temperature range of −10 to +85 °C with ±0.5 °C accuracy. Each DS18S20 has unique 64-bit serial code which allows multiple DS18S20s to function on same 1-wire bus. Thus, making it simple to use one microprocessor to control many DS18S20s. The DS18S20 Temperature Sensor is shown in Fig. 4.4. In our proposed system it will measure the body temperature and send the data to the controlling device which is Beaglebone black.

4.4.2.3 REES52 Pulse Sensor Amped

The REES52 pulse sensor amped is a greatly improved version of the original pulse sensor. It is a plug and play heart rate sensor for Beaglebone compatible projects as shown in Fig. 4.4. The pulse sensor amped works with a 3 or 5 V supply and consist of 24 in. color coded cable with standard male header connections. The REES52 pulse sensor amped adds amplification and noise cancellation circuitry to the hardware. It is noticeable faster and easier to get reliable pulse readings. In our proposed system it monitors heart rate of the user and the recorded data is sent to the controlling device which is Beaglebone black.

4.4.2.4 Software Requirement

1. Python programming language
2. Databases
   (a) MYSQLdb
   (b) SQLite
3. LAMP Server
4. HTML, CSS
5. Bootstrap Framework
6. PHP.

4.5 Simulation and Result

First of all each child of the Anganwadi needs to be registered. The registration is done by the help of our website which has a form to be filled. The form contains details like First Name, Last Name, Blood Group, Gender, Father's Name, Mother's Name, Phone number, Pin Code, Address, Date of Birth etc. After the form is filled and successfully submitted, the user becomes a registered valid user. Once the user is registered, a table is generated to hold his/her health details on a regular basis. A unique user id and a password is generated for each user using which he can monitor his record present in the table as shown in Fig. 4.5.

On a daily basis when the device is powered ON first of all users need to be authenticated. The authentication is done using SQLite database present in the device.

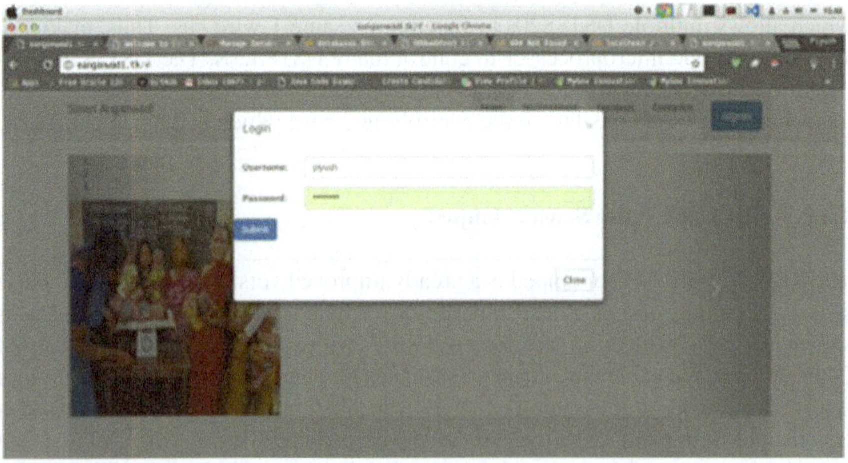

Fig. 4.5 Proposed model running in local host

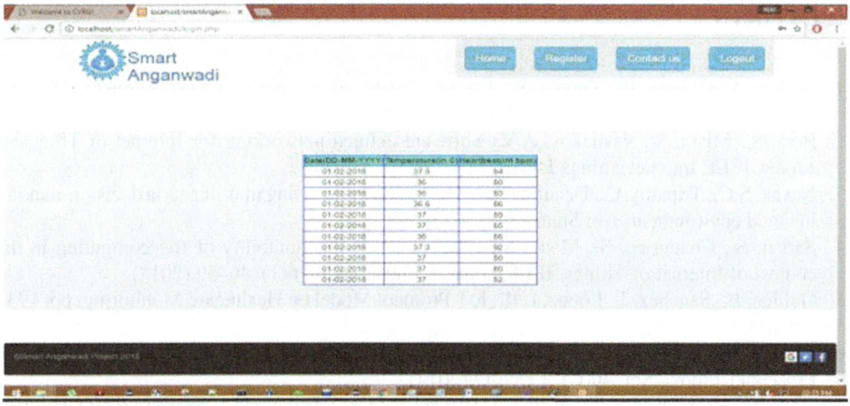

Fig. 4.6 Health monitoring with sample data

The SQLite database contains the table and details of each registered child in that Anganwadi. After successful authentication the user is required to hold temperature sensor first for few seconds so that correct data can be recorded. After that, the user is required to hold the pulse rate sensor for few seconds. After the data has been recorded, it is now pushed to the central server in the corresponding user table and concurrently the web server will be updated. After the data is successfully stored, a message will be sent to the registered mobile number of the parent which will contain information about the recorded data (for e.g. Temperature = 36 °C, Heart Rate = 74 bpm) as shown in Fig. 4.6.

4.6 Conclusion

In this work, we have designed a working model for monitoring the health care of children of "Anganwadi" with the help of this model. The wearable device also designed along with its communication system. The health parameters are also transmitted to the hosted server for further use. Health parameters of each child will be observed on daily basis. Entire health details of each child will be maintained in the database and doctor as well as their parents can see the required information by logging in the website with the proper credentials. The work will be focussed on a mobile android application which can provide a good administrative to monitor the health issues in the rural areas and the government could provide the extra resource to "Anganwadi Center" if required.

The Future work of the proposed system is very essential in order to make the design system more advance. Internet of Things is expected to rule the world in various fields but more benefit could be taken in the field of healthcare. In the designed system the enhancement would be connecting more sensors to the existing device which measures various other health parameters.

References

1. Gómez, J., Oviedo, B., Zhuma, E.: Patient monitoring system based on Internet of Things. Procedia Comput. Sci. **83**, 90–97 (2016)
2. Bera, S., Misra, S., Vasilakos, A.V.: Software-defined networking for Internet of Things: a survey. IEEE Internet Things J. **4**(6), 1994–2008 (2017)
3. Nayak, S.C., Tripathy, C.: Deadline based task scheduling using multi-criteria decision-making in cloud environment. Ain Shams Eng. J. (2018)
4. Sarkar, S., Chatterjee, S., Misra, S.: Assessment of the suitability of fog computing in the context of Internet of Things. IEEE Trans. Cloud Comput. **6**(1), 46–59 (2018)
5. Guillén, E., Sánchez, J., López, L.R.: IoT Protocol Model on Healthcare Monitoring, pp. 193–196 (2017)
6. Maia, P., et al.: A web platform for interconnecting body sensors and improving health care. Procedia Comput. Sci. **40**(C), 135–142 (2014)
7. Khan, S.F.: Health care monitoring system in Internet of Things (IoT) by using RFID. In: 2017 6th International Conference on Industrial Technology and Management, pp. 198–204 (2017)
8. Hassanalieragh, M., et al.: Health monitoring and management using Internet-of-Things (IoT) sensing with cloud-based processing: opportunities and challenges. In: Proceedings of 2015 IEEE International Conference on Services Computing SCC 2015, pp. 285–292 (2015)
9. Li, C., Hu, X., Zhang, L.: The IoT-based heart disease monitoring system for pervasive healthcare service. Procedia Comput. Sci. **112**, 2328–2334 (2017)
10. Chandan, S., Parida, S., Tripathy, C., Kumar, P.: An enhanced deadline constraint based task scheduling mechanism for cloud environment. J. King Saud Univ. Comput. Inf. Sci. (2018)
11. Nayak, S.C., Parida, S., et al.: Multicriteria decision-making techniques for avoiding similar task scheduling conflict in cloud computing. Int. J. Commun. Syst. 1–31 (2019)

Chapter 5
Secured Smart Hospital Cabin Door Knocker Using Internet of Things (IoT)

Lakshmanan Ramanathan, Purushotham Swarnalatha, Selvanambi Ramani, N. Prabakaran, Prateek Singh Phogat and S. Rajkumar

Abstract In the present age, Internet of things (IoT) has entered a golden era of rapid growth. The Internet of things is an idea that broadens the advantages of the normal Internet steady availability, remote control capacity, and information sharing. Every day, things are getting connected with the internet. The main aim of this paper is to monitor the visitor of the hospital. If a person knocks or presses the push button, the image of the person is captured and stored in a database. The captured image is converted into bytes in order to reduce the size of the memory and also it's more secured. The server will check the details of the person such as whether the person is authorized or not. If the person is known, the server will send the notification to the owner or else it will send the notification along with the image and video of the unknown person.

Keywords Internet of things · Raspberry pi · Push bullet server · Secure byte conversion · Face detection · Hospital door

5.1 Introduction

In this modern world crime has become ultra-modern too! In this current era a lot of incident occurs like theft, stealing, and unwanted entry abruptly into the hospital violating the privacy of people. So the security is of prime importance in the life of

L. Ramanathan · P. Swarnalatha · S. Ramani · N. Prabakaran · P. S. Phogat · S. Rajkumar (✉)
School of Computer Science and Engineering, Vellore Institute of Technology, Vellore, India
e-mail: rajkumars@vit.ac.in

L. Ramanathan
e-mail: lramanathan@vit.ac.in

P. Swarnalatha
e-mail: pswarnalatha@vit.ac.in

S. Ramani
e-mail: ramani.s@vit.ac.in

N. Prabakaran
e-mail: prabakaran.n@vit.ac.in

P. K. Pattnaik et al. (eds.), *Smart Healthcare Analytics in IoT Enabled Environment*, Intelligent Systems Reference Library 178,
https://doi.org/10.1007/978-3-030-37551-5_5

people. Nowadays people run a very busy life, at the same time they also want to ensure their safety as well as the safety of their belongings. Sometimes they forget to look after their necessary things like keys, wallet, credit cards etc. Without these necessities, they are unable to access their hospital cabin or any place they want. Major inconvenience is faced when the owner is not at his hospital cabin. Such sort of inconvenience also extends to our friends and relatives who may visit the hospital cabin without intimation. In shortly, many of the smart devices will be communicating over IoT [1]. The analyst firm Gartner predicts that by 2020 there will be more than 20 billion devices connected to the Internet of Things.

The problem identified is that there is no smart means through which the owner of the hospital cabin is notified about the visitor in case he is outdoors or unable to hear the bell or anyone knocking at the door.

To identify the person who is standing in front of a door, security is more essential. If any visitors are knocking at the door or waiting in front of the door we need to intimate the owner of the hospital cabin. Our system customized using microcomputer and Raspberry Pi to communicate to the user through smart phone internet.

In this paper, the image capture is initiated by pressing the doorbell button or knocks at the door. Indeed, an integrated camera will capture image of the visitor. The face recently scanned will be verified in the present database. In case of an unknown face, a notification will be generated with image and video and it will be sent to the owner. If the visitor is known, then the actual image is matched with stored image in the database. Furthermore, the owner will be notified, through SMS on his mobile phone, about the visitor details. The legal user can pass command to open or close the door [2]. If an image is not clear then the legal user can pass command as snap to retake an image. Comparing to old face recognition systems that are already commercialized, this system is more efficient in real time response with better recognition rate. This strategy is very efficient in detecting criminals and thieves.

5.2 Related Work

In the existing work done by Ayman Ben et al., Enhanced smart door bell system that mainly focuses on face recognition using ARMv7 core text-A7 that consumes less power and high processing speed is used. It uses a PCA algorithm to check whether the person is authorized or not. Images are sent via e-mails. Since every time the users want to reload the image content if it is not loaded properly, there was a need for betterment or an alternative system of security [3].

Jaychand et al. proposed a Smart Door bell system based on face recognition, Image processing is done using ARMv7 core text-A7 in order to reduce the processing time. This type of security system sent only the notification to the user. The captured image of the visitor can be viewed only in websites. It uses the Eigen faces algorithm using opencv library to perform face recognition. The main disadvantage is that the recognition rate decreased. The experiment is tested only with a uniform Background [4].

G. Sowjanya and S. Nagaraju designed and implemented door access control and security system based on IoT [5]. The system is implemented by using biometric scanner, password and security question with IoT. Remote operating of door access can be done by IoT with a smart indication.

Aman and Anitha proposed model Motion Sensing and image capturing based smart door system on android [6]. It can eliminate the concept of lock system as here the security is provided to the door itself. The motion sensors are used to detect any movement in front of the door.

H. Singh, V. Pallagani, V. Khandelwal and U. Venkanna proposed solution uses the sensor and detects the presence or absence of a human object in the housework accordingly [7]. It also provides information about the energy consumed by the house owner regularly in the form of message. Also, it checks, the level of gas in the gas cylinder.

M. L. R. Chandra, B. V. Kumar and B. Suresh Babu proposed system for home security [2]. The planned system captures the picture of the intruder and sends it to the authorized mail through internet over Simple Mail Transfer Protocol (SMTP).

M. S. Hadis, E. Palantei, A. A. Ilham and A. Hendra designed of smart lock system for doors with special features using bluetooth technology [8]. The system uses bluetooth technology with low power and is available on almost all gadgets.

5.3 Proposed Model

To solve these problems, a smart doorbell which will identify the person who triggers it and then notify the user via mobile phone was devised as shown in Fig. 5.1. The following five stages represent the basic operation of the system:

A. *Stage 1*: *Action*

If a person visits the house he/she will knock the door or presses the push button.

B. *Stage 2*: *Capture*

If any of the action is performed, then the image of the visitor is captured via Web Camera and sent to the centralized server database.

C. *Stage 3*: *Processing*

The captured image will process in the processing unit. The processing unit gets the image and it is an unknown person the image will be sent to push bullet server where it is processed to identify the visitor.

D. *Stage 4*: *Notification*

Once the visitor is identified, if he/she is a known person then it will send only the notification or else it will send the notification along with image and video via

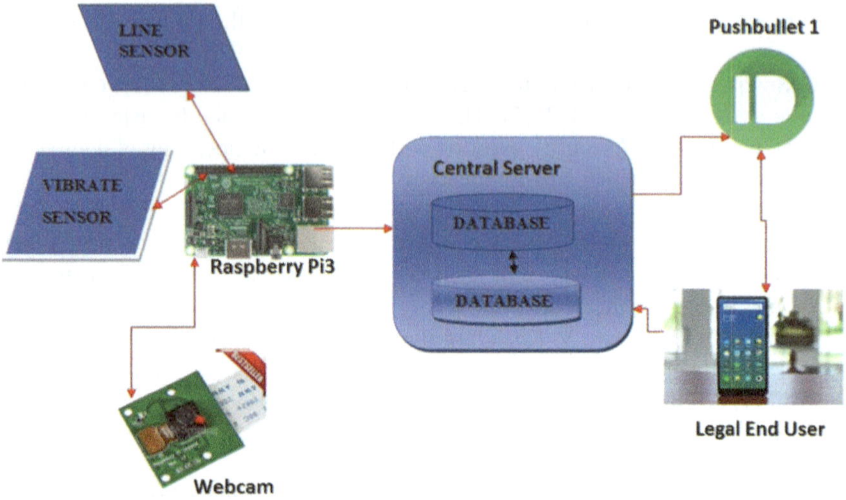

Fig. 5.1 Proposed system architecture

application to the owner. In case the image is not clear, the legal user can retake the image by passing the command "Snap".

E. *Stage 5*: *Response*

Once the notification is received, then the owner will send a command to open or close the door automatically.

5.4 Module Description

5.4.1 User Hardware Module

5.4.1.1 Line Sensor

Figure 5.2 Shows Line Follower sensor, it is an extra for your RedBot that enables your system to identify lines or close-by objects. The sensor works by distinguishing reflected light originating from its own infrared LED. By estimating the sum of reflected infrared light, it can distinguish advances from light to dim (lines) or even questions specifically before it [9].

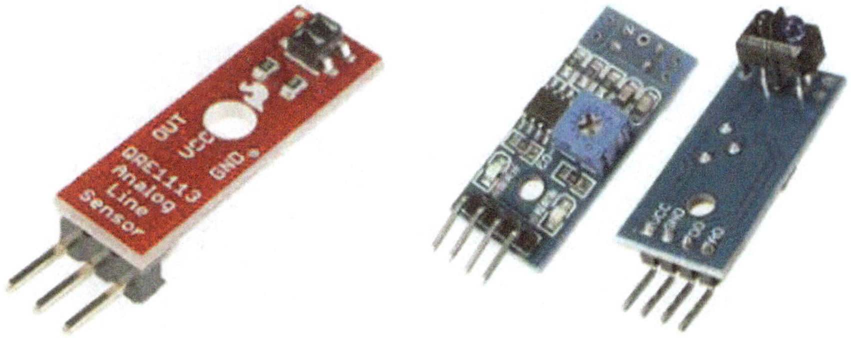

Fig. 5.2 Line follower sensor

5.4.1.2 Vibrate Sensor

Figure 5.3 Shows Vibration sensor switch which is used for vibration detection. This sensor has two contact pins. When an external force is acted upon either by movement or vibration, the sensor's two contact pin are closed and contact is made between the two pins. When the force is removed the sensor terminals returns back to open contacts [10].

Fig. 5.3 Vibrate sensor

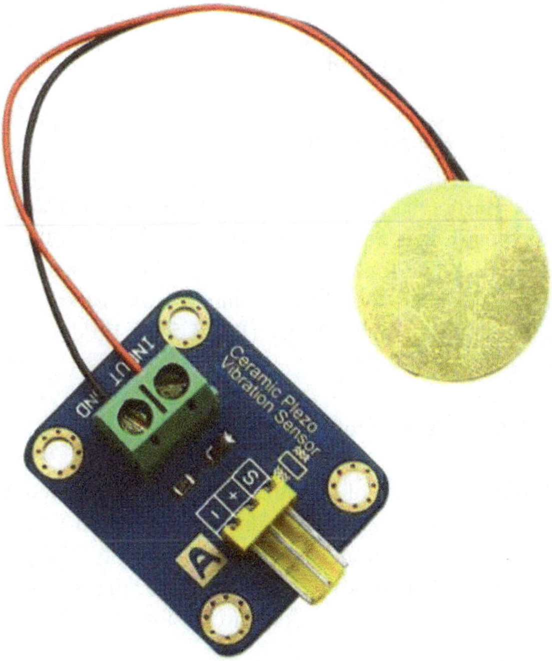

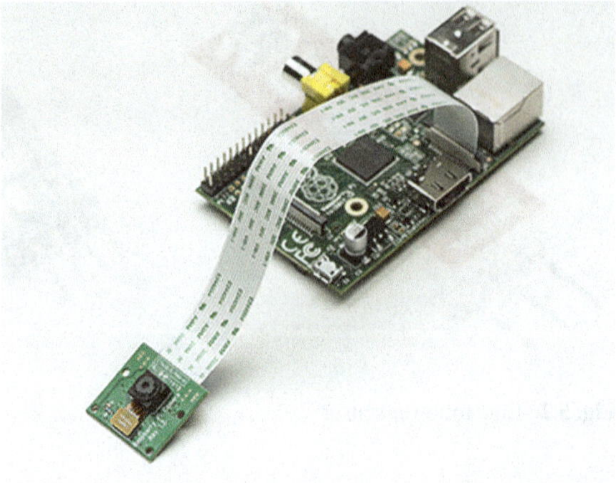

Fig. 5.4 Web camera

5.4.1.3 Web Camera

Figure 5.4 Shows a webcam, it is a camcorder that feeds or streams its picture continuously to or through a PC to a PC organizes. Whenever "caught" by the PC, the video stream might be spared, seen or sent on to different systems by means of frameworks for example, the web, and messaged as an attachment [11].

5.4.2 Processing Module

5.4.2.1 Raspberry Pi

The Raspberry Pi is a charge card estimated PC that fittings into your Tv and a Keyboard. It is a proficient little PC which can be utilized as a part of Electronics Activities, and for a considerable lot of the things that your Desktop Pc does, similar to Spreadsheets, Word Processing, Browsing the Web and Playing Games. It likewise plays High-definition Video (Fig. 5.5).

5.4.2.2 Pushbullet

Pushbullet is one of the quickest and least demanding approach to get links, notes, records, documents, and addresses both from your PC to your cell phone and the other way around and is shown in Fig. 5.6. The greater part of this is done from the Pushbullet Android application, the administration's Web website, or one of the program augmentations for Chrome Firefox [12].

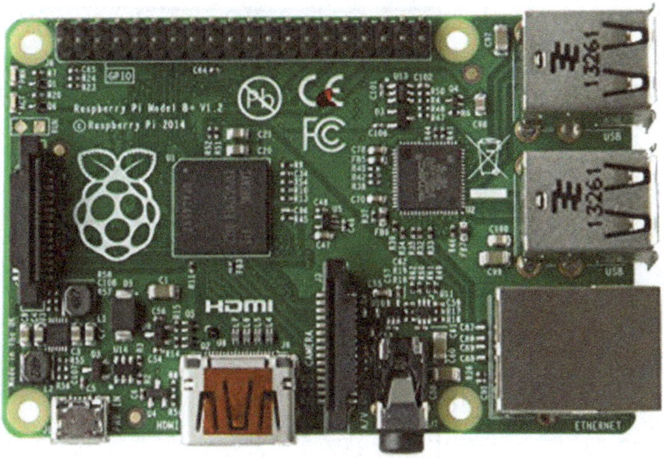

Fig. 5.5 Raspberry Pi 3

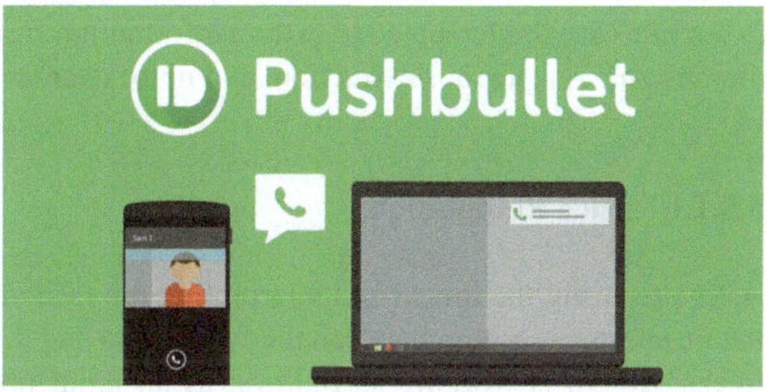

Fig. 5.6 Pushbullet server

5.5 Implementation Technologies

5.5.1 *Face Detection and Face Recognition*

The fundamental role of this section is to resolve the images in order to determine whether visitor is authorized or not. The location of faces is prepared for cropping. The resulting output of this process are patches characterizing each face image, to improve the effectiveness of the algorithm, face alignment and scaling filters are applied to the input image. Face detection is also used for region-of-interest detection, video classification, retargeting images, etc. By applying the Haar-like features, the device could recognize the authorized or not.

In order to retrieve all faces present in the picture, a loop all around the image with conditional structures comparing the image with database. Figure 5.7. Shows, as an example, Haar-Like features applied on picture. After detecting the face in the image, human-face patches are extracted from images. To avoid environmental

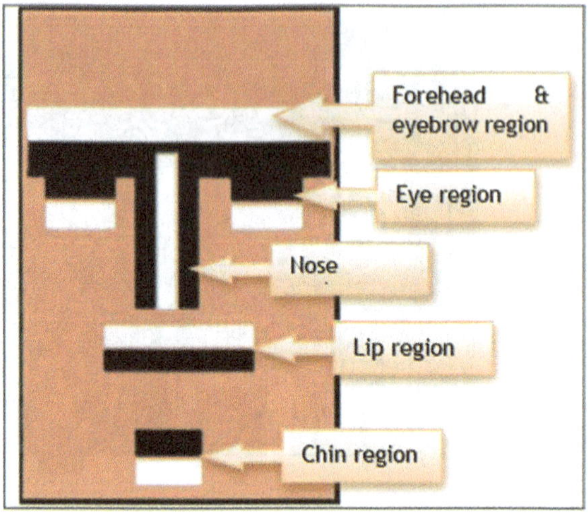

Fig. 5.7 Haar features for face detection

deficiencies like illuminations, face expressions, occlusion and clutter [13], feature extractions are implemented to extract information from the image in order to reduce dimension, conspicuous extraction, and noise decreasing.

5.5.1.1 Face Recognition

After preparing the image and interpreting the face vector, the next step is to apply the matching algorithm between the stored data and the input image [2]. The process of the system is working as follows: as an input image comes in, face detection will pinpoint the traits of a face, then feature extraction will apply the filters to extract only the face and then compare the traits extracted to the ones available in the database, majority of the previous works were infirm with low recognition rate or with undefined time response. In this branch two main applications are established: the first is identification [14] and the second one is verification.

On one hand, using face identification, the system could recognize the person through store in database image, to determine the real unique traits of a face, this may have important implications for the use of identification tools such as Eigen face [8], the algorithm represents every image as vector, compute the mean of all images, eigenvectors, and then represent each face with a linear combination of the best eigenvectors calculated. On the other hand, systems using face verification could differentiate if a capture image matches or not with an authorized list to improve the verification [15]. Steps of face recognition are shown in Fig. 5.8.

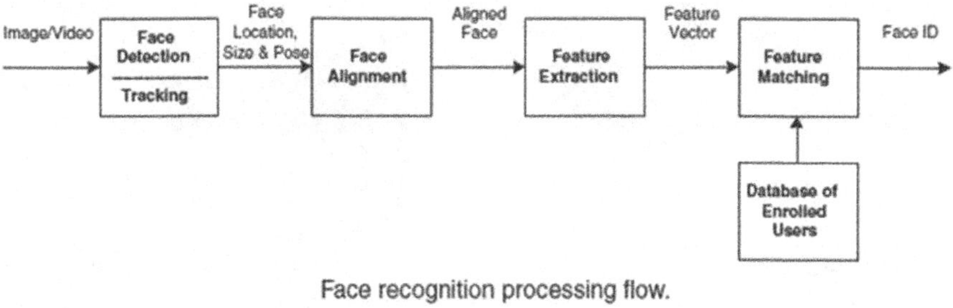

Fig. 5.8 Face recognition stages

5.5.2 *Base 64 Algorithm*

To substitute each pixel of image into encrypted format using Base64 encode table [16].

Encryption Algorithm In this section, we are going to discuss procedure of the algorithm.

```
Input  : Capture image
Output  : Byte format
1. Get the input as image.
2. Convert the image into pixels.
3. Calculate the input length.
4. Then output length = 4 * ((input length + 2) / 3)
5. if (data == NULL) then
        return NULL;
   else:
     for (int i = 0, j = 0; i less than input length;):
          a = i less than input length ?(unsigned char)data[i++] : 0;
          encoded data[j++] = encoding table[(tripl ** 3 * 6) & 0x3F];
    for (int i = 0; i less than mod table[input length % 3];i++):
          encoded data [*output length - 1 - i] = '=';
```

5.6 System Implementation

Figure 5.9 depicts the hardware implementation of our proposed work. All the components and sensors are connected according to system architecture. When line sensor

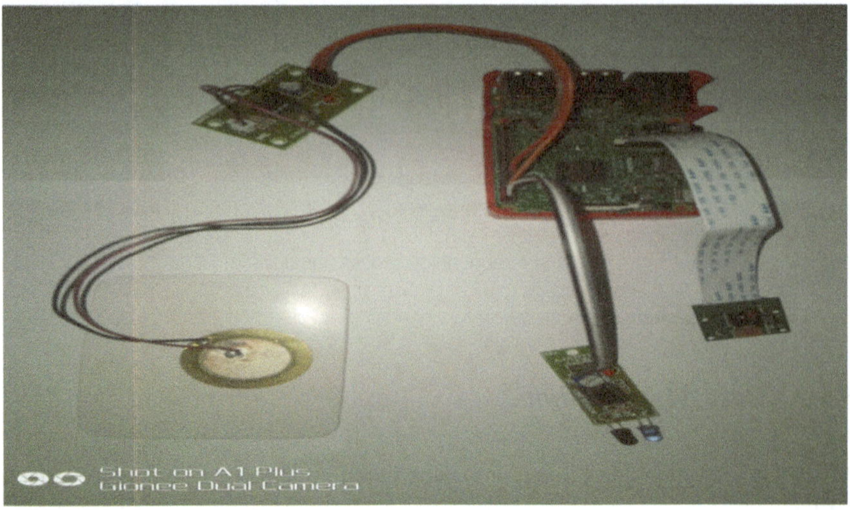

Fig. 5.9 System hardware implementation

or vibrate sensor is interrupted then webcam takes a snap and send the picture taken, as an attachment to the respective application and also notifies the user. The user can see the visitor image and pass the command such as "open" or "close". In case the image is not clear then the user can pass the command "snap" to capture the image again.

Figure 5.10 shows the flow of our working model. If any person knocking at the door or ringing the bell at the door, then our system will take a picture of the person standing in front of the door. After taking picture it will send it to central server for processing. If it is an unknown person it will intimate to pushbullet server. The image will be sent to the authorized user. If it is known person then notification alone will be sent to the user.

5.7 Results and Discussion

This section presents experiment and evaluation of the proposed approach.

5.7.1 Computational Time

Here we compare the time required for sending the image to user with various methods and various network speeds are shown in Fig. 5.11.

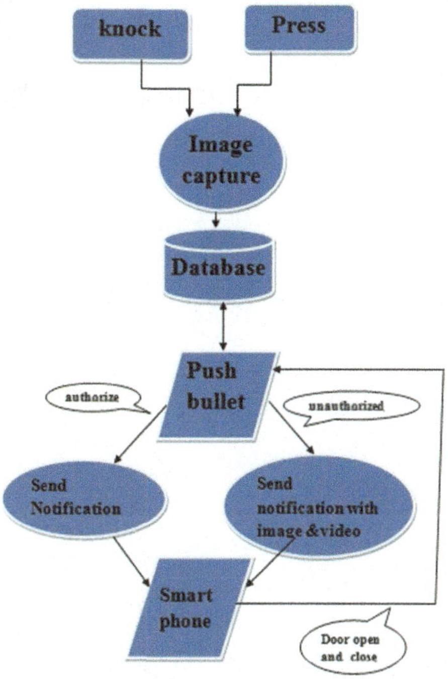

Fig. 5.10 System flow diagram

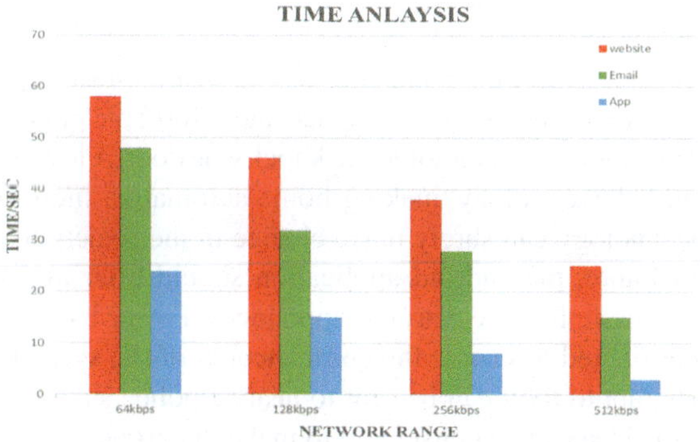

Fig. 5.11 Computational time

5.7.2 Results

Figure 5.12 shows the notification message received by the user when the unknown person knocks or press the push button. The notification message contains the current date and time. Once the picture is received by the push bullet server it will be transmit the image to an authorized person.

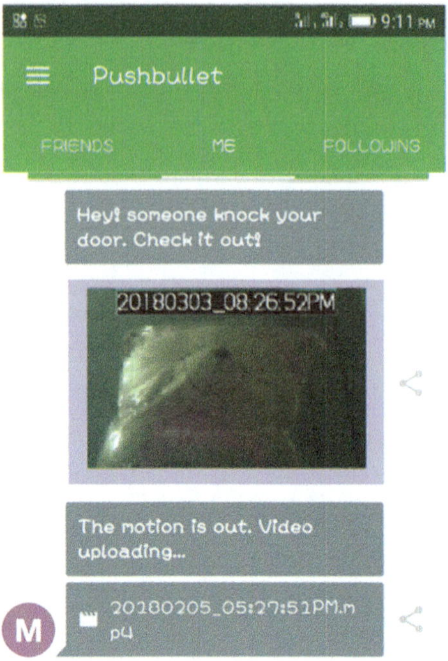

Fig. 5.12 Notification message along with the picture

5.8 Conclusion and Future Work

Secured smart door knocker is one of the most popular digital consumer devices because of the user convenience and affordable price. Users can remotely access the information's when someone knocks the door. A low cost authentication system based on IoT technology, making home automation more secure and cost efficient. This technology can surely make change in the society to drop the percentage of crime. In future, the android application should offer assistance in controlling windows and basic home electronic appliances. Power backup of the system should also be considered to ensure the completeness of the system. An auto trigger report of the attempt to theft can be sent to nearest police station along with residential address. This idea can be considered to make the proposed system better.

References

1. Madakam, S., Ramaswamy, R., Tripathi, S.: Internet of things (IoT): A literature review. J. Comput. Commun. **3**(05), 164 (2015)
2. Chandra, M.R., Kumar and B.V., SureshBabu, B.: IoT enabled home with smart security. In: 2017 International Conference on Energy, Communication, Data Analytics and Soft Computing (ICECDS), Chennai, 1193–1197 (2017)

3. Thabet, A.B., Amor, N.B.: Enhanced smart doorbell system based on face recognition. In: 2015 16th International Conference on Sciences and Techniques of Automatic Control and Computer Engineering (STA), Monastir, 373–377 (2015)
4. Upadhyay, J., Rida, P., Gupta, S.: Smart doorbell system based on face recognition. 2017 Int. Res. J. Eng. Technol. (IRJET). **4**, 2840–2843 (2015)
5. Sowjanya, G., Nagaraju, S.: Design and implementation of door access control and security system based on IOT. In: 2016 International Conference on Inventive Computation Technologies (ICICT), Coimbatore, 1–4 (2016)
6. Aman, F., Anitha, C.: Motion sensing and image capturing based smart door system on android platform. In: 2017 International Conference on Energy, Communication, Data Analytics and Soft Computing (ICECDS), Chennai, 2346–2350 (2017)
7. Singh, H., Pallagani, V., Khandelwal, V., Venkanna, U.: IoT based smart home automation system using sensor node. In: 2018 4th International Conference on Recent Advances in Information Technology (RAIT), Dhanbad, 1–5 (2018)
8. Hadis, M.S., Palantei, E., Ilham, A.A., Hendra, A.: Design of smart lock system for doors with special features using bluetooth technology. In: 2018 International Conference on Information and Communications Technology (ICOIACT), Yogyakarta, 396–400 (2018)
9. Viola, P., Jones, M.: Rapid object detection using boosted cascade of simple features. In: IEEE Conference on Computer Vision and Pattern Recognition, 2001
10. Nassif, H.H., Gindy, M., Davis, J.: Comparison of laser doppler vibrometer with contact sensors for monitoring bridge deflection and vibration. NDT E Int. **38**(3), 213–218 (2005)
11. Tan, L., Wang, N.: Future internet: The internet of things. In: 2010 3rd International Conference on Advanced Computer Theory and Engineering (ICACTE), 2010
12. http://www.pushbullet.com
13. Zhou, H., Huang, T.S.: Tracking articulated hand motion with Eigen dynamics analysis. In: Proceedings of International Conference on Computer Vision, vol. 2, 1102–1109 (2003)
14. Li, Y., Gong, S., Liddell, H.: Support vector regression and classification based multi-view face detection and recognition. In: International Conference on Automatic Face and Gesture Recognition, March 2000
15. Wang, Z., Xie, X.: An efficient face recognition algorithm based on robust principal component analysis. In: ICIMCS '10 Proceedings of the Second International Conference on Internet Multimedia Computing and Service, 2010
16. Ortega-Garcia, J., Bigun, J., Reynolds, D., GonzalezRodriguez, J.: Authentication gets personal with biometrics. Sig. Process. Mag. IEEE **21**(2), 50–62 (2004)

Chapter 6
Effective Fusion Technique Using FCM Based Segmentation Approach to Analyze Alzheimer's Disease

Suranjana Mukherjee and Arpita Das

Abstract The integration of complementary information from multimodal images is called fusion. In this study an efficient fusion technique is proposed to extract salient features from the segmented images of human brain that helps to study the prognosis of Alzheimer's disease. The significant information of each RGB component of low resolution functional PET image has been picked up by fuzzy clustering technique using appropriate membership functions. Intelligent choice of membership functions captures the salient features and spatial structures of the investigated region and does not incorporate any artifacts. To integrate each RGB component of the segmented PET image with MRI is done using principal component analysis approach as there is a possibility of losing relevant information in the conventional simple averaging process. Principal component approach is applied for weighted averaging scheme which is capable to extract important features of each color plane of PET with MRI. The experimental results show that the fused images are the successful combination of anatomical and functional information.

Keywords Alzheimer's disease · Anatomical image · Functional image · Segmentation technique · Fuzzy clustering · Fusion

6.1 Introduction

Medical imaging plays a vital role in diagnostic procedure for detecting any kind of neural degeneration. Loss, damage and death of neurons is responsible for neurological dementia like Schizophrenia, Manic depression, Parkinson's disease, Alzheimer's disease and so on. In this study we have focused on multimodal brain images which are affected by Alzheimer's disease (AD) [1–3].

In AD loss of neurons affects the regions which are involved in memory functioning, such as entorhinal cortex, hippocampus, gray matter and white matter shrinking [2–5]. White matter is built up by bundles of axons, which has a coat of myelin, a composition of proteins and lipids, which help in conduction of neurons and protect

S. Mukherjee · A. Das (✉)
Department of Radio Physics and Electronics, University of Calcutta, Kolkata, India
e-mail: adrpe@caluniv.ac.in

P. K. Pattnaik et al. (eds.), *Smart Healthcare Analytics in IoT Enabled Environment*, Intelligent Systems Reference Library 178,
https://doi.org/10.1007/978-3-030-37551-5_6

the axons. The function of white matter is to build connection in gray matter areas of brain and carrying nerve impulses between neurons. Gray matter is responsible for human perception like seeing, hearing, memory, emotions, capacity of decision making and ability of self control. Due to loss of brain volume, excess cerebrospinal fluid deposited in the ventricles, making the ventricles noticeably large. In later stages of AD, cerebral cortex which is responsible for language, reasoning and social behavior is affected severely.

In detection and treatment planning of AD various imaging techniques are there. Imaging modalities are classified in two categories as *anatomical* and *functional* [4–10]. Some of the popular anatomical imaging techniques are X-ray and digital subtraction angiography (DSA), computed tomography (CT) which is computed narrow beam of X-ray, magnetic resonance imaging (MRI) and ultrasound (US) primarily provides the morphological structure of the investigated region [4]. CT is very useful for locating tumors or any other kind of abnormalities in electron density map for calculation of accurate dose for radio therapeutic treatment. Ultrasound (US) provides the detailed soft tissue structure of blood vessels [5]. MRI provides detailed anatomical structure of brain and spinal cord. The most commonly used MRI sequences are T1-weighted and T2-weighted scans. The detailed anatomical structure is well visualized utilizing MR T1 type imaging procedure whereas the MR T2 prominently highlights the differences of usual and unusual structure of tissues [6, 10]. On the other side, functional imaging techniques like PET and SPECT reveals the functionality of tissues like flow of blood, food activity and metabolism of organ with a low space resolution [7–10]. Combined data from various imaging techniques may assist the physician to gather complete information of the focused tissues or organs under investigation. Integration of multimodal images assists the diagnosis and treatment planning of AD and other kind of neurodegenerative disorder.

The CT scan for diagnosis of AD gives the detailed information of cerebral atrophy with enlargement of cortical sulci and enlarged size of ventricles [4, 6]. It helps to diagnose vascular dementia. The detailed anatomical structure like shrinking of gray matter and white matter, enlargement of ventricles in AD is viewed prominently from MRI [6].

The cause of dementia in AD is destruction of a protein called amyloid which is build up on the walls of the arteries in the brain. Amyloidal precursor protein is expressed in many tissues and accumulated in the synapses of neurons. The exact primary function of amyloidal precursor is not known. But there are some implication of its functioning as a regulator of synapse formation, neural plasticity and iron export. From PET scan of brain image, red and dark blue colour signify the presence/absence of amyloid respectively and as we move blue to green the amount of amyloid increases gradually [8–10]. The amount of amyloid decreases significantly as a result reduced blood flow in those areas and affected by gradual death of neurons with the progression of dementia of AD. The PET scan of healthy brain and AD affected brain is shown in Fig. 6.1.

Image segmentation plays a crucial role to extract the relevant features of the region of interest. The segmentation is a process of partitioning an image into a set of disjoint regions depending on some attributes like intensity, various tone of

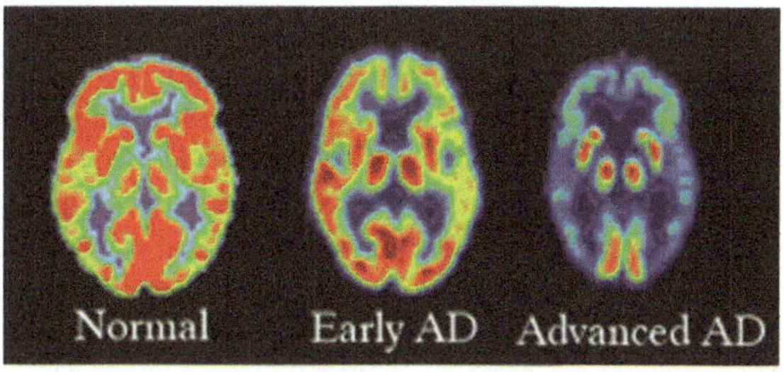

Fig. 6.1 PET scan of healthy brain, brain affected in early and advanced stage of AD

colour or texture [11]. There are three categories for image segmentation. They are thresholding, clustering, edge detection. We will focus on clustering [12]. Among various clustering approach fuzzy logic based method is most popular as it overcomes the limitation of binary logic [13].

After the segmentation, there is a process to combine two or more than two multimodal images into a single composite frame is called fusion. The accumulation of relevant information of PET and MRI is incorporated in the fused image is shown in Fig. 6.2, by indication of arrow marks. The integrated fused images provide finer detailed features of the edges, curves, notches, region boundaries of soft tissues, shape of ventricles, and information of cerebral atrophy which may be very much informative for analyzing AD in early stages as indicated in Fig. 6.2 [10].

In this study we have proposed a FCM based segmentation method followed by effective fusion technique to combine MRI and PET data in a single frame. The

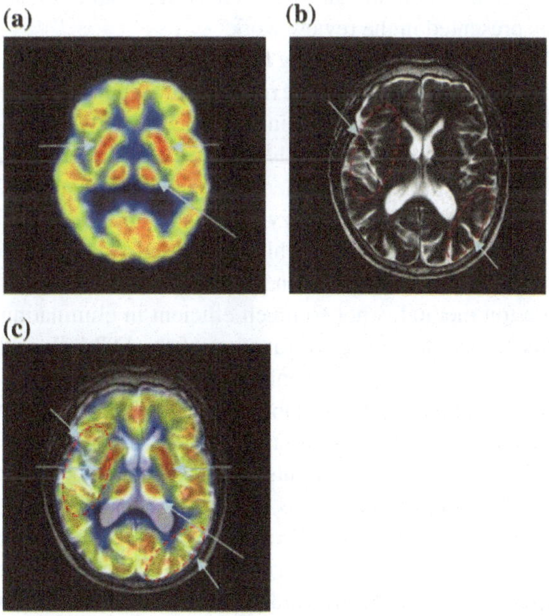

Fig. 6.2 **a** PET, **b** MRI and **c** fused image

fused image can be useful in improving clinical analysis of AD. The presence of noise can lead to misinterpretation of tissue structures which are known as artifacts. Proposed FCM approach can efficiently extract relevant information of PET image and eliminate the artifacts. The proposed fusion rule integrates the relevant details of PET and MRI. The acquisition of complimentary information is useful to study the prognosis of AD. The proposed method improves the quality of the fused image, which is also replicated in the experimental results.

This article is organized as follows. Section 6.2 presents some related fuzzy logic based image segmentation process followed by fusion procedure to study brain images. Proposed methodology is to study the prognosis of AD, which is described in details in Sect. 6.3. Experimental results and its analysis are given in Sect. 6.4 and finally we have drawn some conclusions in Sect. 6.5.

6.2 Review Works

Fusion is the process of combining multiple images of different modalities in a single frame to extract more fine details. The relevant information in the composite fused image plays a significant role in improving the clinical accuracy. In various studies, following the image segmentation approaches, fusion procedure is implemented. This is because segmentation approaches can retain the significant detail features efficiently that are hidden in the whole images. After the segmentation of the image effective fusion rules are imposed on them to integrate information from the multimodal images. Few related technique for segmentation and fusion scheme is presented in the review work.

The segmentation using fuzzy logic control based filter [13] as conventional filtering method may lose some relevant information. Fuzzy logic is the multi-valued logic which can successfully eliminate the impulsive noise and white Gaussian noise and preserves the image details effectively. Fuzzy if then rules give the actual anatomical information of segmented region and intensity of every pixel. Ahmed et al. has proposed a novel fuzzy segmentation approach to estimate the inhomogeneous intensity of MRI data, which is caused from imperfection in the radio-frequency coil during the acquisition process [14]. The conventional intensity based classification method is not so much efficient in eliminating the artifacts. In the proposed technique, the objective function of the FCM algorithm is modified in such a way that can compensate the inhomogeneties by allowing the labeling of a pixel (voxel) to be influenced by the labels of the immediate neighborhood. The effect from the neighborhood is acting as a regularizer and brings piecewise-homogeneous labeling. The segmentation of impulsive or salt and pepper noise, affected scan is also done by such regularization. Tolias and Panas proposed a neighborhood enhancement based fuzzy clustering scheme to impose spatial constraint for the purpose of incorporation of the multiresolution information [15]. In another approach, Noordam et al. has proposed a geometrically guided FCM to segment multivariate image [16]. They have proposed an approach in which condition of each pixel is determined by the membership values of immediate adjacent pixel and then is either incorporated of eliminated from the cluster [15, 16]. Later, a regularization term has been incorporated into a Kernel-based fuzzy clustering mean algorithm (KFCM) by Zhang et al. [17]. KFCM is utilized for noise handling and clustering of incomplete data. Chuang et al. has proposed a segmentation approach in which spatial information is introduced in the membership function as conventional FCM algorithm is not smart enough to do so [18]. Membership function is formed by adding or subtracting the spatial information which is determined by the neighborhood of every pixel. This method is capable of removing noisy dots, spurious blobs and yields more homogeneous regions than those of other methods. Han and Shi proposed ant colony based optimized algorithm inspired by the food-searching behavior of ants, is used for fuzzy clustering in image segmentation [19]. They have concentrated on three major features like gray value, gradient and adjacent pixels, which are extracted for the purpose of searching and incorporation of them in the membership function of the cluster. To speed up the searching process, there is an improved way in which the centre of the cluster is initialized and the heuristic function is enhanced. Halder et al. proposed an automated evolutionary genetic algorithm approach for segmenting a gray scale image into its constituent parts [20]. It is an efficient approach for precise segmentation of an image depending on its intensity information around the neighboring pixels. In this approach FCM helps in the process of generating population of genetic algorithm by utilizing an automatic segmentation technique. It is able to pick up single or multiple feature data with spatial information. Cai et al. proposed a fast as well as robust FCM framework to incorporate local spatial and gray information together. It can successfully nullify the disadvantages of spatial constraints, associated with conventional FCM approach. At the same time it enhances the clustering method [21]. Krinidis and Chatzis proposed a novel FCM approach for incorporating local spatial and gray level information. Their newly proposed algorithm enhances the clustering performance utilizing a fuzzy based local similarity measuring technique [22].

In some cases before the fusion approaches, segmented images are analyzed using similarity measuring matrices [11, 12, 23]. To achieve improved clinical accuracy in segmentation of anatomical structure, *multi-atlas patch-based label* fusion method is useful to obtain detail and accurate appearance of the tissues [23]. The state-of-the-art label fusion method is used in earlier days which may not capture the complex tissue structure in patch based similarity measurement approach. Hence, the previous process is made advanced by addition of three new hierarchical labels of fusion to improve the accuracy in capturing the detail of local and semi-local information.

In the recent years, many types of pyramid and wavelet based decomposition scheme has been studied [24–30] for fusion procedure. An image pyramid represents a number of decreasing resolution images. As we move upward to the pyramid resolution of the image is half of the previous. In the apex level, the resolution of the sub image is lowest. In pyramidal decomposition operation, most common operators are Gaussian pyramid and Laplacian operator [24–26, 31]. In the Gaussian pyramidal approach a Gaussian Kernel is used to convolve the original image. Gaussian Kernel is described as a low pass filtered version of the original image. The cut-off frequency is inversely proportionate with the bandwidth of the filter. On the other side, Laplacian operator is present to compute the difference between the original image and the low pass filtered image. Hence, Laplacian pyramid is a set of band pass filters, which is used for linking point discontinuities into linear structure.

In wavelet based decomposition method [26–30], to extract the finer details of the source image, it is down-sampled to high and low frequency subbands. To combine the detailed features, various fusion rules have been implemented.

Piella proposed an adaptive, data-driven method of thresholding for denoising image utilizing wavelet based soft-thresholding approach. The proposed thresholding technique is simple and in closed-form and it is adaptive to each subband components as it depends on data-driven estimation of the parameters [29]. Kant et al. had shown that discrete wavelet transform based local-correlation strategy of fusion is able to remove the blurred regions of source images and can integrate smooth, homogeneous information in the fused image [30].

To overcome the shortcomings like shift variance, aliasing and lack of directionality in discrete wavelet transform (DWT) there are many other decomposition methods like dual tree complex wavelet, curvelet, contourlet, ripplet transform are applied on multiscale geometric analysis of images to study the efficient fusion approach [32–36]. In dual tree complex wavelet transform (DTCWT), the scaling is not chosen arbitrarily and wavelet filters used in two trees. It solves the problem of shift variance and low directional selectivity in two and higher dimensions of DWT. Lewis et al. proposed DTCWT decomposition method and extract the significant features of pixel from each level of decompositions which is based on the rule of relative importance calculated from its neighborhood [33].

Curvelet transform is a nonshift invariant down sampling process for representing the accurate information of edges along the curves. It is much efficient decomposition process in comparison to the conventional discrete wavelet transform for a given accuracy of reconstruction [34]. But contourlet transform has shown increased efficiency in directional multiresolution expansion which inherits the rich wavelet theory. It has shown better performances in representing the finer details like lines, edges, curves and contours than wavelet and curvelet transform because of its directional and anisotropic property [35]. The contourlet transform consists of two steps which are subband decomposition and directional transformation [35, 36]. The expansion of the image is done by using the basic operations like contour segmentation, hence it is named so. In contourlet transformation, the directional filter bank is used with fixed length and because of this it cannot handle the representation of spatial structures in multi direction efficiently. Hence a computationally efficient, shearlet transform is used in which there are no restrictions on the number of directions for shearing and the size of supports [36]. Ganasala et al. proposed a multi scale shift invariant multi-dimensional decomposition technique like nonsubsampled shearlet transform. Low frequency subband components are combined on the basis of the fusion rule using sum of variations in squares. In selection of coefficient, there is a decision map which is subjected to morphological opening and closing operation, having structural element of square shape. The function of opening operator is to remove the stray background pixels of initial decision map followed by closing which remove the hole in the foreground [36]. Hence there is uniformity in the selection process. High frequency components are selected using activity level measurement of coefficients in horizontal, vertical and diagonal direction in particular location.

After multilevel fusion scheme, different fusion rules are implemented for integrating all possible significant information of source images. Zheng et al. proposed the fusion rule of simple averaging process for approximation images of low frequency subbands and select 'Max' or 'Min' for detail image of high frequency subbands in multi level decomposition [37]. But, combination of low frequency subbands using simple averaging process (SAP) may loss relevant features. Das et al. has shown the advanced approach of principal component analysis (PCA) is to determine the weighted average to avoid the loss of relevant data loss in SAP. PCA is able to integrate information of low frequency sub sampled images of PET in RGB and MRI as well as it can retrieve the inconsistent information [10]. In another study it is observed that wavelet approaches is able to remove the white Gaussian noises obtained from PET and Radiography images in different color spaces [24]. Zhang and Blum has reviewed some fusion rules like point, window and region based activity level measurement to achieve better result [38]. Hence by this short review, we can conclude that fusion methodology plays very crucial role to study the prognosis of AD.

6.3 Methodology

The main objective of this study is to integrate relevant information in a composite frame, which is helpful to observe the dementia and treatment planning of AD. The fundamental methodologies used in the proposed technique are fuzzy logic based clustering and PCA based weighted averaging scheme for integration of PET data with MRI in a single frame.

Fuzzy clustering method is useful for collecting significant data from each color plane of PET. In this study, extraction of relevant information of PET images is performed using fuzzy clustering based segmentation technique. This approach is appropriate to resolve the uncertainties and impreciseness present in the low-resolution functional images like PET. Since AD is the consequence of a gradual degeneration of neurons which affect neurological functions, fuzzy clustering scheme can capture the salient features and spatial structures of different color plane of PET. Fuzzy clustering technique is based on the concepts of membership functions (MFs). Proper and intelligent choice of MFs is the backbone of the proposed fuzzy clustering approach. In Fuzzy logic based clustering approach; the required MFs are determined by optimizing the objective function of dissimilarity. In dealing with smooth and gradual changes of image features, fuzzy clustering technique removes artifacts/misrepresentation of soft tissue structure in the fused images. After that, to prevent data loss in the simple averaging technique, PCA is there to fuse the salient features of PET with MRI. The fused image contained the functional data of PET in

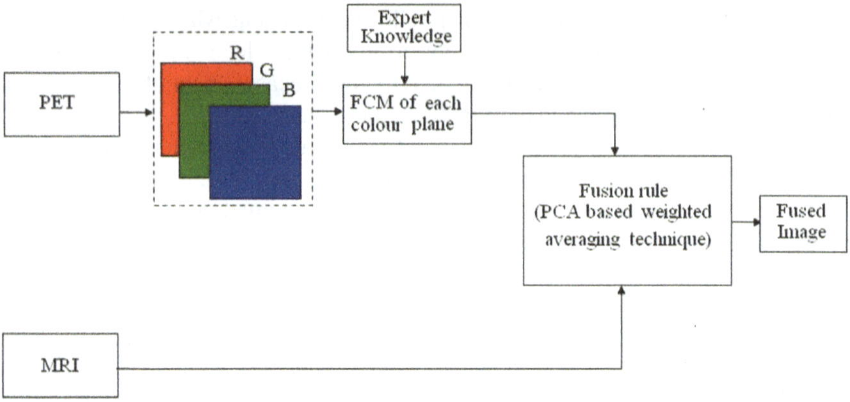

Fig. 6.3 Brief overview of the proposed approach

RGB scale with edge related structural information of MRI. A brief overview of the proposed methodology is shown in Fig. 6.3.

The details of every step like fuzzy logic approach, fuzzy clustering technique and PCA based weighted averaging scheme are described in the following sections to present an overview of the proposed method.

6.3.1 Fuzzy Logic Approach

Fuzzy logic is a multi-valued logic to provide a systematic calculus to interpret incomplete and imprecise sensory information linguistically. Fuzzy set is a set without a crisp boundary. Hence it is the transition from 'belong to set' and 'not belong to set'. This smooth transition of fuzzy set is determined by membership function which has the flexibility to represent in between attributes of two specific conditions like 'hot' and 'cold'. In binary logic there are only two conditions 0 and 1 which are represented as either hot or cold. But in fuzzy logic, there are so many conditions in between 'hot' and 'cold' like too hot, pleasant, warm, cold, too cold.

Say, X is a space of points and a generic element of X is represented by x. Hence $X = \{x\}$. Membership function (MF) $\mu(x)$ determines the fuzzy set Ã in X. The membership function is mapping each point in X in between the interval of [0, 1], with the values of $\mu(x)$, denoting the 'degree of membership' of x in $\tilde{A}$. Thus the 'higher degree of membership' is signifying greater value of the MF.

In the proposed methodology, significant information of each color plane of PET image is collected efficiently by fuzzy logic approach. For this purpose, fuzzy c-mean clustering technique is utilized for the fuzzification of relevant information of each color plane.

Hence, salient features of the RGB color plane are picked up efficiently according to the specification of membership values and membership functions. This fuzzy membership function based clustering approach of integration does not incorporate any additional artifacts or blocking effects in the final results. In the following section, details of fuzzy c-mean clustering technique are described.

Fuzzy C-Mean (FCM) Clustering Algorithm

FCM is a method of partitioning n, number of data elements, $X = \{x_1, \ldots x_j, \ldots x_n\}$ into a cluster or groups, c known as fuzzy groups, and finds a cluster centre in each group in such a way that a cost function for dissimilarity measurement is minimized. FCM is based on fuzzy partitioning technique. So, a given data point can belong to several groups having the degree of belongingness, which is determined by grads of membership lying between [0, 1]. Membership matrix U (U is a $c \times n$ real matrix, $U = [u_{ij}]$ where $i = 1, 2, \ldots, c; j = 1, 2, \ldots n$) allows the accommodation of these in between values.

Normalization stipulates are imposed and the summation of degree of belongingness for a data set is always equal to unity [39], which is denoted as follows.

$$\sum_{i=1}^{c} u_{ij} = 1 \quad \forall_j = 1, \ldots, n \tag{6.1}$$

where c represents the total number of clusters; $2 \leq c < n$.

The objective function for FCM in terms of the cluster centers (c_i) is denoted as follows.

$$J(U, c) = \sum_{i=1}^{c} J_i = \sum_{i=1}^{c} \sum_{j=1}^{n} u_{ij}^m d_{ij}^2 \tag{6.2}$$

where, u_{ij} is between 0 and 1,

$c = (c_1, c_2, c_3, \ldots c_i, \ldots c_{c-1}, c_c)$ = vector of centers, c_i is the ith element, locating in the fuzzy cluster,

$d_{ij} = \|c_i - x_j\|$ is representing the Euclidean distance between ith cluster center and jth data point,

$m \in [1, \infty)$ represents a weighting component to control the relative weights, which is placed on each of the squared errors dij^2.

Significance of weighting exponent: For m = 1, FCM partitions are called as hard c-means partitions. The cost function J approaches inversely to the number of clusters as $m \to \alpha$. The significance of increasing value of m leads to degradation of membership towards the fuzziest state. Hence, no theoretical or computational evidence is there to distinguish an optimal m. It has been observed that for most of the cases 1.5 < m < 3.0. So, m is chosen as m = 2.

The representation of optimal fuzzy clustering of X is as a pair $(\hat{U}, \hat{c})$ which is used for local minimization of the cost function J [40]. For m > 1, for all j and k $\hat{c}_k \neq x_j$ may be locally optimal for J while

$$\hat{c}_i = \frac{\sum_{j=1}^{n} \hat{u}_{ij}^{m} x_j}{\sum_{j=1}^{n} \hat{u}_{ij}^{m}} \tag{6.3}$$

and

$$\hat{u}_{ij} = \frac{1}{\sum_{k=1}^{c} \left(\frac{\hat{d}_{ij}}{\hat{d}_{kj}}\right)^{2/(m-1)}} \tag{6.4}$$

where, $\hat{d}_{ij} = \left\| \hat{c}_i - x_j \right\|$.

The conditions, which are expressed in Eqs. (6.3) and (6.4) are necessary. But they are not sufficient enough for optimizing J via simple Picard iteration, to loop back and forth utilizing Eqs. (6.3) and (6.4) until the iterative sequence exhibits a small changes in successive entries of $\hat{U}$ or $\hat{c}$.

We can describe the whole process as follows:

(a) Initialization of the membership matrix $U = [u_{ij}]$ having random values between 0 and 1 in such a way that should satisfy the condition of constraints of Eq. (6.1).
(b) Calculation of cluster centers of fuzzy data sets, c_i, $i = 1, 2, \ldots c$, Eq. (6.3).
(c) Computation of the cost functions according to Eq. (6.2). End if it is improved in comparison to previous iteration and is lower to a predefined threshold value.
(d) Computation of a membership matrix $\hat{U} = [\hat{u}_{ij}]$ using Eq. (6.4). Return to step-b.

6.3.2 *Expert Knowledge*

In the proposed approach, RGB color space of PET has been fused with MRI. For this purpose, salient features of each the color plane of PET image are picked up by using fuzzy c-means clustering scheme. For the purpose of fuzzification, there is a crucial decision in choosing suitable number of membership functions to cover the universe of discourse that satisfies the conditions of information over-capturing or under-capturing. The requirement of expert knowledge for the purpose of choosing membership functions immensely affects the results of fusion approach. For the present study, this choice is carried out for achieving the best experimental results.

6.3.3 *Fusion Rule Using PCA Based Weighted Averaging*

For the integration of those overall gross features of segmented image are carried out by weighted averaging based fusion rule. To determine the weight factor principal component analysis is utilized. Since in the earlier studies it has been seen that the simple averaging process may suffer from relevant information lose and hence there is significant degradation of contrast in the fused image. To avoid this, we have performed a weighted averaging process to combine the red, green and blue plane of PET image with MRI, which is in gray scale. The proposed approach is shown mathematically in Eq. (6.5).

$$C_F = q_A * C_A + q_B * C_B \tag{6.5}$$

where q_A and q_B are the weighted factors determining the importance of *grayscale image*, C_B and RGB components of the segmented PET image, C_A.

In this study to integrate each of the RGB plane with gray scale MRI, principal component analysis (PCA) is applied [10, 41]. This is because PCA transformation is based on the correlated input data into a set of statistically independent features which are generally arranged by reducing information content. The proposed PCA technique is able to find the significant information component of RGB plane as well as the gray image, which provides the assistance for the determination of weighted factors. In PCA technique, we find the principal axis eigenvalue of the RGB components and MRI image. After that we have to calculate the respective eigenvector implement the fusion rule on them accordingly depending on the principal eigenvector. The procedure of PCA approach is described in detail in the following sections.

- Step 1: We have to calculate the covariance matrix, form the image data vectors. To create image data vectors the matrices are arranged in fore-column-post-row or fore-row-post-column. The covariance matrix is calculated utilizing Eq. (6.6). The respective mean value is subtracted from all the values of each vector to form an image vector whose mean is zero.

$$C = \begin{bmatrix} \mathrm{cov}(A, A) & \mathrm{cov}(A, B) \\ \mathrm{cov}(B, A) & \mathrm{cov}(B, B) \end{bmatrix} \tag{6.6}$$

where $\mathrm{cov}(A, B) = \frac{\sum_{i=1}^{n}\left(A_i - \bar{A}\right)\left(B_i - \bar{B}\right)}{n-1}$.
- Step 2: Calculation of the eigenvectors of the covariance matrix C, which are orthogonal in nature to determine the principal eigenvector. It must be noted that data variables are mainly distributed around one eigen vector in the coordinate graph which is known as principal eigenvector $(x, y)^T$, and it contains the maximum eigenvalue. Basically, most relevant information of the images is associated with principal eigenvector.
- Step 3: The final step is to calculate the weight factors of the images to be fused accordingly to the principal eigenvector. The fusion of segmented components of RGB plane of PET image and MRI is done accordingly to the respective principal eigenvectors $(x, y)^T$. The weight factors of C_A and C_B are determined as follows:

$$q_A = \frac{x}{x + y} \text{ and } q_B = \frac{y}{x + y}$$

6.4 Experimental Results

Proposed fusion approach combines both functional and anatomical imaging details like preservation of color information as well as accumulation of fine curvatures of gray matter, white matter, ventricles and cerebral cortex in the fused image. Fusion scheme is implemented on different sagittal slices of PET and brain MRI (T1 and T2 weighted) images of a 70 years old man, who is suffering from mild AD as described by Harvard University (www.med.harvard.edu/aanlib/home.html). MRI and PET images reveal the widened hemispheric sulci and abnormality in regional cerebral metabolism respectively. In the proposed method, fuzzy clustering is applied on the each RGB plane of PET scan of the patient to extract those significant features and PCA based fusion rule integrates the effective complementary information. Experimental results obtained by this method provide the complete information to study further investigation and progression of AD. Some fused images of different sagittal slices of brain MRI (T1 and T2 weighted) and PET images as shown in Figs. 6.4, 6.5, 6.6 and 6.7.

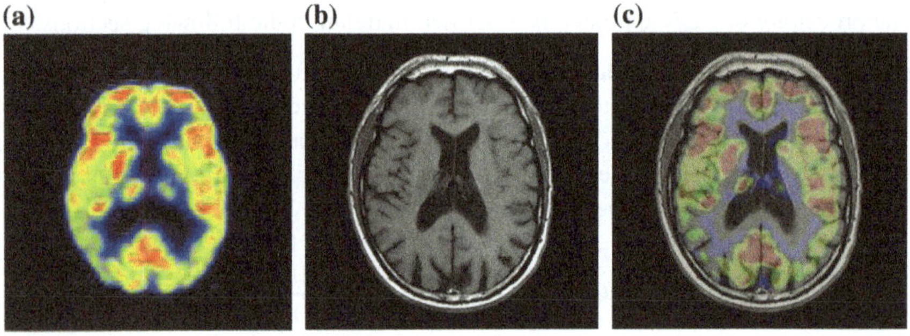

Fig. 6.4 Set-I: Fusion of PET and MRI images: **a** PET, **b** MR-T1 and **c** fused image

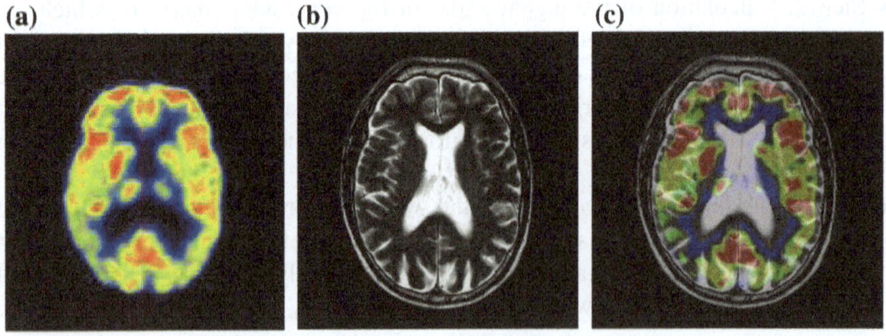

Fig. 6.5 Set-II: Fusion of PET and MRI images: **a** PET, **b** MR-T2 and **c** fused image

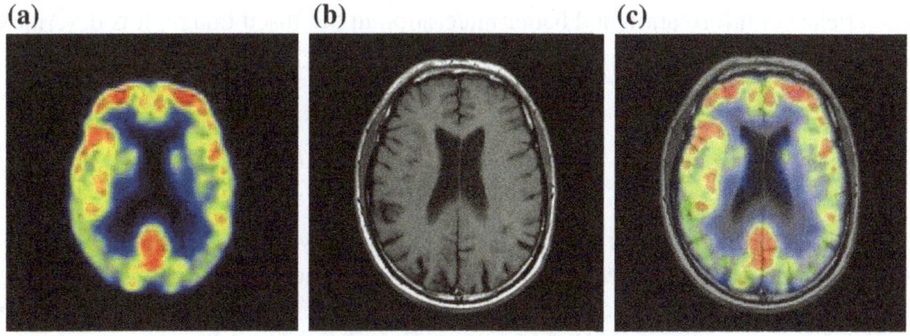

Fig. 6.6 Set-III: Fusion of PET and MRI images: **a** PET, **b** MR-T1 and **c** fused image

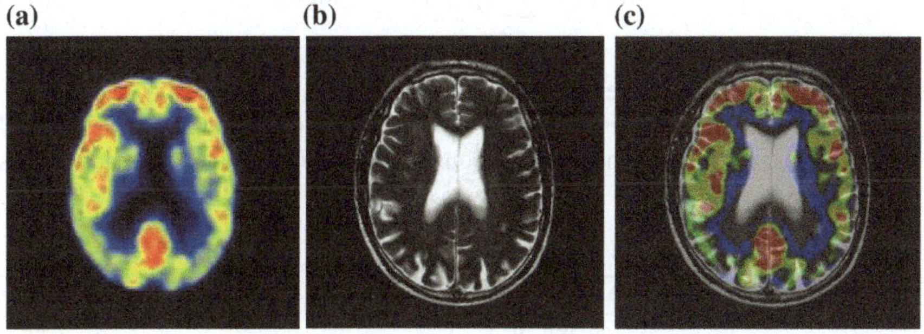

Fig. 6.7 Set-IV: Fusion of PET and MRI images: **a** PET, **b** MR-T2 and **c** fused image

Analysis of Fusion Results

For the assessment of image fusion algorithm, there are two performance indices—objective and subjective. Subjective analysis of proposed fusion scheme shows the detailing of the soft tissue regions surrounding the ventricles from MRI and preservation of color information from PET revealing the metabolism of those regions. The PCA based weighted averaging procedure is able to capture relevant information of PET and MRI. Hence it is found that the proposed approach provides the more informative, integrated fused image, having better contrast and clarity.

However, subjective analysis is based on the comprehensive ability of human experts. On the other hand in objective analysis, there are some mathematical parameters like *Entropy, Standard deviation (STD), Average gradient (AG)* and *Variance*.

To evaluate the salient feature of fused images, mathematical parameters are measured. In this study, we have evaluated (*i*) *Entropy*, (*ii*) *Standard Deviation (STD)*, (*iii*) *Average Gradient (AG)* and (*iv*) *Variance* of the images to study the efficiency of the proposed approach [10, 42]. These parameters are explained as follows.

(i) *Entropy*: This parameter is to evaluate the course information content present in the image and its texture distribution. Grater entropy value corresponds to richer in information and better integration in the fused image. It is described mathematically as:

$$Entropy = \sum_{I=0}^{255} p(z_i) \log_2 p(z_i) \tag{6.7}$$

where $p(z_i)$ represents the probability of randomly variable intensity z_i.

(ii) *STD*: It has significance in exploiting the clarity and visual quality of the image information. The higher value of STD signifies the better visual clarity and rich information content in the fused image. It is defined as follows.

$$STD = \sum_{i=0}^{255} (p(z_i) - m)^2 \log_2 p(z_i) \tag{6.8}$$

where m represents average intensity of image.

(iii) *AG*: It is used to measure the sharpness in the form of gradient values related to edges, curves, notches, region boundaries of images. It can be denoted as follows.

$$AG = \frac{1}{M \times N} \times \sum_{j=0}^{M-1} \sum_{i=0}^{N-1} \sqrt{\left(\frac{1}{2}\left(\left(\frac{\partial z}{\partial x_i}(x_i, y_i)\right)^2 + \left(\frac{\partial z}{\partial y_i}(x_i, y_i)\right)^2\right)\right)} \tag{6.9}$$

(iv) *Variance*: It is an important parameter to evaluate the image contrast. The higher value of *variance* represents better contrast for visualization. It is represented mathematically as follows.

$$Variance = \sum_{i=0}^{255} (z_i - m)^2 p(z_i) \tag{6.10}$$

Those parametric details are depicted in Table 6.1 and the efficiency of the proposed fusion approach is proved.

6.5 Conclusion

In this study, we have applied FCM based segmentation method followed by an effective fusion rule to study and analyze the progression of AD. Selection of salient features from each of the RGB plane of PET image and elimination of artifacts is done by using fuzzy C-mean clustering approach. Application of PCA based averaging rule can determine the weight factors of MRI and each of the RGB planes of PET,

Table 6.1 Objective evaluation of parameters of proposed the fusion techniques

Images	Criteria	PET	MRI	Fused image
Figure 6.4	Entropy	4.2791	4.7025	4.9471
	STD	0.3016	0.2285	0.3096
	AG	0.0176	0.0105	0.0193
	Variance	0.0910	0.0522	0.0973
Figure 6.5	Entropy	4.2791	4.4247	4.7482
	STD	0.3016	0.2508	0.3123
	AG	0.0176	0.01093	0.0206
	Variance	0.0910	0.0629	0.1056
Figure 6.6	Entropy	4.1731	4.5297	4.7595
	STD	0.2810	0.2263	0.2879
	AG	0.0203	0.0185	0.0219
	Variance	0.079	0.0512	0.0810
Figure 6.7	Entropy	4.1731	4.1393	4.5008
	STD	0.2810	0.2308	0.2951
	AG	0.0203	0.0295	0.0298
	Variance	0.079	0.0533	0.0581

as a result the fused image of different sagittal slices of human brain contains the detail anatomical and functional information about AD. The improved information content of the fused image is also reflected in the experimental results. In the proposed method, fused images have better contrast, visual clarity and finer detailing related to edges, curves, tissue structures, region boundaries which help in clinical analyses of AD.

Acknowledgements This work is supported by the Center of Excellence (CoE) in Systems Biology and Biomedical Engineering, University of Calcutta, funded by the TEQIP Phase-III,World Bank, MHRD India. We would also like to thank to Dr. S. K. Sharma of EKO X-ray and Imagining Institute, Kolkata for providing us valuable comments on the subjective evaluation of the proposed fusion scheme.

References

1. Horn, J.F., Habert, M.O., Kas, A., Malek, Z., Maksud, P., Lacomblez, L., Giron, A., Fertil, B.: Differential automatic diagnosis between Alzheimer's disease and frontotemporal dementia based on perfusion SPECT images. Artif. Intell. Med. **47**(2), 147–158 (2009)
2. Fang, S., Raghavan, R., Richtsmeier, J.T.: Volume morphing methods for landmark based 3D image deformation. In: Medical Imaging: Image Processing, Bellingham, WA. SPIE, vol. 2710, pp. 404–415 (1996)

3. Janke, A.L., Zubicaray, G., Rose, S.E., Griffin, M., Chalk, J.B., Galloway, G.J.: 4D deformation modeling of cortical disease progression in Alzheimer's dementia. Int. Soc. Magn. Reson. Med. **46**(4), 661–666 (2001)
4. Hill, D.L.G., Hawkes, D.J., Crossman, J.E., Gleeson, M.J., Cox, T.C.S., Bracey, E.E.C.M.L., Strong, A.J., Graves, P.: Registration of MR and CT images for skull base surgery using point-like anatomical features. Br. J. Radiol. **64**(767), 1030–1035 (1991)
5. Kagadis, G.C., Delibasis, K.K., Matsopoulos, G.K., Mouravliansky, N.A., Asvestas, P.A., Nikiforidis, G.C.: A comparative study of surface- and volume-based techniques for the automatic registration between CT and SPECT brain images. Med. Phys. **29**(2), 201–213 (2002)
6. Bhattacharya, M., Das, A., Chandana, M.: GA-based multiresolution fusion of segmented brain images using PD-, T1- and T2-weighted MR modalities. Neural Comput. Appl. **21**(6), 1433–1447 (2012)
7. Chang, D.J., Zubal, I.G., Gottschalk, C., Necochea, A., Stokking, R., Studholme, C., Corsi, M., Slawski, J., Spencer, S.S., Blumenfeld, H.: Comparison of statistical parametric mapping and SPECT difference imaging in patients with temporal lobe epilepsy. Epilepsia **43**(1), 68–74 (2002)
8. Mayberg, H.S.: Clinical correlates of PET- and SPECT-identified defects in dementia. J. Clin. Psychiatry (1994)
9. Gigengack, G., Ruthotto, R., Burger, B., Wolters, C.H., Xiaoyi Jiang, X., Schafers, K.P.: Motion correction in dual gated cardiac PET using mass-preserving image registration. IEEE Trans. Med. Imaging **31**(3), 698–712 (2012)
10. Das, A., Bhattacharya, M.: Effective image fusion method to study Alzheimer's disease using MR, PET images. In: IEEE International Conference on Bioinformatics and Biomedicine (BIBM), pp. 1603–1607 (2015)
11. Pal, N., Pal, S.: A review on image segmentation techniques. Pattern Recogn. **26**, 1277–1294 (1993)
12. Bezdek, J.C., Hall, L.O., Clarke, L.P.: Review of MR image segmentation techniques using pattern recognition. Med. Phys. **20**, 1033–1048 (1993)
13. Russo, F., Ramponi, G.: A fuzzy filter for images corrupted by impulse noise. IEEE Signal Process. Lett. **3**(6), 168–170 (1996)
14. Ahmed, M.N., Yamany, S.M., Mohamed, N., Farag, A.A., Moriarty, T.: A modified fuzzy C-means algorithm for bias field estimation and segmentation of MRI data. IEEE Trans. Med. Imaging **21**, 193–199 (2002)
15. Tolias, Y.A., Panas, S.M.: Image segmentation by a fuzzy clustering algorithm using adaptive spatially constrained membership functions. IEEE Trans. Syst. Man Cybern. Part A Syst. Humans **28**(3), 359–369 (1998)
16. Noordam, J.C., Van Den Broek, W.H., Buydens, L.M.: Geometrically guided fuzzy C-means clustering for multivariate image segmentation. Proc. Int. Conf. Pattern Recogn. **1**, 462–465 (2000)
17. Zhang, D.Q., Chen, S.C., Pan, Z.S., Tan, K.R.: Kernel-based fuzzy clustering incorporating spatial constraints for image segmentation. In: International Conference on Machine Learning and Cybernetics, pp. 2189–2192. IEEE (2003)
18. Chuang, K.S., Tzeng, H.L., Chen, S., Wu, J., Chen, T.J.: Fuzzy c-means clustering with spatial information for image segmentation. Comput. Med. Imaging Graph. **30**(1), 9–15 (2006)
19. Han, Y., Shi, P.: An improved ant colony algorithm for fuzzy clustering in image segmentation. Neurocomputing **70**(4–6), 665–671 (2007)
20. Halder, A., Pramanik, S., Kar, A.: Dynamic image segmentation using fuzzy c-means based genetic algorithm. Int. J. Comput. Appl. **28**(6), 15–20 (2011)
21. Cai, W., Chen, S., Zhang, D.: Fast and robust fuzzy c-means clustering algorithms incorporating local information for image segmentation. Pattern Recogn. **40**(3), 825–838 (2007)
22. Krinidis, S., Chatzis, V.: A robust fuzzy local information C-means clustering algorithm. IEEE Trans. Image Process. **19**(5), 1327–1337 (2010)
23. Wu, G., Kim, M., Sanroma, G., Wang, Q., Munsell, B.C., Shen, D.: Hierarchical multi-atlas label fusion with multi-scale feature representation and label-specific patch partition. NeuroImage **106**, 34–46 (2015)

24. Zhao, H., Li, Q., Feng, H.: Multi-focus color image fusion in the HIS space using the sum-modified-Laplacian and a coarse edge map. Image Vis. Comput. **26**(9), 1285–1295 (2008)
25. Amolins, K., Zhang, Y., Dare, P.: Wavelet based image fusion techniques—an introduction, review and comparison. ISPRS J. Photogramm. Remote Sens. **62**(4), 249–263 (2007)
26. Pajares, G., De La Cruz, J.M.: A wavelet-based image fusion tutorial. Pattern Recogn. **37**(9), 1855–1872 (2004)
27. Li, H., Manjunath, B.S., Mitra, S.K.: Multisensor image fusion using the wavelet transform. Graph. Models Image Process. **57**(3), 235–245 (1995)
28. Piella, G.: Adaptive Wavelets and Their Applications to Image Fusion and Compression. CWI & University of Amsterdam, Amsterdam (2003)
29. Kant, S., Singh, P., Kushwaha, M.: A new image enhancement technique using local-correlation based fusion using wavelet transform. Int. J. Curr. Trends Sci. Technol. **8**(05), 20601–20610 (2018)
30. Hamdi, M.: A comparative study in wavelets, curvelets and contourlets as denoising biomedical images. Image Process. Commun. **16**(3–4), 13–20 (2011)
31. Heeger, D.J., Bergen, J.R.: Pyramid-based texture analysis/synthesis. In: Proceedings of the 22nd Annual Conference on Computer Graphics and Interactive Techniques, pp. 229–238. ACM (1995)
32. Lewis, J.J., O'Callaghan, R.J., Nikolov, S.G., Bull, D.R., Canagarajah, N.: Pixel- and region-based image fusion with complex wavelets. Inform. Fusion **8**(2), 119–130 (2007)
33. Nencini, F., Garzelli, A., Baronti, S., Alparone, L.: Remote sensing image fusion using the curvelet transform. Inform. Fusion **8**(2), 143–156 (2007)
34. Do, M.N., Vetterli, M.: Contourlets: a directional multiresolution image representation. In: Proceedings of IEEE International Conference on Image Processing, vol. 1, pp. 357–360 (2002)
35. Yang, S., Wang, M., Jiao, L., Wu, R., Wang, Z.: Image fusion based on a new contourlet packet. Inform. Fusion **11**(2), 78–84 (2010)
36. Ganasala, P., Kumar, V.: Multimodality medical image fusion based on new features in NSST domain. Biomed. Eng. Lett. **4**(4), 414–424 (2014)
37. Zheng, Y., Hou, X., Bian, T., Qin, Z.: Effective image fusion rules of multi-scale image decomposition. In: Proceedings of the 5th International Symposium on Image and Signal Processing and Analysis (2007)
38. Zhang, Z., Blum, R.S.: A categorization of multiscale-decomposition-based image fusion schemes with a performance study for a digital camera application. Proc. IEEE **87**(8), 1315–1326 (1999)
39. Das, A., Bhattacharya, M.: A study on prognosis of brain tumors using fuzzy logic and genetic algorithm based techniques. In: International Joint Conference on Bioinformatics, Systems Biology and Intelligent Computing, IJCBS'09, pp. 348–351. IEEE (2009)
40. Bhattacharya, M., Das, A.: Discrimination for malignant and benign masses in breast using mammogram: a study on adaptive neuro-fuzzy approaches. In: Proceedings of Indian International Conference on Artificial Intelligence (IICAI-07), Pune, India, pp. 1007–1026. Springer (2007)
41. Li, B., Lv, H.: Pixel level image fusion scheme based on accumulated gradient and PCA transform. J. Commun. Comput. **6**, 49–54 (2009)
42. Gonzalez, R.C., Woods, R.E., Eddins, S.L.: Digital image processing using MATLAB. Pearson-Prentice-Hall, Upper Saddle River, New Jersey (2004)

Chapter 7
Application of Machine Learning in Various Fields of Medical Science

Subham Naskar, Patel Dhruv, Satarupa Mohanty and Soumya Mukherjee

Abstract With some unique aspects, Machine Learning is now a trending part in today's world. The ability of these machine learning models to independently adapt to data they are being exposed to make them unique. Just like the brain these models are able to produce reliable decisions with minimal human intervention from computations and calculations done previously. In the era where wearable sensors and devices can provide real time data about a patient's health, machine learning is really taking over traditional approach of diagnosing and predicting tumors, polyps, cardiac arrests, hemorrhages, and even cancer. Medical professionals teaming up with data analyst and scientists can analyze data to extract it's features which will lead to a better understanding of the disease symptoms and increase the efficiency of diagnosing. This article discusses the application and some of the case studies of machine learning in various medical fields like diagnosing diseases of brain and heart.

Keywords K nearest neighbour classifier · Genetic algorithm · Regularized logistic regression · Semi-supervised learning · Machine learning

7.1 Introduction

Machine learning approach provides the ability of automatically learning and improving with the experience without being explicitly programmed. This section briefly introduces the various machine learning approaches in the medical field.

S. Naskar · P. Dhruv · S. Mohanty (✉)
KIIT Deemed to Be University, Bhubaneswar, India

S. Mukherjee
Government College of Engineering and Ceramic Technology, Kolkata, India

P. K. Pattnaik et al. (eds.), *Smart Healthcare Analytics in IoT Enabled Environment*, Intelligent Systems Reference Library 178,
https://doi.org/10.1007/978-3-030-37551-5_7

7.1.1 KNN (K Nearest Neighbor Classifier)

K KNN is one of the simplest supervised machine learning algorithms used in classification and regression problems. Using proximity, distance function and basing on similarity measures KNN determines the new data. The value of k is directly proportional to the number of the nearest neighbors [1]. Being a supervised learning model KNN learn a function from input data and produce an output when unlabeled test data is introduced. The Euclidean distance between the unknown and the dataset points is calculated by KNN. The general formula is:

$$d(p,q) = d(y,x) = \sqrt{(y_1 - x_1)^2 + (y_2 - x_2)^2 + \cdots + (y_n - x_n)^2}$$

where y_1 to y_n and x_1 to x_n are the values of different observations.

The data is loaded, and K is initiated to the neighbors. Distance between the present example and the train example is determined, added and indexed to an ordered collection. Then after sorting the collection in an ascending order the K entries are picked and their corresponding labels are obtained. Regression returns the mean while classification returns the mode of the K labels. The training dataset is memorized by KNN but the discriminative function is not learnt by it, so it is termed as lazy learner [2].

7.1.2 Genetic Algorithm

Preferably through a biological process of natural selection, both constrained and unconstrained optimization problems can be solved by genetic algorithm. This algorithm proves to be useful in spaces that can be specified combinatorically and there are separate dimensions to contribute to different to the overall fitness value. Analogies with biological evolution can be established via this optimization algorithm [3]. A generation of laws are parametrized by a sequence of numbers, each of which has a performance and cost function contributing to the associated fitness. This is also related to the probability of selection, which constitutes to the formation of future generations via certain genetic operations. This whole procedure is a targeted optimization that improves selectively from one generation to the other and helps a generation to get more and more control laws [4]. Figure 7.1 demonstrate the lock in structure demonstration genetic function.

Thus, it can be defined as a set of optimization technique for high dimensional search spaces of parameters if a lock in structure like Fig. 7.1 is provided with the parameters given as K_P, K_I, K_D. These defined set of parameters are being optimized to define the cost of a high dimensional landscape; genetic algorithm only helps to effectively find these hotspots of best performance in a way that's faster than conventional search methods. Figure 7.2 demonstrates the flow of the process of genetic algorithm.

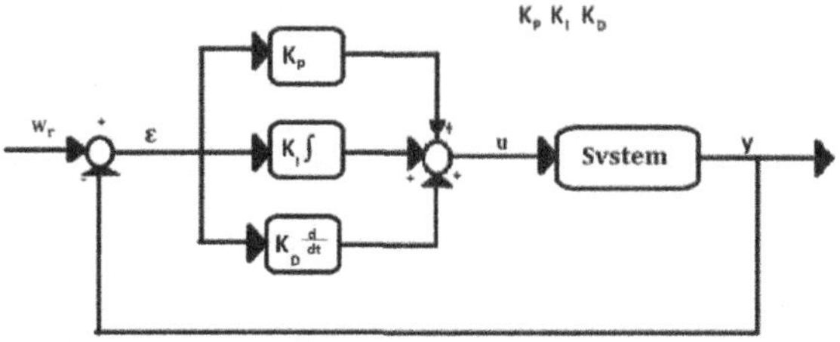

Fig. 7.1 A lock in structure demonstration genetic function [16]

7.1.3 *Regularized Logistic Regression*

In case when several regularization parameters are used the logistic regression, curve will be prone to overfitting, to avoid that a regularized parameter is introduced (lambda) which can decrease the overfitting. But with higher value of lambda the curve will underfit. The high values of the parameters eliminated by tweaking the cost function of logistic regression. The cost function minimized in regularized logistic regression is:

$$j(\theta) = -\frac{1}{m}\sum_{i=1}^{m}\left[y^{(i)}\log\left(he\left(x^{(i)}\right)\right) + \left(1 - y^{(i)}\right)\log\left(1 - he\left(x^{(i)}\right)\right)\right] + \frac{\lambda}{2m}\sum_{j=1}^{n}\theta_j^2$$

Regularization factor is λ.

Models can be trained to generalize on unseen data in a better way using regularization. Generalization error can be diminished using Laplace, L1 and L2 and Gauss. Bayesian approach of regularization can assume prior probability density of the coefficients and the maximum a posteriori estimate approach is used. The coefficients are Gaussian expressions with mean 0 and variance $\sigma 2$ or Laplace distribution of variance $\sigma 2$. The smaller values of these coefficients can produce smaller outputs, but with small values of σ2 it can lead to underfit.

Gauss prior = L2 if $\lambda = 1/\sigma 2$

Laplace prior = L1 if $\lambda = \sqrt{2}/\sigma$

So, regularization doesn't increase the performance on the dataset, but it can regulate the bias factor if the model is suffering from overfitting.

7.1.4 *Semi-supervised Learning*

Semi-supervised learning is becoming most popular in past few years. Semi-supervised learning is the middle ground between supervised learning and unsupervised learning. Before going to semi-supervised learning let's talk briefly about Supervised learning and unsupervised learning. Supervised learning is the learning in which data of dataset are labeled and Unsupervised learning is the learning in which data of dataset are unlabeled. Semi-supervised learning dataset is collection

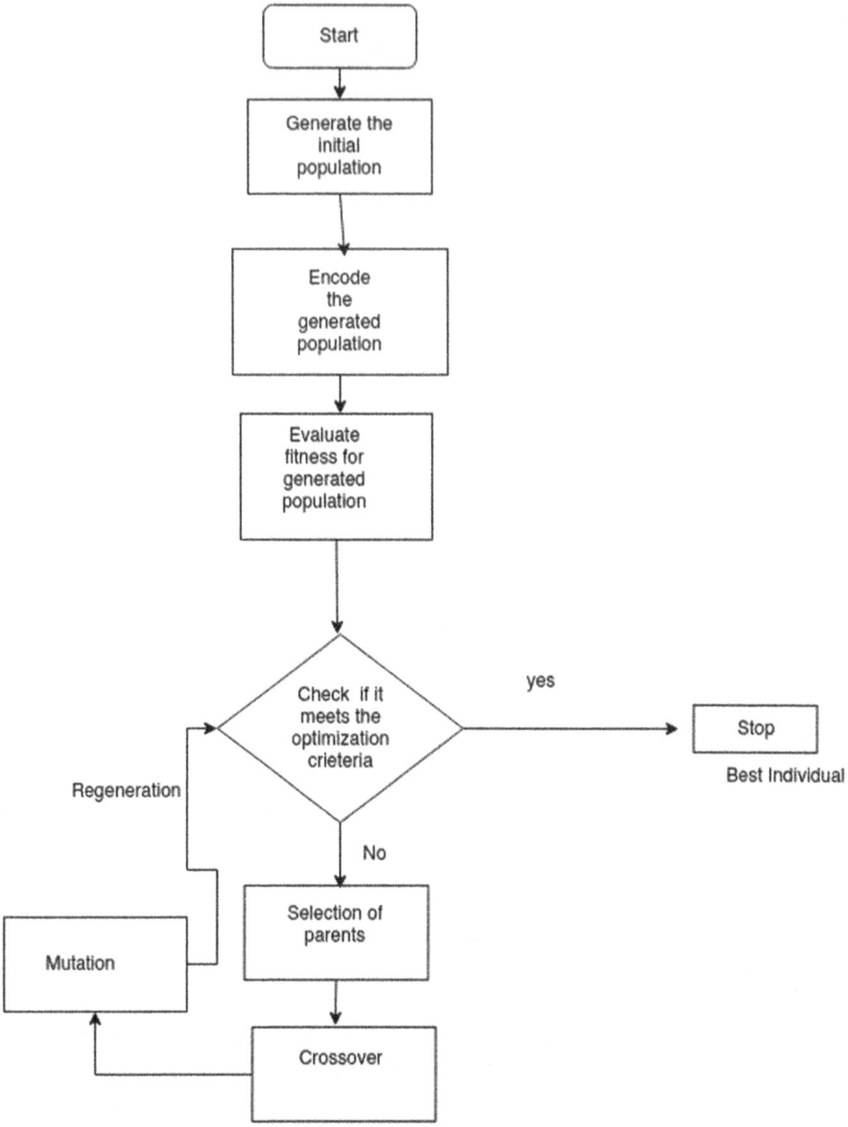

Fig. 7.2 A flowchart demonstrating the genetic algorithm [16]

of labeled data in small amounts and unlabeled data in large amounts. Semi- supervised learning uses unlabeled data for training purpose and the goal is to classify unlabeled data using given labeled data [5]. Semi-supervised Learning is widely applicable in real world:

1. Web mining: classifying web pages.
2. Text mining: identifying names in text.

3. Video mining: classifying people in the news.

To classify unlabeled data of Semi-supervised learning 'Clustering' is very important approach for classification. There are many algorithms used for Semi-supervised learning:

i. *Self-training*: As per name self-training refers to training in which trainer trains data itself. Self-training algorithm is semi-supervised learning algorithm that repeat training base classifiers and labeling unlabeled data of training set [6]. In self-training before applying Procedure is given below:

   1. Find out classifiers using labeled data.
   2. Train model using classifiers and label the unlabeled data.
   3. Most confidently labeled data are added to training set.
   4. Repeat step (1), step (2) and step (3) until no data remain unlabeled.

ii. *Graph-based methods*: Graph based algorithm is old and simple algorithm. It is easy to understand and show higher accuracy for classification. Graph contain nodes and edges, where node represents unlabeled or labeled sample and edge represents similarity between labeled and unlabeled sample [6]. Procedure for Graph-based method is given below:

   1. Graph construction.
   2. Injecting seed labels on a subset of the nodes.
   3. Inferring labels on unlabeled nodes in the graph.

iii. *Co-Training*: Co-Training divides each problem into two feature sets and these sets provide different and complementary information about instance. It is used in classify web pages [6]. Procedure is given below:

   1. Using labeled data find out each attribute and build a model for each attribute.
   2. Use each model to assign labels to unlabeled data.
   3. Select each unlabeled data that were most confidently predicted by models.
   4. Add those data to the training set.
   5. Go to procedure no (1.) until data exhausted.

iv. *Semi-supervised SVM*: Recently Standard Vector Mechanism (SVM) and Semi-supervised learning incorporated with each other and Semi-supervised SVM is came into existence. Semi-supervised SVM is better than SVM. This method is not able to handle large data set due to huge space and time requirements [7].

v. *Low density separation*: Low density separation is the method used to place boundaries where there are few labeled and unlabeled points. Transudative support vector machine is most commonly used algorithm to classify Semi-supervised data whereas Support vector machines is used to classify supervised data [8].

7.1.5 Principal Components Analysis

Principal component analysis (PCA) is a statistical procedure that uses an orthogonal (i.e. linearly independent) transformation to convert a set of observations of possibly correlated variables into a set of values containing linearly uncorrelated variables called principal components. This transformation is defined in such a way that the first principal component has the largest possible variance and each succeeding components successively has the highest variance possible provided that it is orthogonal to the preceding component. The resulting vectors are an uncorrelated orthogonal basis set. Thus, it is implied that PCA is sensitive to the relative scaling of the original variables. To calculate PCA the covariance matrix X of data points, eigen vectors and their corresponding eigen values have to be calculated. Then eigen vectors are sorted according to their eigen values in decreasing order. First K eigen vectors are chosen to give new K dimensions. Then the original n dimensional data points are transformed into K dimensions [9].

7.1.6 Support Vector Machine

K Support vector machine (SVM) is a very popular method used for supervised learning algorithm that analyze data and used for classification and regression analysis. SVM is used for separating different outputs by a hyperplane. For a set of labelled training data, an SVM algorithm outputs an optimal boundary which clearly separates one category different from the others, making it a non-probabilistic binary linear classifier. If parameters of problem change than hyperplane is also changing. When working in the 2D, a hyperplane is a line that divides the plan into two different part. Most of the times the SVM algorithm gives higher accuracy than other any other supervised learning algorithm. When we do not have an idea about the type of data then SVM should be the first choice to apply because SVM also works with semi-structured and unstructured data [10].

7.1.7 Random Forest Classifier

We create multiple random subsets where data may or may not overlap. Then we create randomized decision tree based on random selection of data and random selection of variables. One important property is that trees protect each other from their individual error if the data is taken unbiased. Subsequently we rank the classifiers according to their votes. This provides class of dependent variables based on many trees. Thus, random trees create a random forest. We take two assumptions: Most trees can provide correct class prediction for most part of the data & the trees is making errors at different places. Each tree in the random forest gives a prediction. The class with maximum votes is taken as our model's prediction. To create an uncorrelated forest of trees, we use two methods Bagging or Bootstrap Aggregation, & Feature Randomness. However, to ensure that our random forests make reasonably accurate class predictions, we need to have features that will have some predictive powers and those predictions need to be uncorrelated.

7.2 Application of Machine Learning in Heart Diseases

Essential, and knowledgeable information is extracted from the databases of medical sciences using several data mining techniques. These techniques help in developing models and classify different data classes and attributes. The construction of the classifiers is conducted by these class attributes. This whole new mechanism has been utilized in the Heart disease classification. For pattern detection a sophisticated algorithm called KNN is used. Medical Databases are sometimes huge and may also contain irrelevant data which might hinder the efficiency of the whole process. Cardiovascular diseases cause 45% of the deaths in Europe and about 37% in the European union, 35% in Canada and USA totaling up to 6.5 million deaths worldwide as in reports of 2017 [11, 12].

There are several types of heart diseases which have been classified depending on their symptoms: Heart failure, Arrhythmia, Valvular Heart disease, Hypertensive heart disease, Ischemic heart disease, Aortic aneurysms, Inflammatory heart disease.

The various risk factors which affect heart condition may vary from one patient to another and is a debatable issue: Smoking, High or low HDL, Abnormal blood lipids, Gender and age, High C-reactive protein, Physical inactivity, Obesity (BMI over 25), Uncontrolled stress anger, Diabetes, Use of tobacco [13], Alcohol use, family issues [14].

7.2.1 Case Study-1 to Classify Heart Diseases Using a Machine Learning Approach

An approach on how the accuracy of the classification of heart diseases can be improved using KNN and genetic algorithm has been discussed. Genetic search has been used to rule out the irrelevant parameters and sort the useful attributes depending on their contribution to the classification. Only the evaluated attributes play a role to build the classification algorithm. The procedure is described as follows:

Part 1. using genetic search attributes are evaluated.
Part 2. The classifier is built and measuring accuracy is dealt here.

Procedure: The data set is loaded, genetic search is implemented, the subsets having attributes of higher rank are selected. KNN and genetic algorithms are applied to maximize the accuracy of the classification. Finally, the ability of the classifier is tested with unknown sample.

$$Accuracy = \frac{Total\ numbers\ of\ samplesclassified\text{in}testdata}{Total\ number\ of\ samples}$$

7.2.1.1 Results and Discussion

The data sets have been collected from UCI data repository [15] and the disease data is generated from some hospitals in Andhra Pradesh. Table 7.1 contains the attribute name followed by number of instances and number of attributes. The comparison of the performance of KNN + GA and other algorithms is given in Table 7.2. With increasing value of K the precision of the data sets was decreasing. The difference of precision between the datasets with or without GA has also been mentioned in Table 7.3. A 5% increment in accuracy of heart diseases is found using GA. Breast cancer and primary tumor still could not be determined by the approach of KNN + GA because of the redundancy of the attributes present in the given data-set. A lower mutation rate of 0.033 was preferred. Overall, this approach benefited the purpose

Table 7.1 Description of various data sets

Dataset	Instances	Attributes
Weather	14	5
Pima	768	9
Hypothyroid	3770	30
Breast cancer	286	10
Liver disorder	345	7
Primary tumour	339	18
Heart stalog	270	14
Lymph	148	19

Table 7.2 Comparison between different models

Name of dataset	KNN + GA	NN + PCA	GA + ANN
Weather data	100	100	100
Heart stalog	100	98.14	99.6
Hypothyroid	100	97.06	97.37
Breast cancer	94	97.9	95.45
Lymphography	100	99.3	99.3
Heart disease A. P	100	100	100
Primary tumour	75.8	80	82.1

Table 7.3 Comparison of accuracy of training dataset with and without using GA

Dataset	With GA			Without GA		
	K = 1	K = 3	K = 5	K = 1	K = 3	K = 5
Weather data	100	100	100	85.71	85.71	85.71
Breast cancer	94.05	94.05	94.05	90	90	82.5
Heart stalog	100	90.7	87.03	100	90.74	83.3
Lymphography	100	100	100	99.32	99.32	84.4
Hypothyroid	100	96.18	95.75	100	95.62	94.69
Primary tumor	75.8	66.3	60.7	75	65.48	61.35
Heart disease A.P	100	95	95	95	75	83.3

The KNN parameters are
1.K=1,2,3…..n
2.Debug=True
3.Distance weighing=weight by 1 dist.
4.mean square=true
5.no normalization =false

Parameters of genetic search
Cross over probability=0.6
Mutation probability=0.033
Maximum generations=20
Population size=20
Report frequency=20
Seed=1

Fig. 7.3 KNN parameters, genetic search parameters [16]

of classification of heart diseases [16]. The different parameters of KNN and genetic search have been described in Fig. 7.3.

Attributes of gender, diabetes, hypertension, rural, urban, disease are nominal data types while, age, BP Dialic, BP systolic, BMI, weight height are numeric types.

Through these predictions' doctors can successfully diagnose certain heart conditions effectively with few attributes. With more efficient disease diagnosing techniques the morality factor can be reduced and the patient will receive accurate treatment and surgical procedures.

7.2.2 *Case Study-2 to Predict Cardiac Arrest in Critically Ill Patients from Machine Learning Score Achieved from the Variability of Heart Rate*

Priority based patient treatments is quite a hefty operation for the medical department. Health conditions of the admitted patients are analyzed and priority treatment is established depending on the severity of their condition [17]. Risk assessment for cardiac arrest is the most crucial part in assigning the priority treatment for the patients, quick assessment of this technique can however save a lot of time, effort and lives. Clinical judgments, pulse oximetry, temperature and respiratory rate determine the judgments and establishing a risk factor for the patient [18].

MEWS: Modified Early Score (depends on psychological attributes)
AVPU: (Alert, Reaction to vocal stimuli, Reaction to pain, Unconscious)

MEWS and AVPU scores are used to determine an early score [19]. The MEWS tool has been widely used all over UK, and it can be determined without any test results.

A Machine learning (ML) score can be generated in consideration with heart rate variability (HRV). This score is developed by comparing the sensitivity and specificity of the curve, and the area under it with the 'Modified Early Warning Score (MEWS)'. Patients in a terminally stage with Scale 1 and 2 Acuity Category is observed, from electrocardiogram recording of 5 min. Heart rate vitality(hrv) parameters are generated along with other factors like age. These observations help in developing a definite ML score for the individuals.

According to Singapore health care systems the risk assessment and priority check is made by determining the Patient Acuity Category Scale (PACS). PACS1 patients are critically ill and need to be treated without delay. PACS 2 patients pass the cardiovascular tests done initially and are not in the state of immediate danger. PAC 3 and 4 are however non-emergencies.

Patients classified within PACS 1 and PACS 2 were continuously monitored via ECG monitoring, however patients with disorders like ventricular arrhythmias, complete heart block, supraventricular arrhythmias were not included since HRV metrics were not reliable for them. Certain HRV parameters were obtained in the study, the recordings ranged between 5 and 30 min. The data was collected and processed after getting the consent of the patient and the ethics approval was received from the Sing health Centralized Institutional Review Board.

The ECG data were extracted as text files after being sampled at 125 Hz to filter out the noise, using an ECG extraction software. In order to be accurate and sufficient for the HRV metrics minimum 5 min of recorded data was taken. The QRS complex and the distance between two successive beats helped in determining the Ectopic beats. The height, width and RR interval of the QRS complex was also analyzed.

7.2.2.1 Prediction and Analysis of Machine Learning Score

A multi variate non parametric approach called black box approach is used instead of traditional logistic regression to overcome problems of overfitting and collinearity. The vectors of the vital signs and the HRV parameters represents each patient data which is based on geometrical distances between different feature vectors. An optimal plane was obtained for separating the patterns by mapping the feature vectors into a space having higher dimensions. Support Vector Machines has widely been used in text [20], ECG and EEG classification [21].

Patients suffering from cardiac arrests or death as outcomes are classified as positive samples, and the ones without the outcomes are negative samples [22]. The Euclidean distance is calculated between the data from the patients and both of the cluster centers to produce the score. If the produced outcome be positive then it'll lead to rise in the risk score.

Conventional approach of machine learning algorithms was not preferred here due to the imbalanced database, which might show poor performance and lead to failed generalization on new patients. Majority of the samples in the data set are normal while only a minor portion has abnormal outcomes as cardiac arrests or death. So, the data set is imbalanced.

Basic characteristics of the patients like, Age, Gender, group wise diagnosing (cardiovascular, respiratory, gastrointestinal, renal, endocrine, vascular, trauma, cancer) are considered. Their medical history of having diabetes, hypertension, heart, renal disease, cancer and stroke is considered. Medical therapy done before the admit are considered (digoxin, Amiodarone, calcium channel blockers). Then the patients are classified into the ones who had no cardiac arrests within 72 h. (n = 882) and the ones who had cariad arrests within 72 h. where n = 43. The corresponding P value is determined.

7.2.2.2 Outcomes

As observed 4.6% of the number of patients had cardiac arrests, while 9.3% died within 72 h of admission. The respiratory diagnosis, and cardiovascular groups had primary outcomes at 23.3%. But gastro intestinal and renal group patients did not have any primary outcomes. Most of the secondary outcome of 22.1% was found in the respiratory diagnosis followed by the cardio vascular group having outcome at 20.9%.

Predictor factor with probability of cardiac arrest within 72 h was studied and it was deduced that 9.6, 62.3, 28.1% patients were classified into groups having 'low, intermediate, high' risk groups depending on their machine learning scores. Figure 7.4 demonstrates the risk factor of the patents' in terms of high-risk, moderate-risk and low-risk.

The machine learning score generated by incorporating the vital signs along with HRV parameters was found to be more predictive of cardiac arrest than MEWS with 72 h of observational data. The categorization of the risk factors is made by classifying the patients into groups having low, intermediate and high-risk of cardiac arrest. The ML score can determine the risk factor be useful for the prediction of cardiac arrests causing fatality. Traditional diagnosis by emergency departments is often time consuming and the decisions based from different professionals are independent

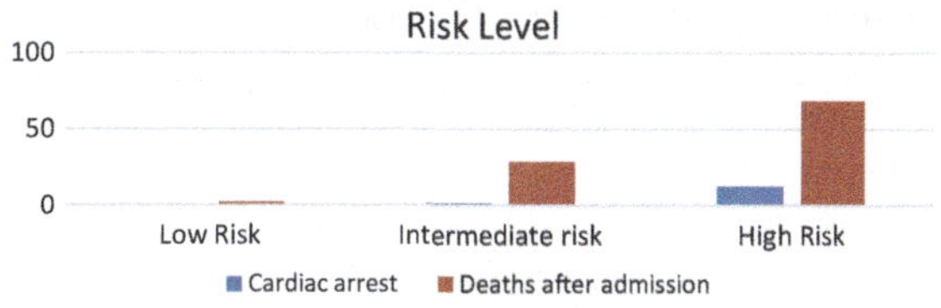

Fig. 7.4 Demonstrating the risk factor in patients

and opinion. High level of priority biased monitoring, complicated management of priority-based classification of patients is a hefty issue for the medical centers so machine learning based risk assessment procedures can save a lot of time effort for the department and lives of the critically ill patients. Traditional statistical approaches were not perfectly applicable in these cases because of the high correlativity between the Heart Rate Variability factors. But these limitations were avoided via the machine learning approach with more precise and perfect sensitivity, specificity, and accuracy of the prediction.

7.3 Application of Machine Learning Algorithms in Diagnosing Diseases of Brain

7.3.1 Case Study 1: Alzheimer's Disease

Alzheimer's disease is a progressive disorder that causes brain cells to waste away and progressively die. Alzheimer's disease is the most common cause of dementia a condition causing continuous decline in thinking, behavioral and social skills that disrupts a person's ability to function independently. It is expected that in near future machine learning technologies and artificial intelligence may assist in the creation of stable and effective diagnostic tests for early-onset Alzheimer's. Thus it would be possible for ML and artificial intelligence (AI) to replace invasive and expensive tests for the disease and provide a low-cost, painless and accurate solutions to early stage Alzheimer detection. Major companies include IBM have made inroads in this area of research [23]. We see an example of a Machine learning framework that predicts MRI-based Alzheimer's conversion from early MCI subjects based on MRI reports [24]. The earliest clinical manifestation of Alzheimer's Disease is selective memory impairment and while treatments are available to help some symptoms, there is no cure currently available for complete recovery. Brain Imaging via magnetic resonance imaging (MRI), is used for evaluation of patients with suspected Alzheimer's Disease. Findings from MRI do include both, local and generalized shrinkage of brain tissue [25]. Certain studies indicate that MRI features may predict rate of decline of Alzheimer's Disease and may guide pathway for development of therapy in the future. Although in order to reach the stage, clinicians and researchers will have to make use of machine learning techniques that can accurately predict progress of a patient from mild cognitive impairment to dementia. In the cited article, the authors have proposed to develop a model that can help clinicians track the progress and predict early Alzheimer's Disease.

7.3.1.1 Noteworthy Techniques

Semi-supervised learning was run on the data available from Alzheimer's Disease patients and normal controls, (without using MCI patients' data), to help with the stable MCI/progressive MCI classification. Feature selection was performed using Regularized logistic regression. Aging effects was removed from the MRI data before training by the classifier was performed to prevent any incidental confusion between changes reflected due to Alzheimer's Disease and those due to normal aging. An aggregate biomarker was constructed by first learning a separate MRI biomarker. Consequently, data regarding the age and cognitive measures about MCI subjects was combined by running a Random forest classifier algorithm.

7.3.1.2 Information on Type of Datasets Used

Operation was performed a longitudinal MRI data of 150 subjects aged 60–96, every subject being scanned at least once. All subjects taken were right-handed. 72 subjects were grouped as 'Nondemented' during the study while 64 subjects were grouped as 'Demented' at the time of their initial visits and remained so throughout the study. 14 subjects were grouped as 'Nondemented' at the time of their initial visit and were henceforth characterized as 'Demented' in a later visit. These fall under the 'Converted' category.

7.3.1.3 Findings

The paper highlights that Mild cognitive impairment (MCI) is the transitional stage between age-related cognitive decline and Alzheimer's Disease. It is noteworthy that MCI patients having high risk for conversion to AD were included. A Magnetic Resonance Imaging MRI-based bio-marker [26] using semi-supervised learning was developed. This biomarker was integrated with age and cognitive data about the subjects using a supervised learning algorithm which gave another bio-marker. Data used was made available from the Alzheimer's Disease Neuro imaging Initiative ADNI Database. The paper claims that their aggregate biomarker [26] achieved a 10-fold cross-validation area under the curve (AUC) score of 0.9020 in discriminating between progressive MCI (pMCI) and stable MCI (sMCI). The results presented in this study demonstrate the potential of the suggested approach for early AD diagnosis and an important role of MRI in the MCI-to-AD conversion prediction. Figure 7.5 demonstrates the comparison between survival probability versus time.

Kaplan-Meier survival curve: A non-parametric statistic used to estimate the survival function from lifetime data [25]. Figure 7.6 demonstrates the importance of MRI, age and cognitive measurements calculated by Random Forest classifier.

The importance of MRI, age and cognitive measurements calculated by Random Forest classifier.

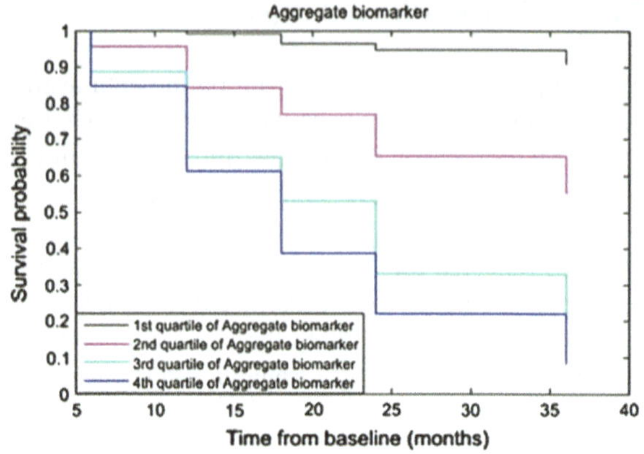

Fig. 7.5 Comparison between survival probability versus time [27]

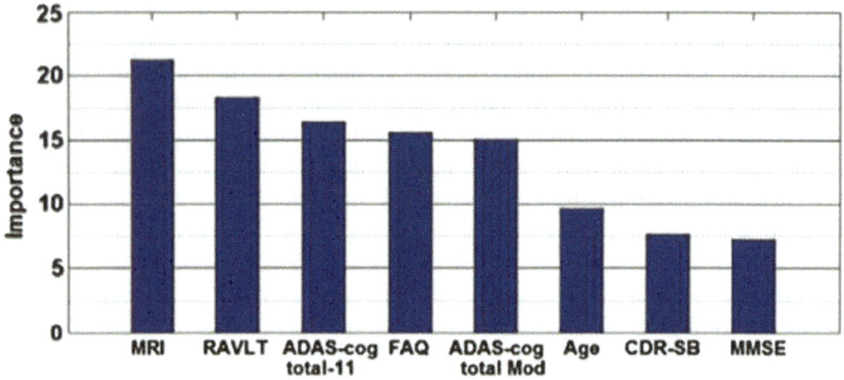

Fig. 7.6 The importance of MRI, age and cognitive measurements calculated by random forest classifier [27]

7.3.2 Case Study 2: Detecting Parkinson's Disease from Progressive Supranuclear Palsy

Parkinson's disease is a progressive nervous system disorder that affects movement of the human body. The symptoms related to the disease start gradually, sometimes starting with a barely noticeable tremor in just one hand. This disorder commonly causes stiffness or slowing of movement of various parts of the body. Speech may become soft or slurred with time. Other symptoms include tremor, slowed movement (bradykinesia), rigid muscles, impaired posture and balance, Loss of automatic movements, speech changes & writing changes. Progressive Supranuclear palsy (PSP) and Parkinson's Disease (PD) have overlapping symptoms but remain difficult to distinguish. Telling these differences apart can be challenging because most patients with PSP do not develop distinctive symptoms such as paralysis or weakness of the eye muscles and episodes of frequent falling until later stages. In the paper [27], machine learning algorithms were run on brain MRI data to differentially diagnose Parkinson's disease and Progressive Supranuclear Palsy. The aim of this work was to determine the feasibility of application of a supervised machine learning algorithm to assist diagnosis of patients with clinically diagnosed Parkinson's disease (PD) and Progressive Supranuclear Palsy (PSP).

7.3.2.1 Noteworthy Techniques and Dataset Used

Morphological T1-weighted [28] Magnetic Resonance Images (MRIs) of 28 PD patients, 28 PSP patients and 28 healthy control subjects was taken. A supervised machine learning algorithm based on the combination of Principal Components Analysis as feature extraction technique and Support Vector Machines as classification algorithm was created and used to run on the MRI data. The algorithm obtained voxel-based morphological biomarkers of PD and PSP. The algorithm does not require a prior hypothesis of where useful information may be coded in the images.

7.3.2.2 Findings

The algorithm allowed individual diagnosis of PSP versus controls, PD versus controls, and PSP versus PD with an accuracy, specificity and sensitivity greater than 90%. Voxels [29] influencing classification between PD and PSP patients included midbrain, pons, corpus callosum and thalamus, four critical regions strongly involved in the pathophysiological mechanisms of PSP.

7.4 A Brief Approach of Medical Sciences in Other Fields

There is a never-ending demand for machine learning to process the data accumulated from each and every field more precisely. Unsupervised learning is used in the manufacture and drug discovery purposes. Therapy for multi-factorial diseases are being introduced by machine learning techniques that can identify patterns in the data without providing any prediction. Inner Eye initiative by Microsoft is utilizing deep learning which works specially on image analysis to boost the unbounded the opportunities of Computer Vision. Even rare disorders or genetical syndromes can now possibly be diagnosed using these machine learning approaches. Tumor based detection is made more perfect by integrating cognitive computation in the diagnosing and tracking techniques. With easily available wearable sensors data accumulation is made by users performing different activities. ML based processes helps in detecting these gestures made regularly and made us aware of our unconscious behavior. As discussed in the topic ML can also save a lot of time and effort of both the department and the patient via predictive analysis to identify possible abnormal conditions.

ANN or artificial neural network plays an important role in computer vision. Data is fed into these ANNs, which compares the data, labels the data depending on their characteristics. ANN is a biologically inspired system having three layers: input, hidden and output layer. At first, values are assigned to every neuron in the input layer, hidden layers are assigned with a random bias. The activation function assigns weights for the neurons in the hidden layer. Finally, after being multiplied by the random bias value an output is generated. The process of back-propagation makes the process better gradually by more of the iterations of this multiplication technique.

ANN helps to predict the presence of cancer; large number of hidden layer neurons are used for the purpose. Several mammographic records are fed into the system as data. Gradually with the process of 'learning' the network can effectively produce the difference between the benign and malignant tumors. These models are effective, more consistent and less error prone than human intervention in the diagnosing process. Cancer survival rates, cancer recurrence can also be successfully until now using these neural networks.

Robust detection of hemorrhages from diabetic retinopathy grading system has also been possible via a machine learning approach [30]. Spat based segmentation algorithm, rule-based mask detection showed impressive result in this process. Pre-trained CNN or convolutional network models are used to extract features from blood smear images for the detection of malarial parasites. So, basically machine learning is gradually revolutionizing the entire emergency healthcare system by inducing more precision, effectivity and less human intervention which might be susceptible to errors [31].

7.5 Conclusion

Essential and knowledgeable information is extracted from the databases of medical sciences using several machine learning techniques and data mining techniques. Initially this article discusses several machine learning techniques and data mining techniques. There are several types of heart diseases which have been classified in the case study depending on their symptoms. Risk assessment for cardiac arrest is the most crucial part in assigning the priority treatment for the patients and this chapter gives a case study on this. Furthermore, the article demonstrate two case studies on the basis of application of machine learning algorithms in diagnosing diseases of brain. The different case studies shows that with more efficient disease diagnosing techniques the morality factor can be reduced and the patient will receive accurate treatment and surgical procedures.

References

1. Korting, T.S.: How kNN algorithm works. https://www.youtube.com/watch?v=UqYde-LULfs&feature=youtube (2014)
2. K-nearest neighbor classification. https://www.youtube.com/watch?v=CJjSPCslxqQ&feature=youtu.be, (2018)
3. Sivanandam, S.N., Deepa, S.N.: Introduction to Genetic Algorithms. book, Springer (2008)
4. Jabbar, M.A., Deekshatulu, B.L., Chandra, B.L.: Heart disease prediction system using associative classification and genetic algorithm, pp. 183–192. Elsevier (2012)
5. Semi supervised learning. https://www.youtube.com/watch?v=tVsVmy6w7FE&t=6s (2018)
6. Semi-supervised learning. https://en.wikipedia.org/wiki/Semi-supervised_learning. last edited on 30 Aug 2019
7. Ying, L.: Online semi supervised support vector machine (2018)
8. Shay, B.D.: Learning low density separators. https://arxiv.org/abs/0805.2891 published on May (2008)
9. Jolliffe, I.T., Cadima, J.: Principal component analysis: A review and recent developments. Philos. Trans. A Math. Phys. Eng. Sci. (2016)
10. Zhang, Y.: Support vector machine classification algorithm and its application. In: Information Computing and Applications ICICA (2012)
11. Breiman, L.: Machine learning. **45**(5), (2001). https://doi.org/10.1023/A:1010933404324
12. Jabbar, M.A., Deekshatulu, B.L., Chandra, P.: Knowledge discovery from mining association rules for heart disease prediction. JATIT. **41**(2), 45–53 (2013)
13. Jabbar, B.L., Deekshatulu, M.A., Chandra, P.: An evolutionary algorithm for heart disease prediction, pp. 378–389. CCIS, Springer (2012)
14. Jabbar, M.A., Deekshatulu, B.L., Chandra, P.: Prediction of risk score for heart disease using associative classification and hybrid feature subset selection. In: Conference ISDA, IEEE, 628–634 (2013)
15. Center for machine learning and intelligent system. www.ics.uci.edu/~mlearn
16. Jabbar, M.A.: Classification of heart disease using ANN and feature subset selection. https://www.semanticscholar.org/paper/Classification-of-Heart-Disease-using-Artificial-Jabbar-Deekshatulu/072cb3f9e9cbef46ed576edad28fed74d351954e published in 2013
17. Goldman, L.: Using prediction models and cost-effectiveness analysis to improve clinical decisions: Emergency department patients with acute chest pain. https://www.ncbi.nlm.nih.gov/pubmed/8608418
18. Peacock, W.F.: Risk stratification for suspected acute coronary syndromes and heart failure in the emergency department. https://www.ncbi.nlm.nih.gov/pubmed/19452341
19. Subbe, C.P.: Validation of physiological scoring systems in the accident and emergency department. https://www.ncbi.nlm.nih.gov/pubmed/17057134
20. Ubeyli, E.D.: ECG beats classification using multiclass support vector machines with error correcting output codes. https://www.sciencedirect.com/science/article/pii/S1051200406001941 published on May, (2017)
21. Liang, N.Y.: Classification of mental tasks from EEG signals using learning machine. https://www.worldscientific.com/doi/abs/10.1142/S0129065706000482?journalCode=ijns
22. Liu, Y.: Comparison of extreme learning machine with support vector machine for text classification. https://link.springer.com/chapter/10.1007/11504894_55
23. Goudey, B.: Using machine learning to develop blood test for key Alzheimer's biomaker. https://www.ibm.com/blogs/research/2019/03/machine-learning-alzheimers/ published on 11 March 2019
24. Elaheh, M.: Machine learning framework for early MRI-based Alzheimer's conversion prediction in MCI subjects. https://tutcris.tut.fi/portal/en/publications/machine-learning-framework-for-early-mribased-alzheimers-conversion-prediction-in-mci-subjects(dda3bf0f-be96-45cb-8586-e81099617cf9).html published on Jan, (2015)
25. Johnson, K.A.: Brain imaging in Alzheimer disease. https://www.ncbi.nlm.nih.gov/pubmed/22474610 published on April, (2012)

26. Strimbu, K., Tavel, J.A.: What are biomarkers. https://www.ncbi.nlm.nih.gov/pmc/articles/PMC3078627/ published on Nov, (2011)
27. Moradi, E.: Machine learning framework for early MRI-based Alzheimer's conversion prediction in MCI subjects. https://www.ncbi.nlm.nih.gov/pmc/articles/PMC5957071/ published on May, (2018)
28. NINDS: Progressive supranuclear palsy sheet. https://www.ninds.nih.gov/disorders/patient-caregiver-education/fact-sheets/progressive-supranuclear-palsy-fact-sheet published on September (2015)
29. Voxel: https://en.wikipedia.org/wiki/Voxel. last edited on 6 Sept 2019
30. Xiao, D., Yu, S.: Retinal hemorrhage detection by rule-based and machine learning approach. published on September, (2017)
31. Sarkar, D.J.: Detecting malaria with deep learning. https://towardsdatascience.com/detecting-malaria-with-deep-learning-9e45c1e34b60 published on April, (2019)

Chapter 8
Removal of High-Density Impulsive Noise in Giemsa Stained Blood Smear Image Using Probabilistic Decision Based Average Trimmed Filter

Amit Prakash Sen and Nirmal Kumar Rout

Abstract The chapter focuses on the removal of salt and pepper noise from the contaminated giemsa stained blood smear image using Probabilistic Decision Based Average Trimmed Filter (PDBATF). The experiments outcomes are recorded and compared with recently reported algorithms. The proposed algorithm provides better accuracy level in terms of peak signal to noise ratio, image enhancement ratio, mean absolute error and execution time.

Keywords Medical image de-noising · Salt and pepper noise · Noise removal · Trimmed median filter · Probabilistic approach

8.1 Introduction

Biomedical Image processing is a promising area of research for enhancing the quality of diagnosis and thereby minimizing human intervention. The giemsa stained blood smear images are often corrupted by impulse noise because of transmission errors, malfunctioning pixel elements in the camera sensors, faulty memory locations, and timing errors in analog-to-digital conversion. With the contamination of impulsive noise in the blood smear images, the diagnosis of the life threatening disease malaria becomes extremely difficult task which can lead to misinterpretation. Therefore noise removal becomes a noteworthy task in biomedical image processing.

Numerous linear [1] and non-linear [2] filtering techniques have been proposed for noise reduction. Linear filters are not able to viably eliminate impulse noise as they tend to obscure the edges of an image. The conventional linear techniques are extremely basic in usage however they experience the ill effects of the loss of image details. They also don't perform well with the variation of signal-dependent noise. To conquer this constraint, nonlinear filters are proposed. Several nonlinear filters [1, 2] dependent on Classical and fuzzy techniques have increased in a preceding couple of years. The Standard Median Filter (SMF) [1, 2] is the basic non-linear filter developed which is the simple basic rank selection filter, used to remove impulse noise

A. P. Sen · N. K. Rout (✉)
School of Electronics Engineering, KIIT University, Bhubaneswar, India

P. K. Pattnaik et al. (eds.), *Smart Healthcare Analytics in IoT Enabled Environment*, Intelligent Systems Reference Library 178,
https://doi.org/10.1007/978-3-030-37551-5_8

by processing the central pixel of the filtering window with the median value of the pixels contained within the window. SMF can extensively reduce impulse noise in an image. The uncorrupted pixel is likewise changed by the SMF. Many variations and improved strategies based on SMF is reported till date such as Adaptive Median Filter (AMF) [3] in which the size of the filtering window is adaptive in nature, and it depends on the number of noise-free pixels in the current filtering window, Adaptive Weighted Median Filter (AWMF) [4, 5] where the weight of a pixel is decided on the basis of standard deviation in four-pixel directions (vertical, horizontal and two diagonals). The detection of the noisy pixel in an image contaminated by random-valued impulse noise, is increasingly troublesome in comparison with fixed valued impulse noise, as the gray value of a noisy pixel may not be substantially larger or smaller than those of its neighbors. Because of this reason, the conventional median-based impulse detection strategies don't perform well if there is an occurrence of random-valued impulse noise. Switching Median Filter (SMF) [6] which identifies noisy pixels, applied with AMF to develop Adaptive Switching Median Filter (ASMF) [7, 8]. It computes the threshold value locally from the image pixel values in the sliding window. These filters work well in de-noising to a certain level of noise density but fail to perform for high noise density due to the use of basic median operations. One of the major concern is the time complexity with the above-reported algorithms. Thereby Trimmed Median Filter (TMF) [9] developed which removes the unwanted pixel elements before processing. In TMF, if the concerned processing pixel is noisy then the pixel elements with intensity value "0" and "255" is removed before applying the median approach. Several algorithms [9–12] are developed and reported with the application of TMF. In Alpha Trimmed Median Filter (ATMF) [9], trimming is symmetric which leads to blurring and loss of image details. This leads to the development of Un-symmetric Trimmed Median Filter (UTMF) [10] where the uncorrupted pixel elements are arranged in increasing or decreasing order in a selected window for the calculation of median after removing pixels with intensity value "0" and "255".

UTMF is applied in many state-of-the-art algorithms like Decision Based Unsymmetric Trimmed Median Filter (DBUTMF) [10], Modified Decision Based unsymmetric Trimmed Median Filter (MDBUTMF) [11], and Probabilistic Decision Based Filter (PDBF) [12]. DBUTMF is developed to overcome the drawback of decision based algorithm (DBA) [10] where the median value after calculation comes to be either "0" or "255". In such cases, DBA replaces processing pixel with a pixel value from the neighbor which leads to streaking effect [13]. DBUTMF [10] fails to operate when all the pixel elements are either "0" or "255" in a selected window which leads to the development of MDBUTMF [11]. MDBUTMF do not perform well in high noise density (ND) due to its fixed window size. Therefore PDBF is reported where TMF is utilized for low ND and a new technique called Patch Else Trimmed Median Filter (PETM) is incorporated for high ND. The algorithm works well in low as well as in high ND when the remaining noise free pixel (NFP) in the trimmed median filter is odd valued. It shows some blurring and loss of image information in case of even valued NFP. This particular issue motivated to develop the proposed Probabilistic Decision Based Average Trimmed Filter (PDBATF) to remove salt and pepper noise from a highly contaminated image. Here two new technique is proposed namely, proposed Average Trimmed Filter (ATF) and proposed Patch Else Average Trimmed Filter (PEATF) to develop the proposed PDBATF. ATF is incorporated for low ND and PEATF is utilized for high ND. Simulation results show that the developed algorithm de-noise an image may it be a normal image or medical image contaminated with salt-and-pepper noise very efficiently and outperforms the recently reported State-of-the-art algorithm.

The rest of the chapter is organized as follows. Section 8.2 discusses the complete procedure of the PDBATF. Section 8.3 discusses the simulation results and Sect. 8.4 concludes the chapter.

8.2 Proposed Algorithm

The PDBATF algorithm is developed by incorporating ATF for low ND and PEATF for high ND. In order to establish various relationship, Z is considered as the original image of size m × n corrupted by noisy density (ND). NI is considered as the noisy image and Z_d be the de-noised image.

8.2.1 Proposed Average Trimmed Filter

With the application of TMF to de-noise an image, it works absolutely fine to retrieve the estimated original information in a selected window when the remaining NFP in the selected window is odd valued after removal of the intensity value "0" and "255". It simply sorts the remaining pixel elements and calculates the median value in order to replace the processing noisy pixel element. The situation becomes troublesome when the remaining NFP in the selected window is even valued. In such a case, after sorting of the pixel elements, the mean of the two center elements are calculated to replace the processing pixel. Mean of the center element is considered as an estimate of the original information. But the major concern with this approach is that the original information of the processing pixel may be at a far distance from the mean of the two center elements after application of the trimming. In most of the cases, it might not be able to estimate properly the original pixel intensity as only the two center elements are utilized to estimate the original processing pixel information. This leads to some probability of getting image detail loss and blur.

So, in order to resolve such an issue Average Trimmed Filter is proposed. The strategy of the algorithm is as follows,

Case 1. Odd value of NFP.

In this case, noisy pixels are removed and the remaining NFP are sorted. Median will be the central element.

Case 2. Even value of NFP.

In this case, the same approach is followed until sorting. Then a probabilistic estimation strategy. Now the two center elements may or may not be adjacent to each other. So instead of taking the mean of the two center elements, the average of the remaining pixel elements is calculated to replace the processing pixel. It will minimize the distance to a maximum extent compared to the original pixel intensity.

The algorithm for ATF is shown in Algorithm 1 as follows:

Algorithm 1: Proposed ATF Algorithm

i. Select the window size of 3×3. Assume that the processing pixel is NI (i , j).

ii. **If** 0 < NI (i , j) < 255 then

NI (i , j) is a NFP and its value is unchanged.

End

iii. **If** NI(i , j)=0 or NI(i, j)=255 then

NI (i , j) is a noisy pixel, then the probabilities are,

If the considered window holds all the pixels as 0's and 255's, then

NI (i , j) is replaced by the mean of the selected window.

Else eliminate 0's and 255's from the considered window. Let the number of NFP be p_1. Again two possibilities occur, they are,

If p_1 is an odd number, then

Sort and find the median value. Replace it with NI (i , j).

Else Follow the below steps,

1. Find the average of the remaining NFP.
2. Replace the obtained average value with NI (i , j).

End

End

End

iv. Repeat the same procedure from i to iii for all the pixels in the image.

8.2.2 Proposed Patch Else Average Trimmed Filter

This algorithm is developed to de-noise an image contaminated with high ND. The Patch Median (PM) can be defined for a matrix of an odd size, as the pixel element obtained at the center of the matrix, after sorting the patch elements in rows and then columns or vice versa either in ascending or descending order. Single sample output is obtained by the Patch Median, whereas there is a probability that average output can be obtained in Trimmed Median. ATF along with PM is incorporated to develop the PEATF. The algorithm of PEATF is shown in Algorithm 2.

8.2.3 Proposed Probabilistic Decision Based Average Trimmed Filter

In order to design the PDBATF, ATF and PEATF is implemented considering the facts arrived from and above sections and from the referred literature [6–9, 11–13] are as follows:

1. ATF and PEATF works approximately equivalent under ND 50%.
2. As the ND increase above 50%, ATF lags behind PEATF.
3. Switching strategy enhances the capability of the proposed algorithm.
4. With the increase in window size, undoubtedly noise removal capability will increase but with the loss of execution time.

The flowchart of PDBATF is set up and shown in the Fig. 8.1.

Algorithm 2: Proposed PEITMF Algorithm

i. Find PM of the selected window.

ii. **If** obtained estimation is NFP then

  Consider this as the final estimate value

iii. **Else** find ATF

iv. **If** obtained estimation is NFP then

  Consider this as the final estimate.

v. **Else** increase the size of the window and go to step 1

  End

vi. Repeat the procedure till the noise free pixel is obtained and stop.

End

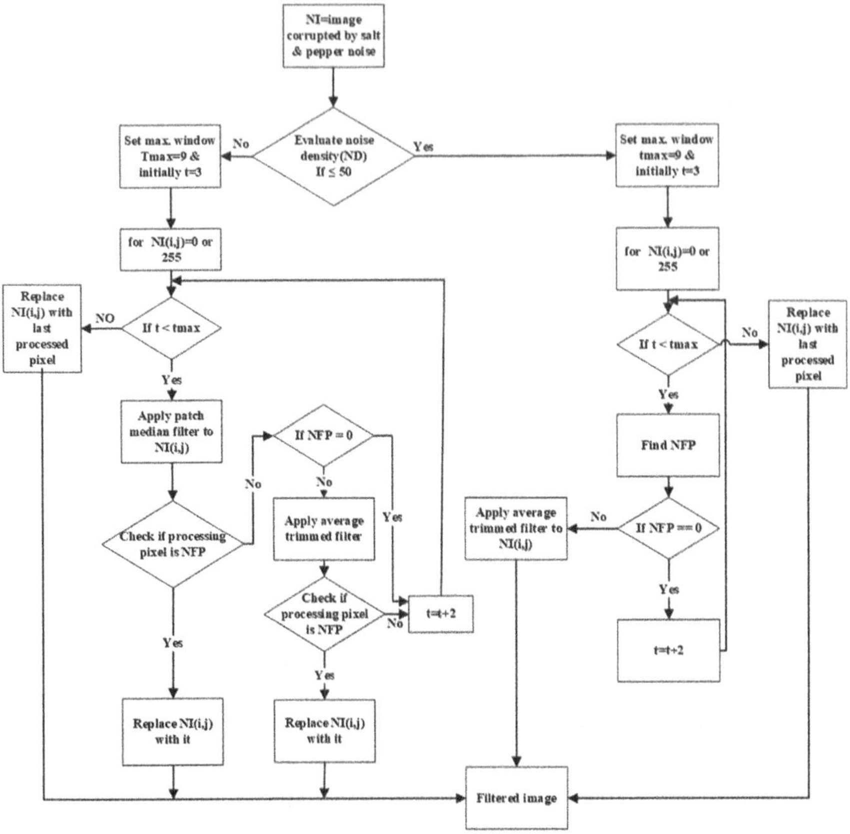

Fig. 8.1 Flowchart of proposed PDBATF

8.3 Simulation Results and Discussion

The PDBATF are examined against some of the recently reported state-of-the-art algorithms like NAFSM-2010, MDBUTMF-2011, PDBF-2016, BPDF-2018 in terms of peak signal to noise ratio (PSNR), image enhancement factor (IEF), execution time (ET), mean square error (MSE) and mean absolute error (MAE). Standard images of giemsa stained malaria-blood-smear images are collected from authentic standard image websites named www.data.broadinstitute.org. The images are of size 256 × 256. The experiments are conducted using Intel(R) Core(TM) i3-7200 central processing unit @ 2.30 GHz, 8 GB RAM with MATLAB R2013b environment.

The above-mentioned parameter can be defined as follows:

$$\mathrm{MSE} = \frac{\sum_{i,j}^{m,n} \left(z_{i,j} - Z_{d_{i,j}}\right)^2}{m \times n} \tag{8.1}$$

$$\mathrm{MAE} = \frac{\sum_{i,j}^{m,n} \left(z_{i,j} - Z_{d_{i,j}}\right)}{m \times n} \tag{8.2}$$

$$\mathrm{PSNR} = 10 \log_{10}\left(\frac{255^2}{\mathrm{MSE}}\right) \tag{8.3}$$

$$\mathrm{IEF} = \frac{\sum_{i,j}^{m,n} \left(z_{i,j} - NI_{i,j}\right)^2}{\sum_{i,j}^{m,n} \left(z_{i,j} - Z_{d_{i,j}}\right)^2} \tag{8.4}$$

For better performance, the PSNR and IEF should be as high as possible, while the MSE, MAE, and ET should be as low as possible. ET is calculated using Matlab command "tic" and "toc".

Tables 8.1, 8.2, 8.3, and 8.4 shows the objective measures of the PDBATF in comparison with the considered state-of-the-art while the graphical representation of the corresponding table is presented in Figs. 8.4, 8.5, 8.6, and 8.7. It can be seen from Table 8.1 and Fig. 8.4 that IEF is comparably high using PDBATF while MAE is comparatively less as can be seen in Table 8.2 and Fig. 8.5 which confirms the superiority of the proposed algorithm. Table 8.3 and Fig. 8.6 compares the proposed algorithm in terms of PSNR. It is analyzed and seen that the PSNR is better while de-noising an image using PDBATF in comparison with the other reported state-of-the-art. The proposed algorithm has a better execution time compared to other algorithms except for PDBF as PDBF calculates the processing pixel using only one pixel for the odd valued case and two-pixel for even valued case while in case of the proposed algorithm it depends on the number of NFP for even valued case and same

Table 8.1 Comparison of proposed PDBATF with the considered algorithm in context to IEF using malaria-blood-smear-1

ND	IEF				
In %	NAFSM-2010	MDBUTMF-2011	PDBF-2016	BPDF-2018	Proposed PDBATF
10	101.46	231.68	218.03	111.40	268.05
20	95.36	226.22	188.12	94.38	248.45
30	84.78	216.16	156.25	72.44	233.28
40	77.75	191.66	127.01	55.45	198.05
50	72.44	147.02	108.25	30.86	184.48
60	62.93	97.55	84.38	23.43	152.50
70	57.20	78.08	83.02	20.64	117.68
80	50.02	47.40	79.22	18.46	96.08
90	28.16	26.52	52.38	16.94	56.10

Table 8.2 Comparison of proposed PDBATF with the considered algorithm in context to MAE using malaria-blood-smear-2

ND	MAE				
In %	NAFSM-2010	MDBUTMF-2011	PDBF-2016	BPDF-2018	Proposed PDBATF
10	0.4436	0.462	0.426	0.361	0.3164
20	0.8518	0.767	0.595	0.544	0.6291
30	1.2956	1.174	1.145	1.039	0.9811
40	1.894	1.777	1.594	1.489	1.4341
50	2.653	2.653	3.156	2.996	1.9803
60	3.997	3.246	4.155	5.353	2.9124
70	4.156	5.246	4.553	6.246	3.6893
80	5.156	8.397	4.907	9.246	4.9804
90	8.246	12.246	6.156	14.246	6.1389

Table 8.3 Comparison of proposed PDBATF with the considered algorithm in context to PSNR using malaria-blood-smear-3

ND	PSNR in db				
In %	NAFSM-2010	MDBUTMF-2011	PDBF-2016	BPDF-2018	Proposed PDBATF
10	37.46	41.28	42.35	41.13	43.96
20	35.51	37.46	40.91	38.13	42.35
30	33.57	34.67	35.77	36.13	40.87
40	32.62	33.53	34.29	34.14	36.85
50	30.34	30.21	33.05	32.15	36.06
60	29.16	28.36	31.93	30.14	32.76
70	27.13	27.69	30.83	26.12	32.05
80	24.17	27.13	27.43	24.21	28.89
90	21.38	25.62	25.32	23.14	25.85

in the odd valued case. Figures 8.2, 8.3, and 8.8 displays the visual representation of image Malaria-blood-smear using considered state-of-the-art in comparison with the PDBATF. It can be seen that the PDBATF retrieves the edges and fine details of the image better in comparison to PDBF and other algorithms in very high ND which confirms the outperformance of the PDBATF.

Table 8.4 Comparison of proposed PDBATF with the considered algorithm in context to ET using malaria-blood-smear-3

ND	T in second				
In %	NAFSM-2010	MDBUTMF-2011	PDBF-2016	BPDF-2018	Proposed PDBATF
10	5.37	3.47	3.23	7.39	3.55
20	6.10	4.66	2.94	8.17	3.59
30	7.62	5.14	3.06	10.29	3.48
40	8.66	5.47	3.69	13.17	4.11
50	10.36	6.94	3.53	15.44	3.85
60	11.60	7.36	3.96	18.33	4.28
70	13.13	7.94	4.81	20.42	5.13
80	14.00	8.68	5.89	21.01	6.29
90	15.56	9.38	6.40	21.47	6.62

8.4 Conclusion

The PDBATF consist of ATF for low noise density and PEATF for high noise density. ATF estimates the processing pixel by finding the maximum relation among the remaining NFP in order to replace the noisy pixel. The PEATF, in case of high ND first tries to find the patch median then if the processing pixel remains noisy then it calculates ATF. The proposed algorithm works excellently in de-noising the giemsa stained image contaminated with salt and pepper noise. It retains the fine details of a blood smear image efficiently in comparison to the recently reported algorithms. The proposed algorithm can be very efficient as a pre-processing tool in the medical image for disease detection and in an application for image identification.

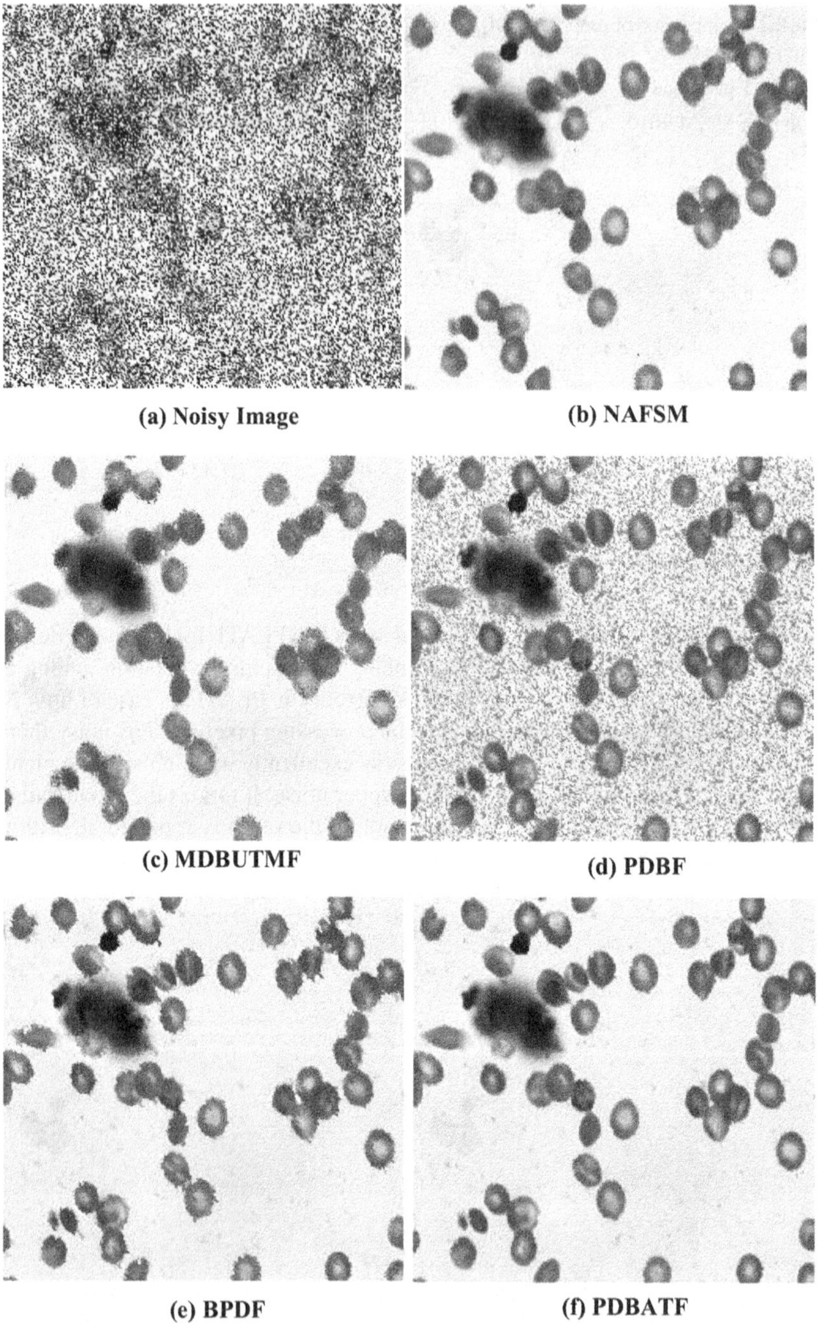

Fig. 8.2 Visual comparison of the proposed PDBATF with considered algorithm using image malaria-blood-smear-1 with ND 60%

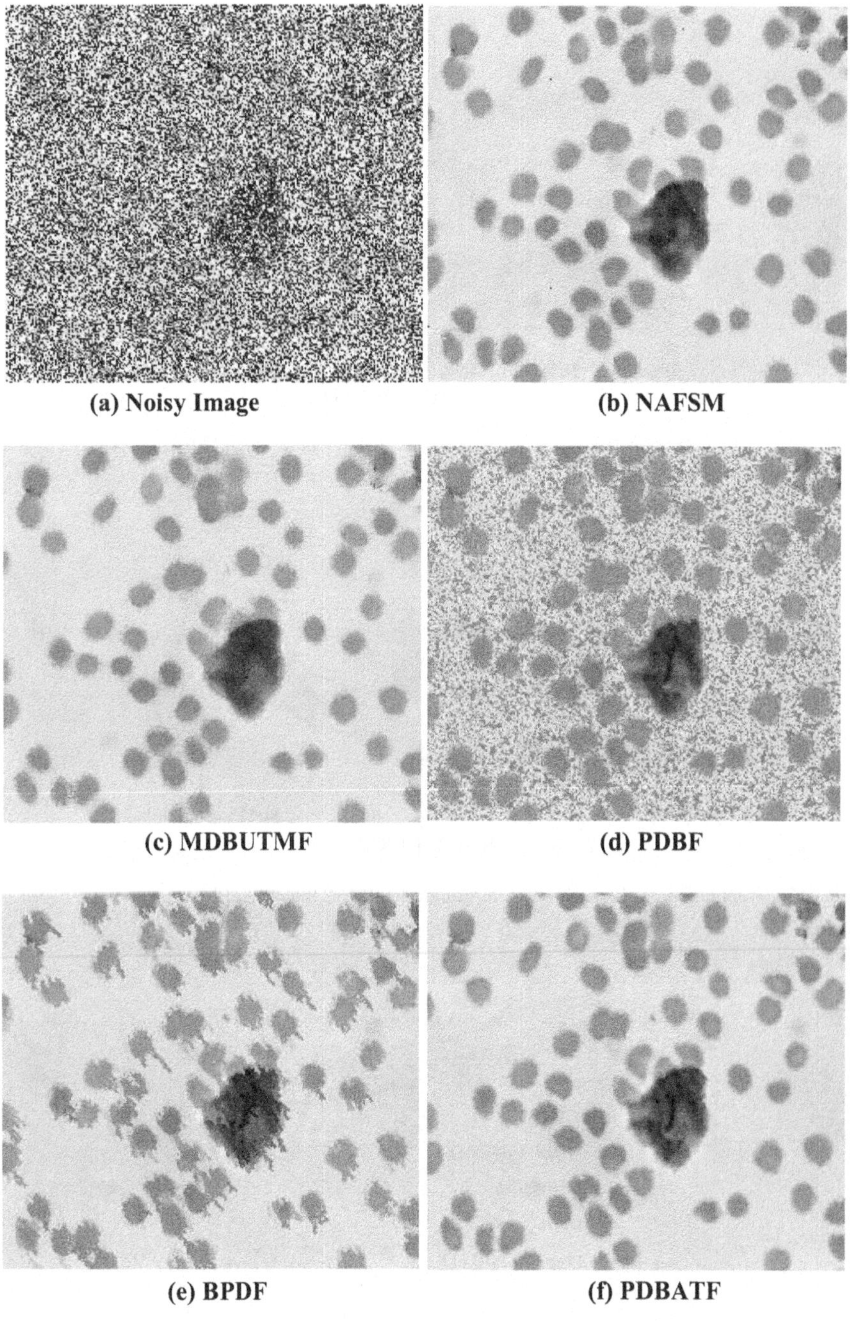

Fig. 8.3 Visual comparison of the PDBATF with considered algorithm using image malaria-blood-smear-2 with ND 70%

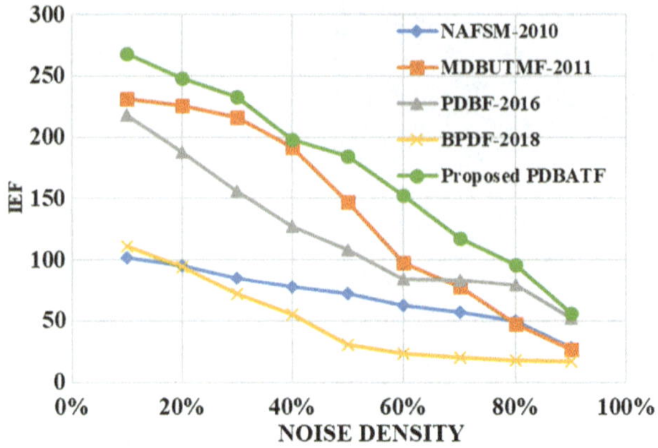

Fig. 8.4 Graphical representation of malaria-blood-smear-1 in terms of IEF

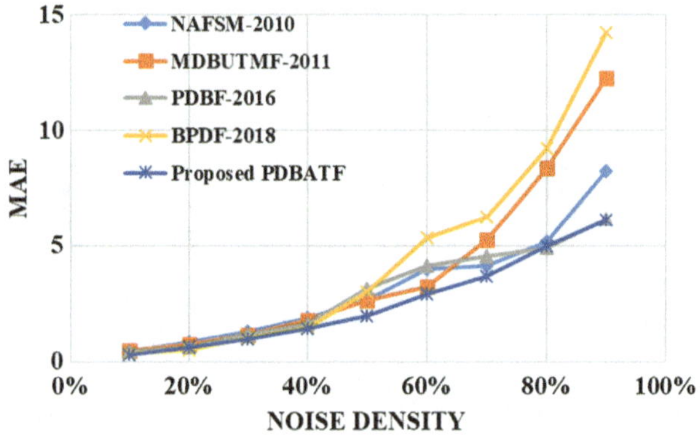

Fig. 8.5 Graphical representation of malaria-blood-smear-2 in terms of MAE

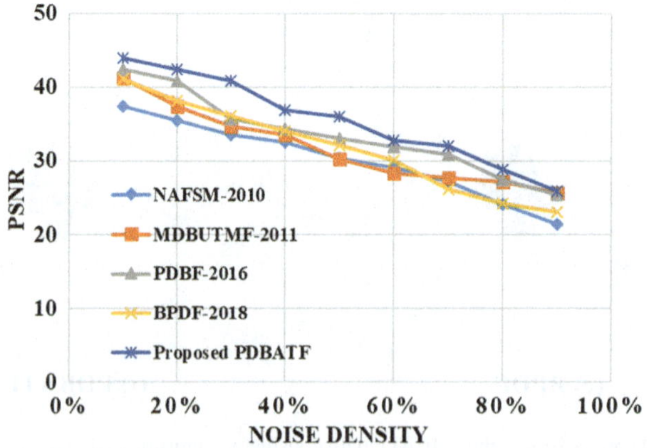

Fig. 8.6 Graphical representation of malaria-blood-smear-3 in terms of PSNR

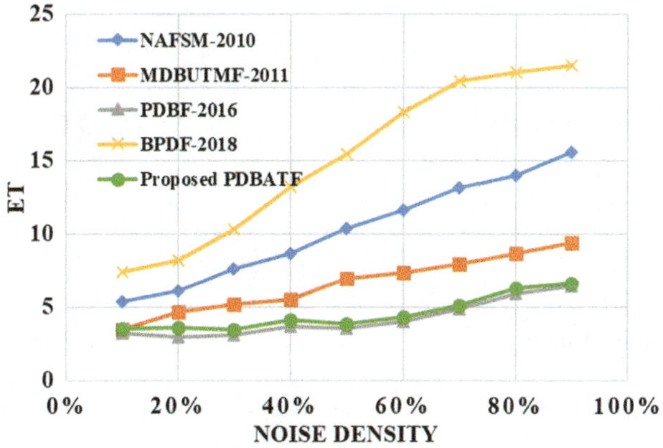

Fig. 8.7 Graphical representation of malaria-blood-smear-3 in terms of ET

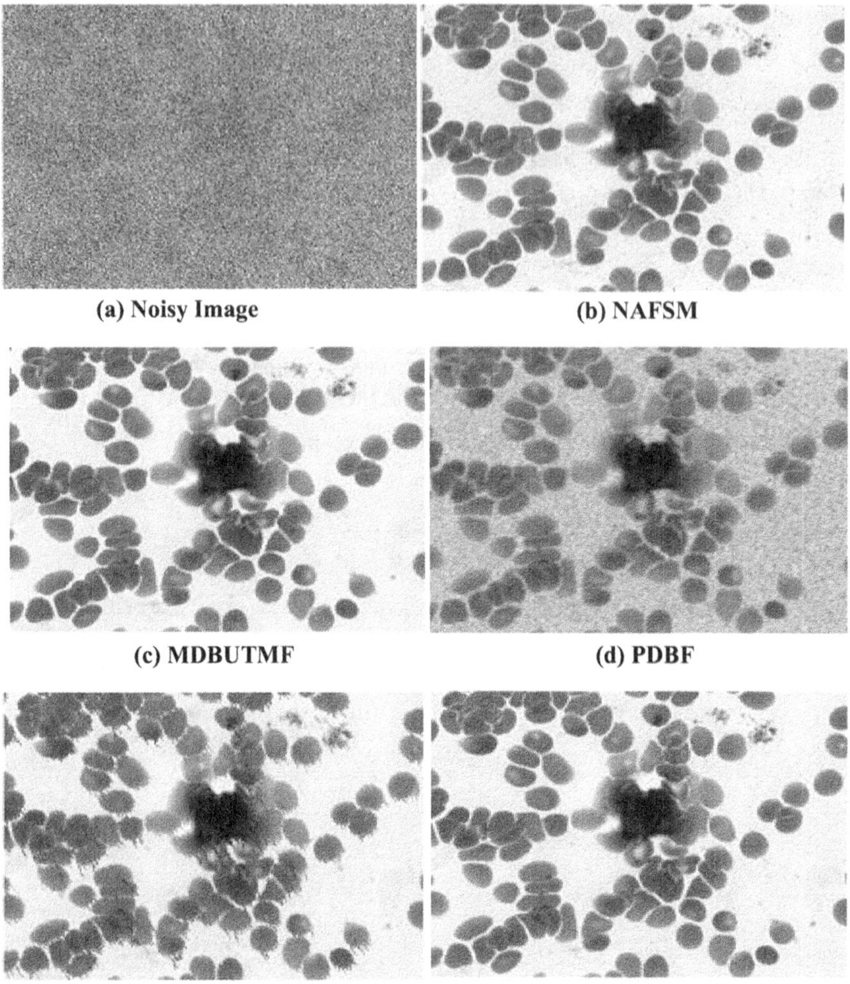

(a) Noisy Image (b) NAFSM (c) MDBUTMF (d) PDBF (e) BPDF (f) PDBATF

Fig. 8.8 Visual comparison of the proposed PDBATF with considered algorithm using image malaria-blood-smear-3 with ND 90%

References

1. Gonzalez, R., Woods, R.: Digital image processing, 2nd edn. Prentice Hall (2002)
2. Poularikas, E.A.D.: Nonlinear digital filtering. Handbook of formulas tables for signal process. Taylor and Francis Group, CRC Press (1998)
3. Hwang, H., Haddad, R.A.: Adaptive median filters: new algorithms and results. IEEE Trans. Image Process. **4**(4), 499–502 (1995)
4. Zhang, P., Li, F.: A new adaptive weighted mean filter for removing salt-and-pepper noise. IEEE Signal Process. Lett. **21**(10) (2014)

5. Khan, S., Lee, D.H.: An adaptive dynamically weighted median filter for impulse noise removal. EURASIP J. Adv. Signal Process. **1**, 2017 (2017)
6. Zhang, S., Karim, M.A.: A new impulse detector for switching median filters. IEEE Signal Process. Lett. **9**(11), 360–363 (2002)
7. Akkoul, S., Lédée, R., Leconge, R., Harba, R.: A new adaptive switching median filter. IEEE Signal Process. Lett. **17**(6), 587–590 (2010)
8. Faragallah, O.S., Ibrahem, H.M.: Adaptive switching weighted median filter framework for suppressing salt-and-pepper noise. AEU—Int. J. Electron. Commun. **70**(8), 1034–1040 (2016)
9. Luo, W.: An efficient detail-preserving approach for removing impulse noise in images. IEEE Signal Process. Lett. **13**(7), 413–416 (2006)
10. Srinivasan, K.S., Ebenezer, D.: A new fast and efficient decision-based algorithm for removal of high-density impulse noises. IEEE Signal Process. Lett. **14**, 189–192 (2007)
11. Esakkirajan, S., Verrakumar Adabala, T., Subramanyam, N., PremChand, C.H.: Removal of high density salt and pepper noise through a modified decision based unsymmetric trimmed median filter", IEEE Signal Process. Lett. **18**(5), 287–290 (2011)
12. Balasubramanian, G., Chilambuchelvan, A., Vijayan, S., Gowrison, G.: Probabilistic decision based filter to remove impulse noise using patch else trimmed median. AEU—Int. J. Electron. Commun. **5**(11), 1–11 (2016)
13. Jayaraj, V., Ebenezer, D.: A new switching-based median filtering scheme and algorithm for removal of high-density salt and pepper noise in images. EURASIP J. Adv. Signal Process. **1**, 2010 (2010)

Chapter 9
Feature Selection: Role in Designing Smart Healthcare Models

Debjani Panda, Ratula Ray and Satya Ranjan Dash

Abstract With the leveraging fields of data mining and artificial intelligence, the data is growing day by day in an exponential manner. In health care sector, huge amount of biomedical data are generated from online hospital management applications, online sites, biomedical devices and sensors, and from various other electronic devices in an innumerous manner. There is a huge demand in the health sector to store this data so that they can be analyzed for future predictions. The process involves storing of high dimensional data and also very high volume of data ("Big Data"), which later needs to be processed to extract the desired information. The important attributes of the data needs to be identified, and then a subset is to be generated which can help in training the prediction model classifiers. This big data needs to be preprocessed to eradicate the unrequited attributes, identifying the essential attributes, then filtering out the noise (irrelevant attributes) from it and minimize its size without affecting its quality, i.e. after filtrating the attributes, there should not be any required attribute missing which will affect the performance of the predictive models. This task of identifying patterns, identifying relevant attributes for prediction of diseases and selecting min. no. attributes from the huge data set so as to achieve the results from predictive models with minimum time and cost is very challenging and requires a lot of expertise. This book chapter explains the importance of feature selection and feature creation related to biomedical data. Actually first a set of features have to be created which will study the hidden behavior and patterns and these features will then in turn be used to identify patterns and assist in prediction of diseases. Feature identification is again a rigorous task and involves lot of expertise. This chapter gives an insight into why feature selection is essential in designing the smart healthcare predictive models for real time data.

D. Panda
School of Computer Engineering, KIIT Deemed to Be University, Bhubaneswar, India
e-mail: pandad25@gmail.com

R. Ray
School of Biotechnology, KIIT Deemed to Be University, Bhubaneswar, India

S. R. Dash (✉)
School of Computer Applications, KIIT Deemed to Be University, Bhubaneswar, India
e-mail: sdashfca@kiit.ac.in

P. K. Pattnaik et al. (eds.), *Smart Healthcare Analytics in IoT Enabled Environment*, Intelligent Systems Reference Library 178,
https://doi.org/10.1007/978-3-030-37551-5_9

Keywords Big data · Feature selection · Feature creation · Patterns · Smart healthcare predictive models

9.1 Introduction

Today's world is overflowing with data and data is increasing in size and variety in almost an exponential manner. Huge amounts of data are generated from online applications, online sites, biomedical devices and sensors, from satellites, and so on and so forth in an innumerous manner. This data is being termed as "Big Data" because of its huge size, its multiple attributes i.e. veracity, rate of increase with time and also in terms of its validity.

This big data needs to be preprocessed to eradicate the unrequited attributes, identifying the essential attributes, then filtering out the noise from it and minimize its size without affecting its quality, i.e. after filtrating the attributes, there should not be any required attribute missing which will affect the performance of the predictive models. Here come the actual challenge of actually identifying patterns, identifying relevant attributes for prediction and selecting min. no. attributes from the huge data set so as to achieve the results from predictive models with minimum time and cost.

The process of feature selection involves in creating those features which will study the underlying behavior and patterns and assist in identifying the patterns for effective prediction of outcomes. Both feature selection and feature transformation is again a rigorous task and involves lot of expertise. In this chapter we will summarize various methods of feature selection and transformation and study the merits and demerits of the methods by giving an insight into why feature selection is crucial in designing of prediction models.

9.1.1 Necessity of Feature Selection

Machine learning follows a thumb rule as any other computer based system—if garbage is put inside then the output will be garbage only. The more is the data stored; the addressing of that huge data is even more. Bellman referred to this phenomenon as the "curse of dimensionality" when considering problems in dynamic optimization [1]. So the quality of data which is considered as input is very much essential in machine learning, where the noise needs to be filtered and redundant features to be removed so as to get meaningful and desired results.

This selection becomes even more essential when the numbers of features are prodigious. The need of the hour is to identify which feature will affect the prediction and will result in more accuracy of the model. Each and every feature is not required to be used as it involved cost and time without yielding desired results. The prediction algorithm can be assisted another algorithm by considering only important features.

These features are mostly subsets of the entire set and help in predicting better and accurate results for the models being trained.

Feature selection is very much essential for predictive models because:

- It reduces the total no. of features [N] to [m] where m < N [2].
- It facilitates the prediction model algorithm to get trained in less time.
- It lessens the intricacy of a predictive model and makes interpretation easier.
- It aids in improving the performance of a model on the basis of the choosing the correct set of attributes or subset.
- It minimizes over-fitting.

9.2 Classes of Feature Selection

9.2.1 Brief of Filter Methods

These types of methods are normally used in preprocessing of raw data. They are used where the classification algorithms are independent of the selected features. On the other hand, the selection of relevant features depends upon the output results/scores, which are obtained from different validating mathematical/statistical methods. These set of features are checked for their inter-dependency with output attribute so that the correct subset is chosen.

The statistical functions which are most commonly used to identify the importance of the feature and considered in this chapter are Linear Discriminant Analysis, Pearson Correlation, Analysis of Variance (ANOVA), Chi-Square Test, IR, Relief, GR, Symmetrical Uncertainty and One R.

LDA: Linear discriminant analysis is used in supervised training models to determine a linear composition of features that can identify different classes separately on the basis of their attribute value. Ideally the value of categorical attribute is used to determine the belongingness to a class. It is helpful in maximizing the distance between two different classes and minimizes the distance between attributes of the same class.

Pearson's Correlation: Pearson Correlation measures the linear dependence between two continuous variables X and Y. Its value varies from −1 to +1.

Pearson's Correlation formula:

$$\rho X, Y = \frac{cov\ X, Y}{\sigma_X\ \sigma_Y} \tag{9.1}$$

Where *cov* is the covariance

σ_X is the standard deviation of *X*

σ_Y is the standard deviation of *Y*

Correlation between the quantitative variables is found by plotting them across X axis and Y axis and if the graph shows a straight line then the variables are strongly associated. If the correlation is positive then increase/decrease of one variable increases/decreases the other and if the correlation is negative then increase of one variable decreases the other and vice versa.

Chi-Square: This test is performed to find whether two categorical variables are correlated or independent. This is a statistical method which aids in identifying the correlation between the groups of categorical features. This is carried out by finding out the probability of belongingness to each class by using their frequency distribution.

To calculate Chi square, the statistic value of each cell needs to be calculated by

$$(\text{Observed freq.} - \text{expected freq.})^2/(\text{expected freq.})$$

And the expected numbers in each cell is of the category variable is calculated by $(\text{row total} \times \text{column total})/(\text{grand total})$.

ANOVA: ANOVA stands for Analysis of variance. The underlying process is exactly the same as LDA except that the variance is calculated between a continuous variable and one or more categorical variable. The dependant feature is the continuous variable. This test compares the mean of different groups are compares them for their equality.

Information Gain (IR): It is the entropy(information gain) of the feature for the output variable and varies from 0 (No information) to 1 (Max. information). The features which have higher IR values are considered to be more related to the output and can be considered for building of the model. Cut-off values can also be given to consider the features above that level of Information gain to minimize the training cost of the models. This is helpful in eliminating the features with less relevance.

RELIEF: This algorithm was developed by Kira and Rendell in 1992. RELIEF is an online algorithm which maximizes the value of an objective function within a given margin. It is very useful in solving convex optimization problems [3, 5]. The margin is decided on the basis of the closeness of a point to its neighboring classifier. RELIEF method of feature selection gives much desired results of selecting the important features. The method is recursive in nature. In each iteration, it calculates the weights of each feature and estimates the distance from its nearest classifier and farthest classifier. Depending upon their capability to distinguish between neighboring patterns the belongingness to a class is decided. With start of every loop [4], randomly a pattern c is chosen and its two nearest neighbors are found. Out of the two neighbors the closest neighbor is assigned as its same class (which is named as nearest hit or NH) and the farther class is assigned as the opposite class (which is named as nearest miss or NM). The weight of the ith feature is then calculated as:

$$\text{wi} = \text{wi} + |\text{c(i)} - \text{NM(i)(c)}| - |\text{c(i)} - \text{NH(i)(c)}|, \quad \text{for } 1 \leq \text{i} \leq \text{I}. \tag{9.2}$$

One-R: This algorithm has been developed by Holte [6]. This method has a rule for every aspect of the input data used for learning and establishes the rule by minimizing the mistakes. This algorithm considers features as continuous if they are having some mathematical charge. It is one of the basic techniques which separate continuous values of data to distinct disjoint values. This type of separation is one of the most ancient techniques which help in getting distinct and disjoint values. Here missing values in data are also considered as a valid value called "missing". This algorithm produces one rule for each feature and is very simple to use. This method can be used as a part of complex classifier algorithms and help in scaling of the problems.

Gain Ratio (GR): Gain ratio (GR) is a modified version of the information gain that further minimizes its bias. It considers the number and size of branches while choosing a feature [7]. The information gain absolutely overlooks how other attributes are related and drops the entropy information of the split branches. Gain Ratio considers the entropy information of the branches (considers additional explicit value needed to be given about the belongingness of that attribute to a desired class). If the information needed is very high then the importance of that attribute is low and vice versa.

$$\text{Gain Ratio (Feature)} = \text{Gain (Feature)}/(\text{Intrinsic value (Feature)}) \quad (9.3)$$

Symmetrical Uncertainty: Symmetry property is important when we are measuring the correlation between the features. As explained above, IR (Information Gain) is inclined in favor of features with more values [8]. The biasness of these variables is addressed by normalizing them so that they can be compared with each other. Symmetrical Uncertainty (SU) is the method which aids in normalizing the values. For two attributes X and Y, it is calculated as

$$\text{SU(X, Y)} = 2 \cdot \text{IG(X|Y)H(X)} + \text{H(Y)} \quad (9.4)$$

SU reduces the bias of information gain towards features with more values and normalizes them in range [0, 1]. The value 1 reflects that information about one attribute solely determines the value of other and vices versa. The value 0 indicates that X and Y are not related to each other.

$$\text{H(X)} = -\text{X i P(xi)log2(P(xi))} \text{ is the entropy of a attribute X.} \quad (9.5)$$

Filter methods fails to deal with multi-colinearity. So, multi-collinearity of features needs to be tackled while training the models for real time data.

9.2.2 *Wrapper Methods*

Wrapper methods are restricted to select a subset of features and train a model based on the subset of attributes. Depending upon the results we obtain, the current subset can either be added with more attributes or some of them can be reduced. The problem is finally converted to a search problem. Wrapper methods are normally time consuming because the steps have to be repeated frequently to get the desired accuracy in results. The above mentioned methods are very much resource hungry.

Some common examples of wrapper methods are forward feature selection, backward feature elimination, recursive feature elimination, etc.

Forward Selection: Forward selection is a recursive method in which we start with empty data subset i.e. with nil features. Relevant features are added to the subset with each iteration, and the method is repeated until the subset accepts no new attribute, which can further enhance its performance.

Backward Elimination: This method is just the opposite of the forward selection method. Here we start with complete set of attributes and start reducing it by the most irrelevant attribute. This is repeated in every iteration. This elimination continues until further reduction does not improve the performance of the model.

Recursive Feature Elimination: This is based on greedy optimization algorithm which aims to identify the best suited attribute of the subset being used to train the model. It recursively generates models and identifies the best one and the least important one and sets them aside after each completion of loop. At the end it assigns ranks to features based on their order of elimination.

9.2.3 Filter Methods Versus Wrapper Methods

The preprocessing of raw data and selection of subset of features follows two different schools of thought. They are supervised and unsupervised methods. In unsupervised methods which are performed on raw data to get the reduced subset of features. The subset obtained may not be the best subset for measuring the performance of training models. Whereas supervised methods include extensive training of models and mostly results in generating the best subset of features. Filter methods are mostly unsupervised whereas wrapper methods are supervised. The major differences between the filter and wrapper methods for feature selection are tabulated in Table 9.1.

Table 9.1 Difference between filter and wrapper methods

Filter methods	Wrapper methods
Measures the importance of features by correlating with output/predicted variable	Measures usefulness of feature subset by training models
Faster in terms of time complexity	Less faster is terms of time complexity
Training model is not required	Training model is required
Computation cost is low	Computation cost is very high
Mostly uses statistical methods	Mostly uses cross validation methods

9.2.4 Embedded Methods

The embedded (hybrid) methods of Feature selection is a consolidated method containing Filter and Wrapper methods. Here algorithms have their own feature selection methods which generate the best suited feature subset with dimensionality reduction for the training models.

This chapter analyses the importance of features with several available methods and justifying the need to perform this step to improve the performance of the models. Most widely accepted techniques under embedded methods include LASSO and RIDGE regression consists of inbuilt penalization functions to reduce over-fitting. Other examples of embedded methods are Regularized trees, Memetic algorithm, Random multinomial logic, etc.

9.2.4.1 Lasso Regression

Lasso stands for Least Absolute Selection and Shrinkage Operator, which is a statistical method used for regression analysis. It performs selection of variable and also helps in regularizing it, so that prediction becomes more accurate. The LASSO method [9] sets a limit on the sum of the absolute values of the features considered in a model. The sum of the model variables has to be less than a fixed value (upper bound). This is achieved by applying a shrinking process wherein the coefficients of the regression variables are reduced and even minimized to 0 in some cases. The resultant variables which are left with non-zero coefficients finally are considered as a subset which is considered to build the model. The main objective of this process is to minimize the prediction error. Hence, Lasso regression performs L1 regularization which adds penalty equivalent to absolute value of the magnitude of coefficients.

$$mimimize\left(||Y - X\beta||_2^2/\mathrm{n}\right) \text{ subject to} \tag{9.6}$$

$$\sum_{j=1}^{k} ||\beta 1|| < t \; where\, t\, is\, upper\, bound\; for\; sum\; of\; coefficients.$$

9.2.4.2 Ridge Regression

Ridge Regression: When multi-collinearity occurs, least squares estimates are unbiased, but their variances are large so they may be far from the true value. By adding a degree of bias to the regression estimates, ridge regression reduces the standard errors. This method helps in reducing the variance which is a resultant of non-linear relationships between two independent variables [10]. It performs L2 regularization by adding a penalty to square of magnitude of coefficients.

Regression equation is written in matrix form as $Y = XB + e$ where Y is the dependent variable, X represents the independent variables, B is the regression coefficients to be estimated, and e represents the errors are residuals.

In ordinary least squares, the ridge coefficient B is calculated as:

$$\underline{\hat{B}} = (X'X)^{-1}X'\underline{Y} \tag{9.7}$$

9.2.4.3 Regularized Trees

This method helps in avoiding in selecting a feature whose gain is lesser than a Max_i (Gain(Xi)) of features in the subset. Supposing F is set of features used in the previous set of the model before splitting and Xi is the feature among the set, which is obtained from splitting without loss of generality, then Gain(Xi) > Max_i (Gain(Xi)), where $Xi \in F$.

A regularized tree model keeps on adding sequentially new features to F if these features provide some additional information about the predicted variable Y. So the final set of features in F contains useful and non-redundant features. The elimination of features is achieved by imposing a penalty to the feature with gain lesser than the maximum gain [11].

$$\mathrm{gain}_R(Xj) = \begin{cases} \lambda \cdot \mathrm{gain}(Xj) & Xj \notin F \\ \mathrm{gain}(Xi) & Xj \in F \end{cases} \tag{9.8}$$

where $\lambda \in [0, 1]$ and λ is called the coefficient. A smaller λ produces a larger penalty to a feature not belonging to F.

9.2.4.4 Memetic Algorithms

Memetic Algorithms: These algorithms are influenced by Baldwin Ian Evolutionary Algorithms, Lamarckian Evolutionary Algorithms, Hybrid Evolutionary Algorithms, and Cultural Algorithms [12]. This algorithm follows principles of both genetic evolution and memetic evolution. The term "meme" refers to a piece of discrete information which carries some pattern resemblance and is inherited. The basic search criteria works on the principle of global search in a population and then finding the local search space so that repeated search in an area can provide a local optimum. These algorithms allow the information from global population to be transmitted, selected, inherited and also variated in memes. The MAs are very good global = local search optimizers [13]. Example is Travelling Salesman Problem.

9.2.4.5 Random Multinomial Logit

This is a multiclass classifier which uses ensemble of multinomial logistic regression models [14]. This classifier has the advantage of using the stability and theoretical concept of multinomial logistic regression along with bagging which is less prone to noise and is generally applicable to more no. of applications. This algorithm is very useful in selecting the useful features through statistical methods of logistic regression which also prevents unnecessary wastage of resources by eliminating unwanted features. In RML selection of relevant features is done by replacing one random attribute in the training model with a new feature. After this step, if this model contains statistically insignificant features then they are removed else the model retains those set of features. The advantages and limitations of embedded methods are summarized in Table 9.2.

9.3 Feature Transformation

This is another important aspect of feature selection. Most of the available data in nature follows a normal distribution and its approximation can be done even if the underlying patterns are unknown. For example like employee age, salary, height, weight, sex, etc. can actually be projected for some unknown cases on the basis of already available data.

Feature Transformation (FT) is a set of algorithms which creates a set of new features from the existing features. The newly created set of features may not resemble the original features or may not have same information content but it aids in increasing performance of classifiers and in discriminating the feature in n-dimensional space as compared the original set. The process of transformation of features actually plays a vital role in dimension reduction.

Feature transformation can be achieved by simple linear combinations of original features or by applying some mathematical function to the set of attributes in the original data. The most common methods of feature transformation include:

9.3.1 Scaling

This is normalizing the features to a range mostly between 0 and 1. The variables which are independent and mostly continuous in nature are limited to a range so that they can be studied and analyzed. The formula which is used for scaling is

$$X' = (X - Xmin)/(Xmax - Xmin) \tag{9.9}$$

where X' is the rescale value, X is the original value, Xmax is the highest limit and Xmin is the lowest value of the range in which they are to be scaled.

Table 9.2 Advantages and limitations of embedded methods

Embedded methods	Advantages	Limitations
Lasso regression	Adaptability to various prediction models is very high. Can work well where no. of instances are very less and give accurate results	1. In small-n-large-p dataset the LASSO selects at most n variables before it saturates. If there are grouped variables (highly correlated between each other) LASSO tends to select one variable from each group ignoring the others
Ridge regression	Effectively reduces features in multi-collinear variables. A small bias is added to correlated variables and the features are distinguished. Reduces over-fitting in models. Effectively reduces variance while feature selection	Selecting the value of k is the major bottleneck. It requires experience and expertise to choose correct value of k. Normal inference procedures are not applicable and exact distributional properties are not known. Ridge regression cannot perform variable selection
Regularized trees	Is very useful in creating a compact feature subset by eliminating feature having redundant information content. The expandability is very high and can easily fit other tree like bagged tree and boosted trees. Can deal with both categorical and numerical values. Can also deal with missing values	Does not capture the desired subset of features when no. of instances are less. The no. of selected features are more than other searches which increases the training and computation time of models
Memetic algorithm	Very flexible and can be easily adapted to optimization problems. Require less extensive tuning for adaptation. Changing the tuning parameter hardly affects the performance. Less computational cost as compared to other Genetic algorithms	Stabilization is needed between local and global search to prevent earlier convergence and unnecessary use of resources. Stopping criterion is needed to get the local optimal satisfying the fitness functions
Random multinomial logic	Resistant to noise. Less prone to over-fitting. Can be scaled to large applications easily	Difficult to deal with Large label bias of data. It is prone to noise when it is used as standalone classifier with difficult data sets

For example we have one data with values [10, 20, 30] and we want to rescale value 20.

Then $X' = (20 - 10)/(30 - 10) = 0.5$.

So, the values of the above variable in new scale or new range are [0, 0.5, 1].

9.3.2 Linear Discriminant Analysis

LDA is a supervised method of dimensionality reduction. This is a transformation technique [15, 16] which determines the directions i.e. "linear discriminants" representing the axes. These axes actually are determined where the points satisfy the condition of maximum distance from these axes. The main aim of LDA is to project variables of higher dimension space to lower dimension space so that they can be easily separated into different classes without loss of class information. This is an effective method with less computation cost and also deals with the problem of over-fitting.

9.3.3 Principal Component Analysis

This is the most commonly used technique which effectively reduces the high dimensional data to meaningful data having lesser dimensions. This is a method of feature transformation where the original variables in higher dimensional space are transformed to a set of new variables [17] without loss of essential information. This is a statistical method of determining the principal component of the data (basically the line), which considers the maximum variance of the plotted points belonging to the variables in the original data. This continues till the principal components are identified for total no. of variables in the original data.

9.3.4 SVM

This method along with recursive feature elimination is very useful in reducing the total number of features [18]. This technique continuously removes the unwanted features and results in the best subset generation. The SVM attempts to find the hyper plane with maximum distance from the two classes. This is done until no. new plane is found i.e. the best set of features have been identified beyond which the performance may degrade.

9.3.5 *Random Projection*

In random projection (RP), the original high-dimensional data [19] is projected onto a lower-dimensional space using a random matrix. This matrix has only one column. Random Projection has emerged as a computationally efficient, yet an adequate method for dimensionality reduction of high-dimensional data sets. It is a very simple method where the original data is projected from d-dimension to k-dimensional subspace through origin where k << d. This random projection to lower subspace preserves the intermediate distance of each point. The dimensions and distribution of random projections matrices are restricted in order to retain the pair wise distances between any two samples in the data.

9.3.6 *Neural Networks*

These networks consist of large no. of neurons which are associated with weights. These weights can be adjusted which varies the input signals. The single neuron of the network consolidates all of its connected input and converts them into a scalar which best describes the inputs' state after a weighted sum and activation [20]. Neural Networks do the same work in a paralleled and complex structure of neurons to transform the inputs into a class representing vector.

9.4 Related Works

Abdar [21]. This research paper implements various algorithms of Decision Tree to find out the best one which give the most accurate results. The Cleveland database [22] has been from UCI. The algorithms used for the study includes C 5.0, C&R Tree which results in creating univariate binary tree, CHAID algorithm (chi-square automatic interaction and detection algorithm) and QUEST. Linear separation method is used in QUEST to create tree with one variable. The performance has been studied with factors like Specificity, Sensitivity, Precision and Accuracy. The C 5.0 Tree has given the highest accuracy of 85.33% after determining important factors to be considered as Cp, Old Peak, Slope, Thalach, Rest ECG, Trestbps.

Beyene and Kamat [23]. This research work is a survey of comparing different prediction algorithms on the basis of their prediction accuracy. The classifiers studied are J48, Naïve Bayes and Support Vector Machine using k-fold cross validation. All three have been used to study the occurrence of heart disease and predict the person is suffering from heart disease or not with less cost and time.

Koul and Chhikara [24]. In this work the feature selection is done using Filter Methods like Correlation and Relief Methods. After applying the methods best subset of 20 features is taken and is considered as the input pool of features for Genetic algorithm. Using Fitness function, the best subset is identified. This subset is again fed as input into the Naïve Bayes classifier to optimally predict the heart disease and in much better manner and lesser cost. This paper uses a hybrid method of selection of features which include filter method, wrapper method and GA.

Ottom and Alshorman [25]. Various feature selection techniques have been used and generated ranks for each feature. They have used the Cleveland database from UCI repository. The generated ranks of the 14 features considered under study were nearly similar which was difficult to identify the most relevant feature. The accumulation of ranks have been performed after adding the ranks of relevant feature and the resultant attributes were selected for study whose accumulated rank was >1 and the rest were eliminated. The prediction algorithms used were KNN, Naïve Bayes, SVM, ANN and Tree J48 which showed better enhanced results with filtrated 9 attributes. KNN gave the best results with 3.7% enhancement with reduced features.

Setiono and Liu [26]. In this paper a neural network is constructed having minimum no. of hidden units. These hidden units accept inputs from relevant units only and this is achieved by applying a network pruning algorithm. The activation values are obtained from hidden unit which contain the information about patterns in the data set. When need arises, these values can be fed as input into a classification method that build decision trees to obtain a set of decision rules such that a user may enjoy the high accuracy of the neural network.

Acharya et al. [27]. This work emphasizes on how to focus on higher-order spectra of ECG signals and identify heart diseases. KNN algorithm and Decision Trees have been used to study the application of the signals and its correlation in predicting the heart disease. The results have been tabulated and accuracy has been predicted by the algorithms as 98.17% (KNN) and 98.99% (Decision Tree) and has been proven to give better results for prediction of the disease.

El-Bialy et al. [28]. The authors have analyzed two types of Decision Trees C4.5 and Fast Decision Tree. The data has been obtained from six databases from UCI.

Using 10-fold Cross Validation, the data has been used for training and prediction of heart disease. Association rules have been used which determines 3 most important features like cp, ca and age using C4.5 Decision Tree and using Fast Decision Trees the important features have been found to be cp, age and thal. The intersection of these features have resulted in features to be considered as ca and age and then the accuracy of the data is calculated for predicting the ailment is 78.54% and 78.55% for 4.5 DT and FDT.

Karpagachelvi et al. [29]. This paper summarizes different techniques used to study information from ECG signals and use it to predict the heart diseases based upon the factors i.e. simplicity and accuracy. Different types of transformations have been discussed to extract important and relevant features from ECG signals. The ECG signals have been discussed in detail containing the PQRST wave and the techniques which have been discussed includes ANN, SVM, Fuzzy Logic, GA and other analysis methods. Emphasis has been made on use of more statistical data for feature extraction from ECG signals and use of transformation techniques that increases accuracy of the prediction.

Saxena et al. in [30]. The paper focuses on efficient composite method for compressing data, retrieving signal from compressed data and extracting features from ECG signals. It has been observed that after the data is compressed, the resultant features extracted are more meaningful as undesired noise has been eliminated during the process. Artificial Neural Network has been used wherein the compression ratio is directly proportional to the ECG cycle. When cycle increases, the ratio also increases. The method proves that the composite method of compression gives much better results for ECG signals as compared to the original signal and is best suited for real time applications.

Zhao and Zhang [31]. This paper focuses on a different method of feature extraction using wavelet transform and Support Vector Machine algorithm. The study involves filtrating the noise from the data in preprocessing, extracting the relevant features and classification of the ECG signals. Two different feature extraction methods have been used and results have been combined to create a vector for features and finally these features are studied with SVM and Gaussian kernel for classification of the heart rhythm. The techniques used are wavelength transform and auto regression for creating the feature vector which can classify the heart rhythm efficiently. The study has given accuracy of 99.68%.

Shardlow [32]. The author has analyzed different feature selection mechanisms with same sample data. Almost every technique that has been discussed includes the filter methods, wrapper methods and hybrid methods. The different methods have been studied with the SVM Classifier and results have been compared. It is observed that when the data for training the model has large no. of dimensions, then feature selection plays an important role in reducing the dimensionality and the training cost of the models and results in giving more accurate results by the classifier. The accuracy of hybrid methods (like Rank Forward Search) is better than wrapper and filter methods used for feature selection.

Singh et al. [33]. The study focuses on a new non-invasive method of detecting coronary heart disease by studying the HRV (heart rate variability) signals. The subspaces of the HRV signals are decomposed using Multiscale wavelet packet (MSWP). The performance has been analyzed using Fisher ranking method, GDA (generalized discriminant analysis) and binary classifier as extreme learning machine (ELM). The useful features are then given ranks and are organized according to their ranks. The top 10 features of utmost importance are taken as used in Extreme Learning Machine which has given 100% accurate results in predicting whether a patient is normal or suffering from heart ailment. The GDA with Binary Classifier has given better results than LDA. In case of the NSR-CAD data set, the ELM classifier achieved approx. 100% accuracy for two features in test data, whereas, in case of Self_NSR-CAD, the max. accuracy of 100% is obtained by ELM with multiquadric and sigmoid hidden node + GDA with Gaussian kernel function for the selected top ten features.

Hira and Gillies [34]. This paper emphasizes different methods of feature subset selection and 'feature extraction. The various types of feature extraction that are filter methods, wrapper methods and embedded methods have been elaborated and implemented on micro array data of cancer patients. The merits and demerits of all these methods have been summarized. The feature selection methods preserve the characteristics of the original set of data and make it easier for interpretability. The demerits of feature selection are its high training time, lower discriminating power and overfitting of samples. Feature extraction techniques have the advantage of high discriminating power and have less overfitting problems when used under supervised algorithms. The demerits of this technique are loss of data interpretability and expensive data transformation.

Dash and Liu [35]. The authors have summarized the different feature selection methods along with various classification methods. They have analyzed a total no. 15 feature selection methods and 3 types of generation function. A comparison has been made with total 32 feature selection methods which have been put into different categories on the basis of how they have been generated and how they have been validated. It shows characteristics of the feature selection methods including the type of data that can be handled, the type of data set (large or small) that can be handled, whether the method is able to identify multiple class, whether it is able to handle noise and the ability to produce an optimal subset from the original one. The authors have generalized the feature selection methods into basically four parts that are generation procedure, evaluation function, stopping criteria and evaluation function.

Dewangan and Shukla [36]. This work emphasizes in comparison of different methods and techniques involved for extraction of features from ECG signals. The survey includes preprocessing and denoising of the ECG signals. The hidden Markov Model combines the structural and statistical methods for detecting low amplitude P waves. Several other techniques like Wavelet Transform, Discrete Wavelet Transform have been summarized with their benefits and improvement in accuracy of prediction using the above methods. Kahunen Loève Transform (KLT) has also been discussed with its benefits of feature extraction and shape recognition. Various classification techniques like Neural Networks, Artificial Neural Networks, Bayesian Neural Networks, SVM, and several others have covered under this study which explicit the benefits of the classification algorithms and their improvement in accuracy after feature selection.

9.5 Our Experiment

9.5.1 Workflow Diagram

The workflow diagram for comparison of classifiers with and without feature selection is attached. See Fig. 9.1.

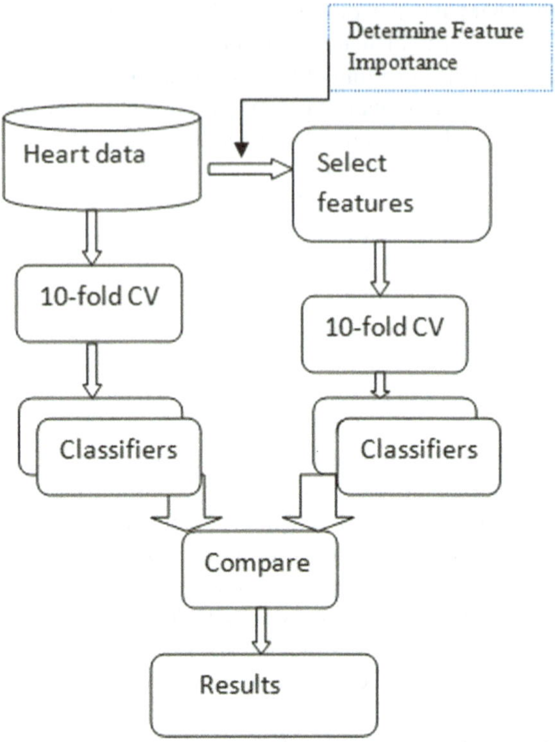

Fig. 9.1 Flow diagram for comparison of classifiers with and without feature selection

9.5.2 Data Set Description

The Statlog heart dataset has been used from UCI database [37]. This database contains 13 attributes (which have been extracted from a larger set of 75) with 270 records. The dataset contains no missing values. The details are as given in Table 9.3.

9.5.3 Results

The dataset contained 270 instances with 13 attributes. The Statlog heart dataset contains no missing values. The implementation has been done in python. The accuracy has been used as a measure to compare the performance of classifications algorithms used for prediction of heart disease.

The experiment was carried out with entire data set of 270 records and 13 attributes for predicting the heart ailments of patients. The feature importance was calculated using in-built function in python and weighted average was taken for each feature importance. Then the features were subsequently ranked according to their weightings and their contribution to the dependant variable given in Table 9.4.

Table 9.3 Dataset detail description

S. no.	Attributes	Type	Values
1	Age	Real	
2	Sex	Binary	
3	Chest-Pain-Type	Nominal	1, 2, 3, 4
4	RestBP	Real	
5	Chol	Real	
6	FBS	Binary	1 for FBS > 120 mg/dl
7	RECG	Nominal	0, 1, 2
8	MaxHR	Real	
9	ExIAng	Binary	0, 1
10	STRest	Real	
11	SlopeEx	Ordered	
12	Mvcol	Real	0–3
13	Thal	Nominal	3 = normal; 6 = fixed defect; 7 = reversible defect
14	Predicted	Output variable	Absence = 1, presence = 2

Table 9.4 Ranking of features based on weighted average of feature importance

Features	DT_Feat_Imp	RF_Feat_Imp	ET_Feat_Imp	Avg.Feat_Imp	Rank
Mvcol	0.1541	0.14152851	0.12266238	0.1541	1
Thal	0.26962812	0.12065559	0.1676	0.1441	2
Chest-Pain-Type	0.0819	0.16928842	0.1297	0.1270	3
Age	0.0919	0.07814107	0.0684	0.0795	4
MaxHR	0.0457	0.09046119	0.1004	0.0789	5
STRest	0.0502	0.12097861	0.0612	0.0775	6
RestBP	0.0833	0.0769499	0.0636	0.0746	7
Chol	0.0850	0.06315875	0.0682	0.0721	8
SlopeEx	0.0280	0.05282374	0.0630	0.0479	9
ExIAng	0.0456	0.02133761	0.0704	0.0458	10
Sex	0.0464	0.03059878	0.0368	0.0379	11
RECG	0.01825	0.025128	0.0336	0.0294	12
FBS	0.0000	0.00894987	0.01431559	0.0078	13

In the subsequent step, the bottom five attributes were dropped to form the new subset with important and relevant features. The new input dataset contained 8 attributes and 270 records.

The accuracy of classifiers has been analyzed before and after applying feature selection method along with 10-fold Cross validation given in Table 9.5. The new

Table 9.5 Performance analysis of classifiers with accuracy before and after feature selection

Classification algo.	Accuracy before (%)	Accuracy after (%)
Decision Tree	74.81	100
Random Forest	81.11	99.62
Extra Trees	78.52	100
Logistic Regression	83.70	100

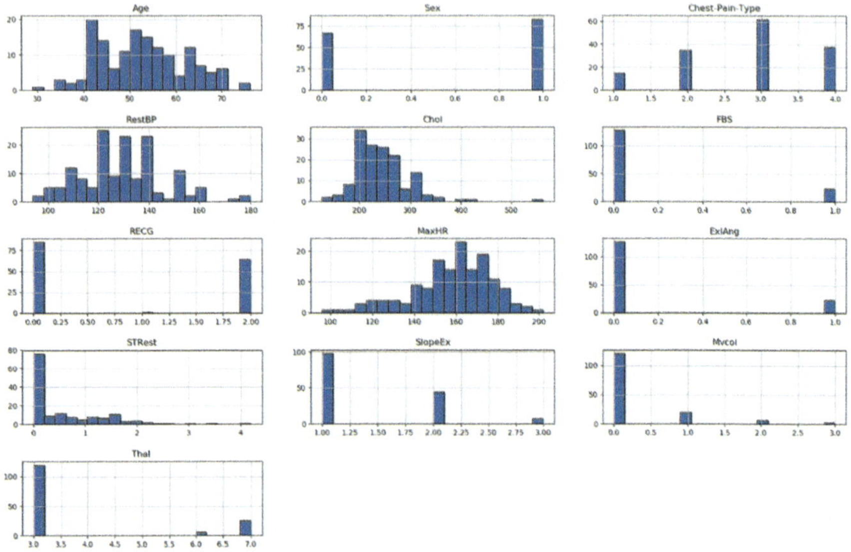

Fig. 9.2 Impact of features on predicted value

subsets of features were then given as input to four classification algorithms: Decision Trees, Random Forest, Extra Trees and Logistic Regression and their results have been tabulated in Table 9.5.

The impact of features on the predicted value has been plotted in graph (Fig. 9.2). The importance of each feature is measured and the relevant features are considered after dropping the less relevant features.

9.6 Conclusion and Future Work

In this chapter the various methods of feature selection methods have been discussed. The advantages and disadvantages of the methods have also been explicitly laid down to guide an appropriate method of feature selection to obtain the desired results from classification algorithms.

Feature selection becomes very much essential when the dimension of data is large and computation time is also huge. In most of the cases the data contains features which are correlated with each other and are also redundant. This makes feature selection very important which removes redundancy and irrelevant features. The data from higher dimensions need to be reduced to lower dimension, which involves creation of new features involving the characteristics of the original attributes, so that interpretation of data becomes easier.

From our experiment, it is observed that prediction accuracy of classifiers have reached 100% in most of the cases. The accuracy of classifiers is better with selected features and gives accurate results with less time and cost. This is a boon to design such smart healthcare systems which predict diseases with more accuracy and are reliable.

The future work can be carried on different data sets with high dimensions and the behavior of prediction models can be studied. The various types of feature selection mechanisms can also be compared to select the optimum set of attributes from the data set to predict the desired results.

References

1. Bellman, R.E.: Adaptive Control Processes. Princeton University Press, Princeton, NJ (1961)
2. Grissa, D., Pétéra, M., Brandolini, M., Napoli, A., Comte, B., Pujos-Guillot, E.: Feature selection methods for early predictive biomarker discovery using untargeted metabolomic data. Front. Mol. Biosci. **3**, 30 (2016)
3. Kira, K., Rendell, L.A.: A practical approach to feature selection. In: Machine Learning Proceedings 1992, pp. 249–256. Morgan Kaufmann (1992)
4. Sun, Y., Li, J.: Iterative RELIEF for feature weighting. In: Proceedings of the 23rd International Conference on Machine Learning, June 2006, pp. 913–920. ACM
5. Sun, Y., Wu, D.: A relief based feature extraction algorithm. In: Proceedings of the 2008 SIAM International Conference on Data Mining, Apr 2008, pp. 188–195. Society for Industrial and Applied Mathematics
6. Holte, R.C.: Very simple classification rules perform well on most commonly used datasets. Mach. Learn. **11**, 63–91 (1993)
7. Priyadarsini, R.P., Valarmathi, M.L., Sivakumari, S.: Gain ratio based feature selection method for privacy preservation. ICTACT J. Soft Comput. **1**(4), 201–205 (2011)
8. Yu, L., Liu, H.: Feature selection for high-dimensional data: a fast correlation-based filter solution. In: Proceedings of the 20th International Conference on Machine Learning (ICML-03), pp. 856–863 (2003)
9. Tibshirani, R.: Regression shrinkage and selection via the lasso. J. Roy. Stat. Soc.: Ser. B (Methodol.) **58**(1), 267–288 (1996)
10. Goap, A., Sharma, D., Shukla, A.K., Krishna, C.R.: Comparative study of regression models towards performance estimation in soil moisture prediction. In: International Conference on Advances in Computing and Data Sciences, Apr 2018, pp. 309–316. Springer, Singapore
11. Deng, H., Runger, G.: Feature selection via regularized trees. In: The 2012 International Joint Conference on Neural Networks (IJCNN), June 2012, pp. 1–8. IEEE
12. Lee, J., Kim, D.W.: Memetic feature selection algorithm for multi-label classification. Inf. Sci. **293**, 80–96 (2015)
13. Neri, F., Tirronen, V.: On memetic differential evolution frameworks: a study of advantages and limitations in hybridization. In: 2008 IEEE Congress on Evolutionary Computation (IEEE World Congress on Computational Intelligence), June 2008, pp. 2135–2142. IEEE

14. Prinzie, A., Van den Poel, D.: Random forests for multiclass classification: random multinomial logit. Expert Syst. Appl. **34**(3), 1721–1732 (2008)
15. Sharma, A., Paliwal, K.K., Imoto, S., Miyano, S.: A feature selection method using improved regularized linear discriminant analysis. Mach. Vis. Appl. **25**(3), 775–786 (2014)
16. Guo, Y., Hastie, T., Tibshirani, R.: Regularized linear discriminant analysis and its application in microarrays. Biostatistics **8**(1), 86–100 (2007)
17. Holland, S.M.: Principal Components Analysis (PCA), p. 30602-2501. Department of Geology, University of Georgia, Athens, GA (2008)
18. Kaur, S., Kalra, S.: Feature extraction techniques using support vector machines in disease prediction. In: Proceedings of IJARSE, May 2016, p. 5
19. Bingham, E., Mannila, H.: Random projection in dimensionality reduction: applications to image and text data. In: Proceedings of the Seventh ACM SIGKDD International Conference on Knowledge Discovery and Data Mining, Aug 2001, pp. 245–250. ACM
20. Liu, Y.H.: Feature extraction and image recognition with convolutional neural networks. J. Phys. Conf. Ser. **1087**(6), 062032 (2018)
21. Abdar, M.: Using decision trees in data mining for predicting factors influencing of heart disease. Carpathian J. Electron. Comput. Eng. **8**(2) (2015)
22. UCI Machine Learning Repository [homepage on the Internet]. http://archive.ics.uci.edu/ml/machine-learning-databases
23. Beyene, M.C., Kamat, P.: Survey on prediction and analysis the occurrence of heart disease using data mining techniques. Int. J. Pure Appl. Math. **118**(8), 165–174 (2018)
24. Koul, S., Chhikara, R.: A hybrid genetic algorithm to improve feature selection. Int. J. Eng. Tech. Res. **4**(5) (2015)
25. Ottom, M.-A., Alshorman, W.: Heart diseases prediction using accumulated rank features selection technique. J. Eng. Appl. Sci. **14**, 2249–2257 (2019)
26. Setiono, R., Liu, H.: Feature extraction via neural networks. In: Feature Extraction, Construction and Selection, pp. 191–204. Springer, Boston, MA (1998)
27. Acharya, U.R., Sudarshan, V.K., Koh, J.E., Martis, R.J., Tan, J.H., Oh, S.L., Chua, C.K.: Application of higher-order spectra for the characterization of coronary artery disease using electrocardiogram signals. Biomed. Signal Process. Control **31**, 31–43 (2017)
28. El-Bialy, R., Salamay, M.A., Karam, O.H., Khalifa, M.E.: Feature analysis of coronary artery heart disease data sets. Procedia Comput. Sci. **65**, 459–468 (2015)
29. Karpagachelvi, S., Arthanari, M., Sivakumar, M.: ECG feature extraction techniques-a survey approach. arXiv preprint arXiv:1005.0957 (2010)
30. Saxena, S.C., Sharma, A., Chaudhary, S.C.: Data compression and feature extraction of ECG signals. Int. J. Syst. Sci. **28**(5), 483–498 (1997)
31. Zhao, Q., Zhang, L.: ECG feature extraction and classification using wavelet transform and support vector machines. In: 2005 International Conference on Neural Networks and Brain, vol. 2, Oct 2005, pp. 1089–1092. IEEE
32. Shardlow, M.: An Analysis of Feature Selection Techniques, pp. 1–7. The University of Manchester (2016)
33. Singh, R.S., Saini, B.S., Sunkaria, R.K.: Detection of coronary artery disease by reduced features and extreme learning machine. Clujul Med. **91**(2), 166 (2018)
34. Hira, Z.M., Gillies, D.F.: A review of feature selection and feature extraction methods applied on microarray data. Adv. Bioinform. (2015)
35. Dash, M., Liu, H.: Feature selection for classification. Intell. Data Anal. **1**(1–4), 131–156 (1997)
36. Dewangan, N.K., Shukla, S.P.: A survey on ECG signal feature extraction and analysis techniques. Int. J. Innov. Res. Electr. Electron. Instrum. Control Eng. **3**(6) (2015)
37. UCI Machine Learning Repository. http://archive.ics.uci.edu/ml/datasets/statlog+(heart)

Chapter 10
Deep Learning-Based Scene Image Detection and Segmentation with Speech Synthesis in Real Time

Okeke Stephen and Mangal Sain

Abstract We present a technique for real time deep learning based scene image detection and segmentation and neural text-to-speech (TTS) synthesis; to detect, classify and segment images in real time views and generate their corresponding speeches. In this work, we show improvement to the existing convolutional neural network approach for a single-model neural text to speech synthesis with an extension to object segmentation features in a given scene. This model, built on top of a high effective and efficient building block of a trained neural network model (masked R-CNN), generates as output, high precision images with bounding boxes and a significant audio signal quality improvement on the corresponding images detected in real time views. We show that a convolutional neural network model combined with neural TTS system can detect, classify and segment multiple objects in a single scene with their various bounding boxes, unique voices and display them in real life time. We applied transfer learning technique on the base model for the image detection, classification, and segmentation tasks. This work introduces a powerful image-to-speech tracking system with instant object segmentation which could be valuable for pixel level image to image measurement in a real time view for easy navigation.

Keywords Deep learning · Image detection · Speech synthesis · Classification

10.1 Introduction

Deep learning method has played significant role in computer vision tasks and thus has recently enjoyed tremendous success in large-scale image and video processing possibly due to the large availability of image repositories to researchers like ImageNet [1], which has played important role in the advancement of deep visual recognition architectures, powerful computing systems, such as GPUs or large-scale distributed clusters [1], algorithms and highly improved network architectures, Fig. 10.1. The most noticeable impact in object-detection is not just from the deep networks

O. Stephen · M. Sain (✉)
Division of Information and Communication Engineering, Dongseo University, 47 Jurye-Ro, Sasang-Gu, Busan 47011, Republic of Korea

P. K. Pattnaik et al. (eds.), *Smart Healthcare Analytics in IoT Enabled Environment*, Intelligent Systems Reference Library 178,
https://doi.org/10.1007/978-3-030-37551-5_10

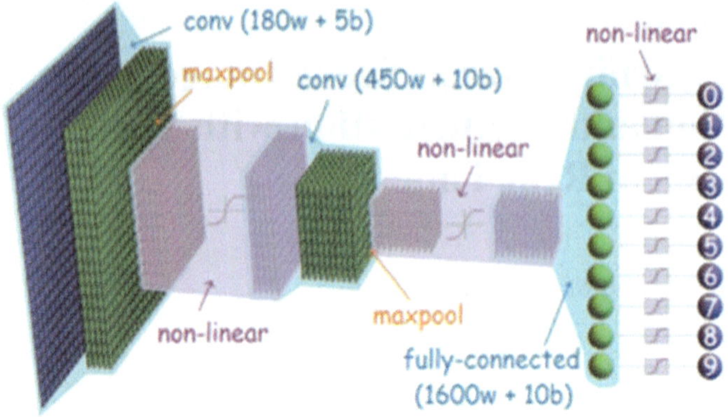

Fig. 10.1 Deep learning model [2]

utilization alone or bigger models, but from the combination of deep architectures and classical computer vision, like the faster R-CNN algorithm. Another important factor to note is that with the ongoing traction of real time object tracking, mobile and embedded computing, the efficiency of deep learning models—especially their power and memory use—has become important. On the other hand, knowledge acquisition through paying attention to sounds is a distinctive property. Speech signal is more effective channel of communication when compared to text-based system because people are more attracted to sound and visualization. This paper aimed at introducing an effective model for real time object detection, classification, recognition and segmentation with corresponding synthesized speech capabilities for easy information acquisition from images and effective object tracking.

10.2 Related Work

The Several object detection methods with text-based systems mainly rely on recurrent neural networks and convolutional neural networks, which are majorly pioneered by the breakthroughs recorded in the application of sequence based computations and convolution operations with neural networks for object detection, classification and machine translation [3]. The analogous conversion of an image into a word or sentence is the main reason image caption generation is the most favorable process for the encoder-decoder framework [3] of machine translation. The initial move to apply neural networks for creating words and captions was recorded in [4], a multimodal log-bilinear algorithm that sorely depends on features from the images was proposed.

An image parsing method for description and production of texts and video contents was proposed by Yao et al. [5]. The major task of their framework was text description and image parsing. The framework creates a graph with the highest probable interpretation of a given image. The parsed graph comprises of a structured object segmentation, components or scene that cover all the pixels in the image. Deep learning based models has been applied to several subcomponents of a single-speaker text to speech synthesis, which includes the fundamental duration prediction, frequency prediction [6], acoustic modeling, and autoregressive sample-by sample audio waveform generation [7].

To achieve a manageable number of candidate object regions [8, 9] and the independent evaluation of convolutional networks [10, 11] on every region of interest (RoI) for a bounding-box object detection is the main objective of region-based CNN object detection approach [12]. To obtain a network with better accuracy and fast speed, R-CNN was extended [13, 14] to operate on RoIs on feature maps by applying RoI Pool. Faster R-CNN [15] extended this process by learning the attention mechanism using a Region Proposal Network (RPN). Faster R-CNN is more robust and flexible when compared to the presiding variants (e.g. [16]), and is one of the leading framework for several object detection benchmarks. Figure 10.2 shows the process of image classification.

5G, for instance segmentation tasks, through the effectiveness of R-CNN, several methods of instance segmentation rely on segment proposals. Previous techniques [12, 14] were based on bottom-up segments [17, 18]. The works on [19, 20] and Deep Mask [21] operate by learning to propose segment candidates, which are then classified by Fast R-CNN. In these methods, segmentation precedes recognition, which is invariably less accurate and slow. A complex multiple-stage cascade method which predicts segment proposals from bounding-box proposals and followed by classification was proposed by Dai et al. [22]. However, Mask RCNN operates by performing parallel prediction of masks and class labels, thus obtaining a more flexible and simpler network. Li et al. [22] combined object detection system and segment proposal system in [23] to perform (FCIS) fully convolutional instance segmentation. The primary idea in [24] is to perform prediction on a collection of position sensitive output channels solely convolutionally. These channels perform object classification, boxes, and masks simultaneously, making the network fast. However, FCIS have systematic errors when operating on overlapping instances and

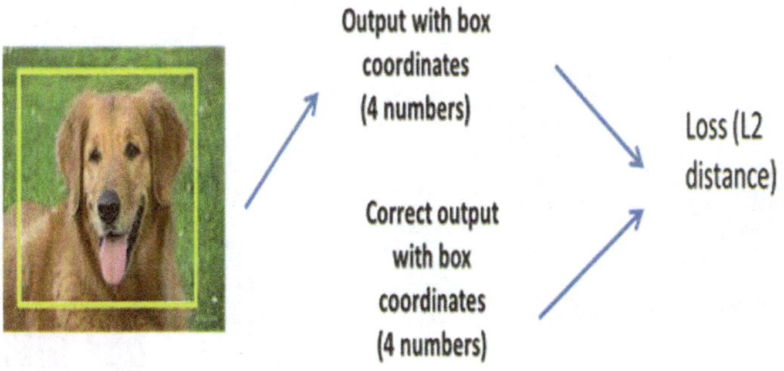

Fig. 10.2 Image classification process

generate spurious edges, indicating that it has difficulties in segmenting overlapping instances. A collection of solutions [24] for conducting instance segmentation are pioneered by the success recorded by semantic segmentation. These systems try to cut the pixels with same category into several instances begging from each pixel classification results as obtainable in FCN outputs. In contrast to the strategy of performing segmentation first, Mask R-CNN works on instance-first method.

The Faster R-CNN object detector [15] is made up of two stages. The first stage is the region proposal network (RPN) which proposes a candidate object for bounding boxes creation and the second is the Fast R-CNN [14], which is responsible for extracting object features by applying the RoI pooling from any candidate box and conducting bounding-box regression and classification tasks. To speed up the inference operation, features from both stages can be shared and used. During the second stage process, Mask R-CNN also generates a binary mask for any RoI which is in parallel to the class and box offset prediction. This contrasts most of the recent systems, where classification solely rely on mask predictions [7].

In concept, Mask R-CNN is simple: Faster R-CNN generates double output for every candidate object. These outputs are the class label, the bounding-box offset and a third branch that generates the object mask was added in the Mask R-CNN network [25] Fig. 10.3. The extra branch that generates the masks is distinct from both the class and box outputs and requires the extraction of more finer spatial layout of an object. Pixel-to-pixel alignment is the key component of Mask R-CNN which embeds the main missing branch of Fast/Faster R-CNN. During Mask R-CNN training a multi-task loss on every sampled region of interest was defined as $L = L\_(c) + L\_(b) + L\_(m)$. Both L_(c) (classification loss) and L_b (bounding box loss) are identical like those described in [14].

The mask branch generates a $(Km)^2$ dimension for every sing RoI, which perform the encoding of K binary masks with $m \times m$ resolution, which is one for each of the K classes. A per-pixel sigmoid was used, and L_(m) define as the average binary cross-entropy loss [25]. For any region of interest that is associated with the ground-truth k class, L mask is only defined on the k-th mask (other mask outputs do not contribute to the loss). The definition of L_(m) permits the network to create masks for all the classes without the classes competing among each other and applied dedicated

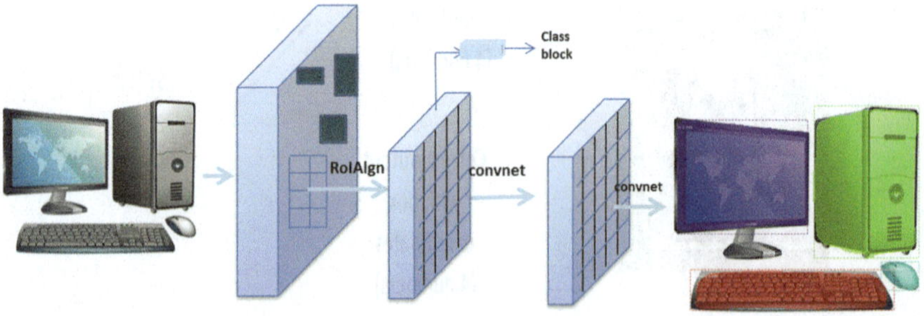

Fig. 10.3 Mask R-CNN network

classification section for predicting Mask Representation. Unlike the box offsets or class labels that are inevitably fused into short output vectors with the fully-connected (fc) layers, pixel-to-pixel correspondence created by convolutions naturally extracts the spatial structure of masks.

The Mask R-CNN specifically predicts an m × m mask from every region of interest by applying an FCN. This enables each layer in the mask section to explicitly maintain an m × m object spatial layout without necessarily embedding it into a vector representation that has no spatial dimensions. The mask R-CNN's fully convolutional representation needs smaller parameters unlike previous techniques that requires fully connected layers for mask prediction operations [21], and produced more accurate results through experiments. This pixel-to-pixel system need region of interest features which are small feature maps for proper alignment in order to conserve the explicit per-pixel spatial correspondence.

The standard operation for small feature map extraction from each RoI is obtained with the RoIPool [11]. A floating-number RoI is first quantized by the RoIPool to a discrete granularity of the feature map, spatial bins are then obtained by subdividing the quantized RoI and they themselves are equally quantized in the process and values from features covered by each bin are summed up usually with a max pooling operation [25]. Quantization is carried for example, on a continuous coordinate x by calculating x/16, where [•] is rounding operation and 16 is a feature map stride; also quantization is conducted when dividing for example 7 × 7 into bins. However, the quantization operation causes misalignments between the extracted features and RoI. While this may not have influence during classification, it has enormous negative impact in predicting pixel-accurate masks. To mitigate this impact, RoI Align layer was deployed to eliminate the harsh quantization of RoIPool thereby aligning the extracted features properly with the input.

10.3 The Model

The model consists of five sub units, the real time scene image acquisition unit, the object detection, classification and segmentation through the base model stage, score prediction stage, text-to-speech section and the output unit respectively as shown in Fig. 10.4.

The object acquisition section takes in streams of images or live images from the real world views and passes them to the base model which performs detection, classification and segmentation tasks and finally, the text-to-speech module converts the labels associated to the scene images into their corresponding speeches.

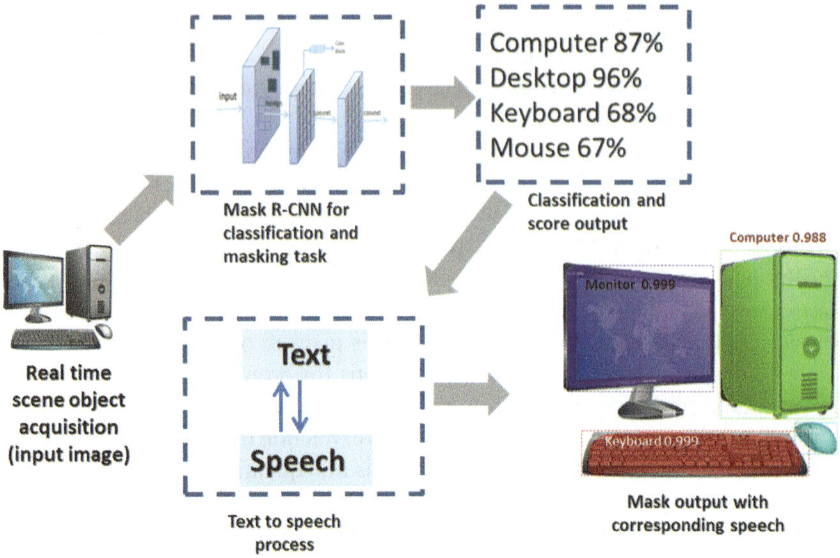

Fig. 10.4 The work flow of the model

10.4 Experiment

There In this work, we applied the model proposed in [25] as our base model which has the capability to detect, classify and segment objects in scenes. Due to the heavy size of the model, we down-sampled and set the input image stream before inferencing to image minimum dimension equal to 800 and image maximum dimension to 1024 respectively. We applied transfer learning to obtain the knowledge in the base model to perform the classification and detection task and then forward the output label to the text-to-speech module to generate their corresponding speeches. We set other parameters such as the learning rate (0.001), learning momentum (0.9), mask pool size (14), pool size (7), number of classes to 7, weight decay (0.00010), batch size to 1 and validation steps to 50. We used one GPU and tensor flow module as our backbone module. On the text-to-speech module, we used the pyttsx3 which loops over the labels generated from the base model to produce speeches.

10.5 Results

In addition to basic LTE capabilities, another important aspect to consider in the future is the spectrum that will be used to deploy these new technologies and the availability of new frequency bands. A quick scan of the proposed frequency bands reveals that the new TDD spectrum is universally available in the range of 3–6 GHz (LTE 6 GHz or less) for LTE Advanced Pro and 5 G NR Phase 1. For the fifth generation phase 2, the plan is to use mm Wave with high bandwidth frequency. Figure 10.5 shows the Mask RCNN framework for instance segmentation [25], and Figs. 10.6 and 10.7 shows the normal segmentation with the base model without speech.

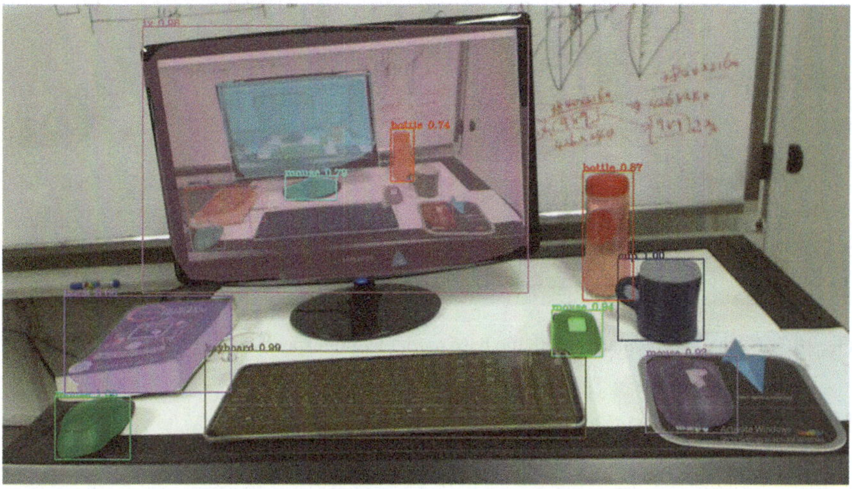

Fig. 10.5 The mask RCNN framework for instance segmentation [25]

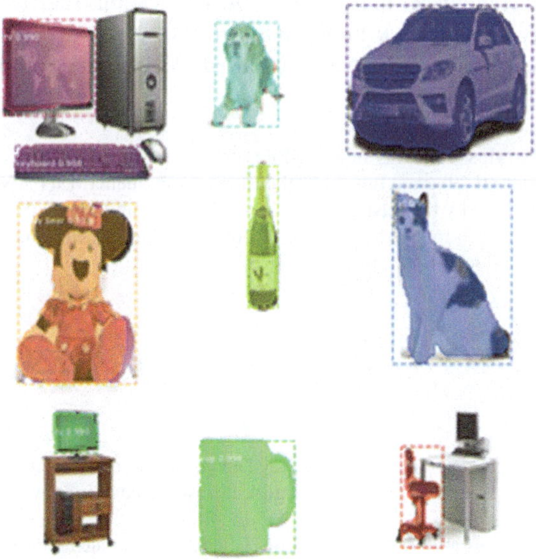

Fig. 10.6 Normal segmentation with the base model without speech

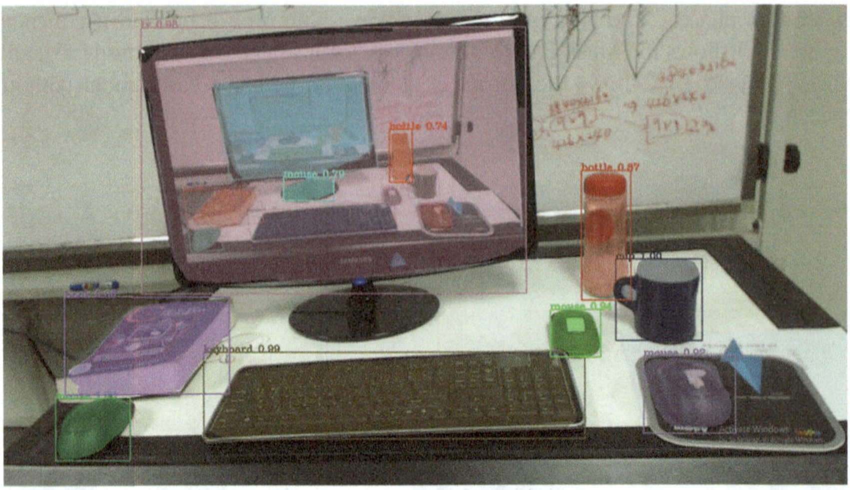

Fig. 10.7 Normal segmentation with the base model without speech

10.6 Conclusion

We have demonstrated how to use the model [25] to detect, classify and segment streams of objects in real time. This work can be further extended to more challenging task such as pixel-level-based object-to-object distance estimation and measurement in a scene, which could usher in more real time applications such as object to object tracking with speech, machine to human interactions, independent language learning, and may also, be useful to the visually impaired. We also look further to extending it to multilingual base system.

Acknowledgements This work was supported by Institute for Information and Communications Technology Promotion (IITP) grant funded by the Korea government (MSIT) (No. 2018-0-00245), And it was also supported by the Basic Science Research Program through the National Research Foundation of Korea (NRF) funded by the Ministry of Education, Science, and Technology (grant number: NRF2016R1D1A1B01011908).

References

1. Dean, J., Corrado, G., Monga, R., Chen, K., Devin, M., Mao, M., Ranzato, M., Senior, A., Tucker, P., Yang, K., Le, Q. V., Ng, A.Y.: Large scale distributed deep networks. NIPS, pp. 1232–1240 (2012)
2. https://leonardoaraujosantos.gitbooks.io/artificialinteligence/content/convolutional_neural_networks.html
3. Cho, K., van Merriënboer, B., Gulcehre, C., Bahdanau, D., Bougares, F., Schwenk, H., Bengio, Y.: Learning phrase representations using RNN encoder-decoder for statistical machine translation. EMNLP, October 2014

4. Kiros, R., Salakhutdinov, R., Zemel, R.: Multi-modal neural language models. In: International Conference on Machine Learning, pp. 595–603 (2014a)
5. Yao, B.Z., Yang, X., Lin, L., Lee M.W., Zhu, S.C.: I2T: image parsing to text description. In: IEEE Conference on Image Processing (2008)
6. Ronanki, S., Watts, O., King, S., Henter, G.E.: Median-based generation of synthetic speech durations using a non-parametric approach. arXiv:1608.06134 (2016)
7. Oord, V.D., Dieleman, S., Zen, H., Simonyan, K., Vinyals, O., Graves, A., Kalchbrenner, N., Senior, A., Kavukcuoglu, K.: Wavenet: a generative model for raw audio. arXiv:1609.03499 (2016)
8. Hosang, J., Benenson, R., Doll´ar, P., Chiele, B.: What makes for effective detection proposals? PAMI (2015)
9. Uijlings, J.R., van de Sande, K.E., Gevers, T., Smeulders, A.W.: Selective search for object recognition. IJCV (2013)
10. LeCun, Y., Boser, B., Denker, J.S., Henderson, D., Howard, R.E., Hubbard, W., Jackel, L.D.: Back propagation applied to handwritten zip code recognition. Neural Comput. (1989)
11. Krizhevsky, A., Sutskever, I., Hinton, G.: ImageNet classification with deep convolutional neural networks. NIPS (2012)
12. Girshick, R., Donahue, J., Darrell, T., Malik, J.: Rich feature hierarchies for accurate object detection and semantic segmentation. CVPR (2014)
13. He, K., Zhang, X., Ren, S., Sun, J.: Spatial pyramid pooling in deep convolutional networks for visual recognition. ECCV (2014)
14. Ren, S., He, K., Girshick, R., Sun, J.: Faster R-CNN: towards real-time object detection with region proposal networks. NIPS (2015)
15. Shrivastava, A., Gupta, A., Girshick, R.: Training region based object detectors with online hard example mining. CVPR (2016)
16. Hariharan, B., Arbel´aez, P., Girshick, R., Malik, J.: Hyper columns for object segmentation and fine-grained localization. CVPR (2015)
17. Dai, J., He, K., Sun, J.: Instance-aware semantic segmentation via multi-task network cascades. CVPR (2016)
18. Dai, J., He, K., Li, Y., Ren, S., Sun, J.: Instance-sensitive fully convolutional networks. ECCV (2016)
19. Pinheiro, P.O., Lin, T.Y., Collobert, R., Doll´ar, P.: Learning to refine object segments. ECCV (2016)
20. Pinheiro, P.O., Collobert, R., Dollar, P.: Learning to segment object candidates. NIPS (2015)
21. Arbel´aez, P., Pont-Tuset, J., Barron, J.T., Marques, F., Malik, J.: Multiscale combinatorial grouping. CVPR (2014)
22. Li, L., Qi, H., Dai, J., Ji, X., Wei, Y.:. Fully convolutional instance-aware semantic segmentation. CVPR (2017)
23. Long, J., Shelhamer, E., Darrell, T.: Full convolutional networks for semantic segmentation. CVPR (2015)
24. Arnab, A., Torr, P.H.: Pixel wise instance segmentation with a dynamically instantiated network. CVPR (2017)
25. Kaiming, H., Gkioxari, G., Dollar, P., Girshick, R.: Facebook AI research (FAIR). Mask R-CNN. arXiv:1703.06870v3[cs.CV] 24 Jan 2018

Chapter 11
Study of Different Filter Bank Approaches in Motor-Imagery EEG Signal Classification

Rajdeep Chatterjee and Debarshi Kumar Sanyal

Abstract Motor-imagery EEG signal classification is an important topic in the Brain-Computer Interface domain. In this chapter, two distinct variants of filter bank models have been used once in normal mode (filter is applied on the entire input signal) and again with overlapping and non-overlapping temporal sliding windows (filter is applied on the segments of input signal): (a) Filter bank of 4 Hz frequency band with cut-off frequencies 4–24 Hz, (b) Filter bank of five frequency bands- delta, theta, alpha, beta and gamma brain rhythms. Subsequently, the Common Spatial Pattern (CSP) has been implemented both on the each filtered output EEG signal as well as on the combined filtered output to form the final feature-sets for all the filter bank techniques. The traditional bagging ensemble classifier has been improvised using the Differential Evolution (DE)-based error minimization for the model training. The obtained classification accuracies are then compared with one another to examine the performance of the proposed approach. The best classification accuracy obtained from our study is 86.43%.

Keywords BCI · Classification · EEG · Filter bank · Motor imagery

11.1 Introduction

Electroencephalogram (EEG) based Brain-Computer Interface (BCI) technique is an emerging research area which includes subjects such as neuroscience, digital signal processing, machine learning etc [1]. It covers research on the fields of emotion detection, epileptic seizure detection, motor-imagery classification and neuro-rehabilitation as its major focus areas. The applications of EEG-based BCI has significant contributions to the gaming (entertainment) industries to the clinical (medical) diagnosis. EEG has advantages over its other alternative techniques because of its portability, non-invasiveness, low cost and high temporal resolution [2, 3]. Human brain triggers certain and similar brain patterns while performing specific cognitive task either in reality or in imagination. In BCI, these brain signals have been trans-

R. Chatterjee (✉) · D. K. Sanyal
School of Computer Engineering, Kalinga Institute of Industrial Technology
(Deemed to Be University), Bhubaneswar, Odisha 751024, India

P. K. Pattnaik et al. (eds.), *Smart Healthcare Analytics in IoT Enabled Environment*, Intelligent Systems Reference Library 178,
https://doi.org/10.1007/978-3-030-37551-5_11

formed into relevant information to model different brain states [4, 5]. Therefore, the classification of different brain states can be further encoded to instruct a machine to solve a problem or assist a person to perform a task. In this chapter, the motor-imagery EEG signal data has been used to build a better classification framework which includes suitable feature extraction and appropriate type of classifier. In motor-imagery EEG signal classification problem, the different brain states need to be classified efficiently [6, 7]. Motor-imagery is an imagination by a person who thinks that he is moving his limbs while it is not happened physically in reality, rather imagined. This study is appropriate for providing a non-muscular pathway without motor neurons between the brain and the different fully or partially paralyzed limbs of a person. A correct prediction of motor-imagery states can help in moving a wheelchair or controlling the surroundings using Internet of Things (IoT) based smart home [8, 9]. The application is not restricted to these two said topics, but can be extended to various aspects of real-world problems [10, 11].

Past literature shows that researchers have spent a good amount of time to identify the best suited feature extraction technique and classifier model for motor-imagery EEG signal classification [12–14]. Previously in [6, 15, 16], the discrete wavelet transform (DWT) based energy entropy features have been used with support vector machine (SVM) and multilayer perceptron (MLP) classifiers. The classification accuracies have been obtained respectively 85 and 85.71%. The morlet wavelet coefficients as features and Bayes quadratic as the classifier have been used to achieve 89.29% accuracy in [17]. Again, Bashar [18] has used multivariate empirical mode decomposition (MEMD) with short time Fourier transform (STFT) for feature extraction. He has also compared its performance based on different classifiers, but the K-Nearest Neighbor (K-NN with cosine distance) gives 90.71% accuracy. Besides the said best performing classification configurations, other feature extraction techniques such as power spectral density (PSD), adaptive auto-regressive (AAR) model, bandpower and filter bank are the most widely used methods. Similarly, naïve bayes, linear discriminant analysis (LDA) and different ensemble approaches are popular used classifiers [6, 19, 20].

Many researchers have come up with filter bank approaches combined with different feature extraction techniques such as common spatial pattern and multivariate empirical mode decomposition to classify EEG signals more efficiently [21–24]. In [25], a generic regularized filter bank ensemble model has been proposed with common spatial patterns as feature extraction technique which builds the classification model using an universal training-set including signals from other subjects.

The expectation of higher accuracy using less number of features is an essential criteria for BCI applications as it handles health and life critical data and must provide response in real-time (as quick as possible). As there is no single combination which has been accepted unanimously by most of the bio-signal researchers working on the EEG-based BCI applications. It is also observed that acquired signal as well as the embedded relevant information vary based not only on time but also on trials even for the same subject. In this chapter, our main aim is to study different traditional as well as modified filter bank approaches with common spatial pattern (CSP) for feature extraction. Another major contribution of this chapter is a variant of bagging ensemble technique where multiple types of learners are used over multiple learners of single classifier type (it is called mixture bagging or mix-bagging) [19, 26]. It is further improved by differential evolution (DE)-based training error minimization which helps the different bags to choose optimal set of training-set samples so that the test-set accuracy improves significantly [27].

The chapter outline: Sect. 11.2 explains the theoretical concepts. The proposed approach has been explained in Sect. 11.3. Experimental preparation is discussed in Sect.11.4. In Sect. 11.5, the experimental results have been compared and analyzed. Finally, the chapter has been concluded in Sect. 11.6.

11.2 Background

11.2.1 Common Spatial Pattern

The Common Spatial Pattern (CSP) is a widely used feature extraction technique in motor-imagery EEG signal classification [28–30]. The X_a^i is the EEG signal data of the ith trial and decision class a. It has dimensions of size $C \times T$. Here, C and T indicate the total count of used channels and the time domain sample points. In our study, the classes consist of the right hand and left hand motor-imagery movements. The normalized covariance matrix M_a is calculated as:

$$M_a = \frac{\sum_{i=1}^{n_a} X_a^i \times X_a^{iT}}{\sum_{i=1}^{n_a} TR(X_a^i \times X_a^{iT})} \tag{11.1}$$

In Eq. 11.1, n_a indicates the number of total trials available in the decision class a. Again, the normalized covariance matrix M_b for the class b has also been computed. The TR(.) and T(.) are used to denote trace of a matrix and transpose of a matrix.

Hence, the combined covariance matrix M_c is as:

$$M_c = M_a + M_b \tag{11.2}$$

Again, we do the eigen decomposition of M_c,

$$M_c = B_c \gamma B_c^T \tag{11.3}$$

The normalized eigen vectors of the matrix M_c are used to form the matrix B_c. Similarly, the eigen values of M_c have been used to form the diagonal matrix γ. Both the matrices B_c and γ are of dimension $C \times C$. Now, to scale the principle components, a whitening transformation has been applied.

$$V = \gamma^{-0.5} B_c^T \tag{11.4}$$

Then, the M_a and M_b covariance matrices have been transformed as,

$$S_a = VM_aV^T \quad and \quad S_b = VM_bV^T \tag{11.5}$$

Now, the matrices S_a and S_b have the same common eigen vectors. The eigen value decomposition of the matrix S_a has been done to find out the common shared eigen vectors between S_a and S_b using,

$$S_a = E\phi_a E^T \tag{11.6}$$

And with the eigen vector in E,

$$S_b = E\phi_b E^T \tag{11.7}$$

Note that $\phi_a + \phi_b = 1$, the sum of two respective eigen values equals to 1.

Equation 11.8 maximizes The separation between the two motor-imagery decision classes a and b has been maximized using the following Eq. 11.8. The transformed matrix is defined as M_{pro},

$$M_{pro} = (E^T V)^T \tag{11.8}$$

The EEG data of ith trial has been projected as R^i using the matrix M_{pro},

$$R^i = M_{pro}X^i \tag{11.9}$$

Subsequently, the total $2m$ rows, that is, the first m and last m rows have been selected as they contain most discriminating features between decision classes a and b. It is recommended in the literature that the log(.) of variances obtained from each row has been computed instead of using the actual row data as feature vector. The variance of kth row of R^i matrix can be represented as var_k^i. Finally, the logarithm value of normalized variance for the kth component of the ith trial is calculated as,

$$f_k^i = \log\left(\frac{var_k^i}{\sum_{i=1}^{2m} var_k^i}\right), \quad k = 1, \ldots, 2m \tag{11.10}$$

The feature vector $F_i = (f_1^i, f_2^i, \ldots, f_2k^i)^T$ has been used to form the feature matrix which is further used to design the classifier for motor-imagery classification.

11.2.2 Filter Bank

The filter bank is a stacked filters which have been used to extract multiple EEG signals of different frequency bands from a given input signal. The filter bank gives a set of signal outputs from a single trial of motor-imagery signal. Then, a suitable feature extraction technique has been implemented on those outputs separately or combined to transform the output signals into feature vectors. The common notion is that the filter bank helps to generate more features from a same input source in turn captures more discriminating information than the traditional approaches. There are no predefined rules for filters selection. The ranges of filters have been chosen based on EEG signal type and problem domain. A simple example of filter bank which starts at 4 Hz and ends at 24 Hz with a 4 Hz frequency band separation is shown in Fig. 11.5. The CSP is implemented on the combined filtered output signals to form the final feature-set.

11.2.3 Mixture Bagging Classifier

Mixture bagging (mix-bagging) is a variant of traditional bagging ensemble classifier [31, 32]. In mix-bagging, multiple type of base classifiers have been used to build the combined model over usage of multiple bags of same classifier [19, 26, 33]. It introduces diversity to the ensemble model than the normal variants. It uses the advantages of all different type of classifiers and develops a diverse decision boundary by reducing the classification error through a suitable combining technique [31, 34, 35]. Here, majority voting is used to combine the mix-bagging ensemble (see, Fig. 11.1) [36, 37]. A pseudo-code representation of the mix-bagging technique is given in Algorithm 1 and a working model is shown in Fig. 11.2. Each time, a subset of instances (that is, $indx$ of size m_{use}) from the actual training-set are randomly selected with replacement to form the bag. This process means some of the training-set instances are repeated and the remaining are selected as fresh. The random selection with replacement introduces certain exploration property to the model so that it is not

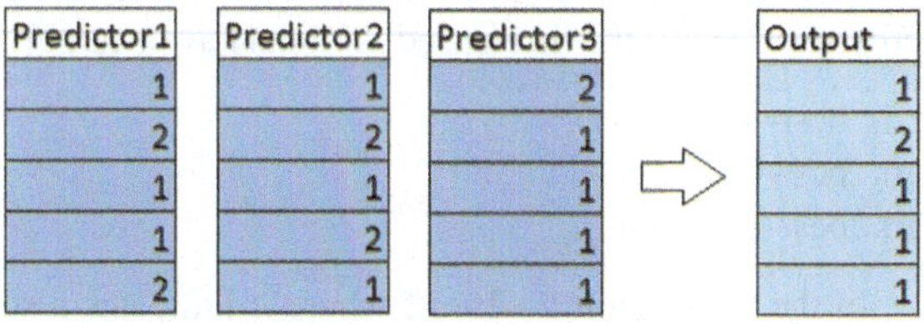

Fig. 11.1 Majority voting

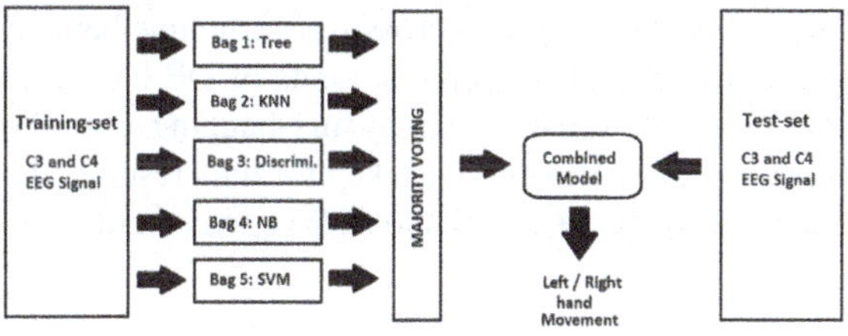

Fig. 11.2 Mixture bagging model diagram

Table 11.1 Mix-bagging ensemble model with 5 different classifiers

Bag #	Classifiers	Parameters
Bag 1	Tree	–
Bag 2	KNN (cosine)	K = 13
Bag 3	Discriminant	Linear
Bag 4	Naïve Bayes	–
Bag 5	SVM	Linear

trapped in local optima. The main aim of the mix-bagging is to *minimize the combined classification error* and provides a higher classification accuracy (Table 11.1).

11.2.4 Differential Evolution

Differential Evolution (DE) is a derivative free optimization technique [27, 38, 39]. Rainer Storn and Kenneth Price introduced this algorithm in the year 1995. F is a positive constant value controlling the amplification of the differential variation. Here, its value is kept as 2. To introduce more diversity of the parameter vector, a suitable crossover value ($Cr = 0.8$) has been used with in [0, 1] range. To generate the trial vector, a *rand* value is generated. If the random value is less than or equal to the crossover value, then the value takes from the mutant vector otherwise it is considered from the parameter vector. Price et al. have given ten different variants of DE and some outlines in implementing those schemes to any given problem [27, 38]. The working principle of DE can be found in details in [38, 40]. These strategies have been derived from the five different DE mutation schemes. Each DE mutation scheme has been combined with either the "exponential" or the "binomial" type crossover. Here, the three used variants have been given:

i. best---1---exp.
ii. best---2---exp.
iii. best---2---bin.

In the expression a---b---c, where a indicates a string denoting the vector to be perturbed, b is the number of difference vectors considered for perturbation of a, and c denotes the type of crossover technique being used (exp: exponential and bin: binomial). The above three variants of DE has been experimented and the best of them (that is, variant i. based mix-bagging gives best classification accuracies in most of the experiments) is taken for final result computation in this study. A simple pseudo-code representation of DE is given below:

Algorithm 1 Modified Bagging (Mix-bagging)

$Inputs : Given(x_1, y_1), \ldots, (x_m, y_m),\ where\ m\ total\ training-set\ instances$
$x_i\ is\ a\ feature-set\ and$
$y_i\ is\ the\ corresponding\ decision-class$
$xtest\ is\ testing-set\ of\ size\ n\ instances$
$-Initialize : m_{bag},\ count\ of\ bags$
$-Initialize : m_{use},\ bootstrap\ sample-set\ size$
$-Initialize : iter,\ number\ of\ independent\ executions$
$-Initialize : prediction^{best}_{final} \leftarrow 0$
for $r \leftarrow 1\ to\ iter$ **do**
  for $t \leftarrow 1\ to\ m_{bag}$ **do**
    $indx,\ bootstrap\ instances\ (m_{use} < m)$
    $X_t \leftarrow \forall\ x_i\ where\ i\ \in\ indx$
    $Y_t \leftarrow \forall\ y_i\ where\ i\ \in\ indx$
    $model_t \leftarrow learner(X_t, Y_t)$
  end for
  for $t \leftarrow 1\ to\ m_{bag}$ **do**
    $predict_{nt} \leftarrow learner(xtest, model_t)$
  end for
  $prediction^r_{final} \leftarrow majority-voting(predict_t),\ for\ n\ test\ instances$
  if $prediction^r_{final}\ >\ prediction^{best}_{final}$ **then**
    $Remember\ the\ bags\ and\ prediction^{best}_{final} \leftarrow\ prediction^r_{final}$
  end if
end for
Return $prediction^{best}_{final},\ for\ iter\ independent\ runs$

Algorithm 2 Differential Evolution (DE)

Initialize population
Evaluate fitness
for i ← 1 to maximum-iteration or it reaches the stopping criteria **do**
  Difference-offspring are generated
  Fitness is evaluated for each offspring
  if an offspring is better than its parent **then**
    Parent vector is replaced by the offspring in the next generation
  end if
end for
Return Best approximate global optima (solutions)

11.3 Proposed Approach

11.3.1 Temporal Sliding Window

Filter bank approach may give more number of features from a single trail EEG signal, but the mental thought of different motor-imagery states varies with time. Therefore, the traditional filter bank model can be further improved by using a overlapping

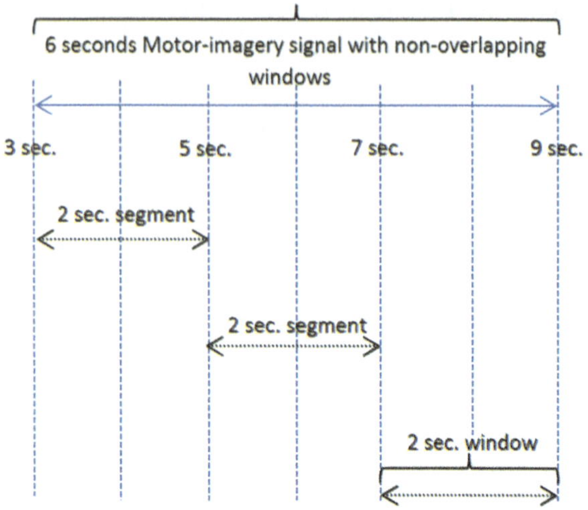

Fig. 11.3 Non-overlapping temporal sliding window technique

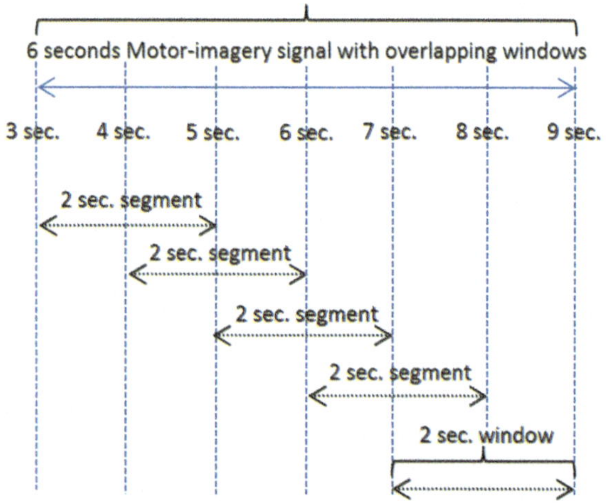

Fig. 11.4 Overlapping temporal sliding window technique

and non-overlapping temporal sliding window to filter multiple output signals from a single input signal using the same filter scheme. That is, the entire 6 seconds input motor-imagery signal is now segmented into 2 s overlapping (128 samples overlap) and non-overlapping multiple input signals as shown in Figs. 11.3 and 11.4. Now, any suitable feature extraction technique can be applied on the obtained output signal to extract appropriate features. Here, CSP has been used for feature extraction. Therefore, same filter can be used to produce more relevant features. Thus, the proposed scheme not only captures the spectral information (filter bank) but also the temporal information (sliding window) from given EEG signal input. This sliding window based filter bank approach has been implemented in three distinct forms: (a) Filter bank of 4 Hz frequency band with cut-off frequencies 4–24 Hz, (b) Filter bank of five frequency bands-delta, theta, alpha, beta and gamma, and (c) Filter bank of only two frequency bands- alpha and beta (as they are the dominant brain rhythms generated while motor-imagery brain activities being triggered). The brief description of the each experiments is given in Table 11.2.

Besides, experiment type (a) (see, Figs. 11.5 and 11.6), another category of filters have been used to extract specific frequency bands corresponding to each brain rhythms in experiment type (b) (see, Figs. 11.7 and 11.8). Lastly, the said filter bank is also used based on only the alpha and beta frequency bands for each input EEG signal (see, Fig. 11.9). It is done with the intuition that these frequency band reflects more relevant information related to the specific brain activities.

11.3.2 Proposed DE-based Error Minimization

DE is a popular optimization technique used in engineering problem solving. It is a novel approach to minimize the overall classification error happened during the model training of the bagging ensemble learning. In step 8 of Algorithm 2, $indx$ is generated from a random subset of instances selection with replacement (explained in the earlier Sect. 11.2.3). It help in exploration of new better solution and to avoid local minima trap. The algorithm is executed $iter$ times and store the best ensemble configuration until a better configuration is found in the next iteration. This process gives us good result but mathematical consistency is missing as $indx$ is formed each time by a random function.

DE can help the training process in optimally reducing the classification error. Initially, each bag starts with a random set of instances ($m_{use} < m$) which is 65% of the total training-set size. The N_{bag} is the used number of bags in the ensemble. Therefore, an initial population of dimension $N_{bag} \times m_{use}$ has been formed. Corresponding to each bag, a classification error from the training is obtained as fitness of the each bag. Now, the DE operators have been applied on these bags (that is, the said population) to form a new set of bag (new population in next generation) keeping in mind that the overall classification error of the model must be reduced. The operations are executed for $iter$ times. It must be noted that the fitness has been calculated from individual bag based on the set of selected m_{use} instances. However, the main objective is to reduce their combined classification error. Thus, the best set of indices are obtained, which provide the best classification accuracy for the unknown test-set data.

Table 11.2 Brief description of the experiments

Experiment	Description	Set size
Exp-1	The filter bank ranges between 4 and 24 Hz with a 4 Hz frequency band has been applied on the entire 6 s input EEG signal. Subsequently, CSP is implemented on the each of the output signal of the filter bank and then combined to form the final feature-set (see model-1 in Fig. 11.5)	4
Exp-2	The filter bank ranges between 4 and 24 Hz with a 4 Hz frequency band has been applied on the entire 6 s input EEG signal. Subsequently, CSP is implemented on the combined output signal of the filter bank to form the final feature-set (see model-2 in Fig. 11.6)	10
Exp-3	The delta, theta, alpha, beta and gamma frequency bands-based filter bank has been applied on the entire 6 s input EEG signal. Subsequently, CSP is implemented on the each of the output signal of the filter bank and then combined to form the final feature-set (see model-3 in Fig. 11.7)	6
Exp-4	The delta, theta, alpha, beta and gamma frequency bands-based filter bank has been applied on the entire 6 s input EEG signal. Subsequently, CSP is implemented on the combined output signal of the filter bank to form the final feature-set (see model-4 in Fig. 11.8)	10
Exp-5	The filter bank ranges between 4 and 24 Hz with a 4 Hz frequency band has been applied on each 2 s non-overlapping segments of the input EEG signal. Subsequently, CSP is implemented on the combined output signal of the filter bank to form the final feature-set	18
Exp-6	The filter bank ranges between 4 and 24 Hz with a 4 Hz frequency band has been applied on each 2 s overlapping segments (that is, 128 overlapping samples) of the input EEG signal. Subsequently, CSP is implemented on the combined output signal of the filter bank to form the final feature-set	30
Exp-7	The delta, theta, alpha, beta and gamma frequency bands-based filter bank has been applied on each 2 s non-overlapping segments of the input EEG signal. Subsequently, CSP is implemented on the combined output signal of the filter bank to form the final feature-set	18
Exp-8	The delta, theta, alpha, beta and gamma frequency bands-based filter bank has been applied on each 2 s overlapping segments (that is, 128 overlapping samples) of the input EEG signal. Subsequently, CSP is implemented on the combined output signal of the filter bank to form the final feature-set	30
Exp-9	The alpha and beta frequency bands-based filter bank has been applied on each 2 s non-overlapping segments of the input EEG signal. Subsequently, CSP is implemented on the combined output signal of the filter bank to form the final feature-set (see model-5 in Fig. 11.9)	18
Exp-10	The alpha and beta frequency bands-based filter bank has been applied on each 2 s overlapping segments (that is, 128 overlapping samples) of the input EEG signal. Subsequently, CSP is implemented on the combined output signal of the filter bank to form the final feature-set	30

Note Elliptic bandpass filter is used to extract different frequency bands from the EEG input signal

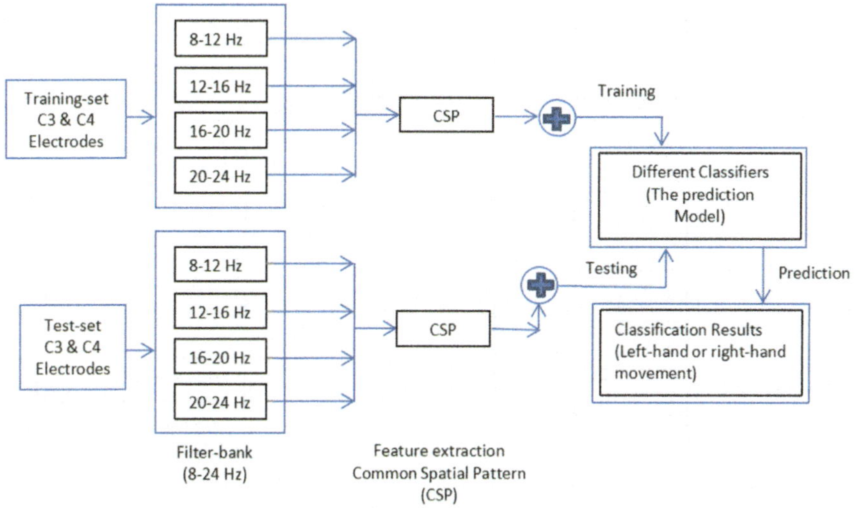

Fig. 11.5 The block representation of the filter-bank model-1

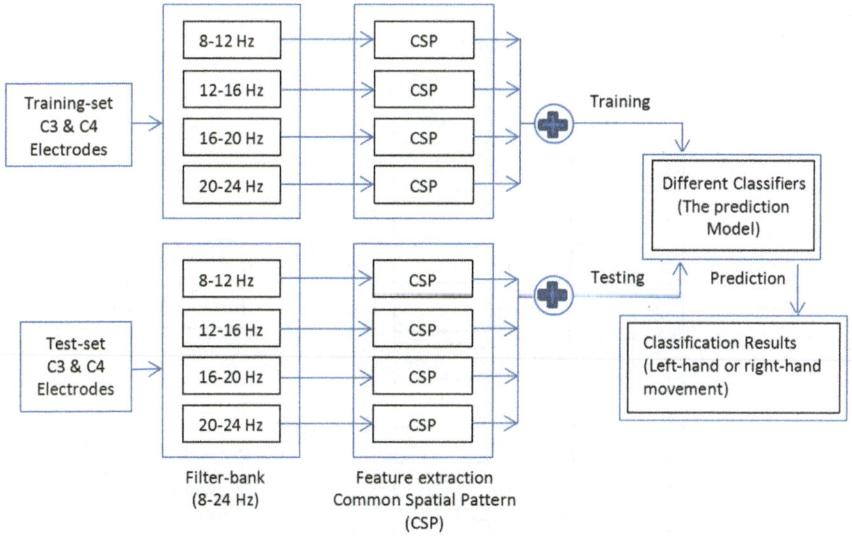

Fig. 11.6 The block representation of the filter-bank model-2

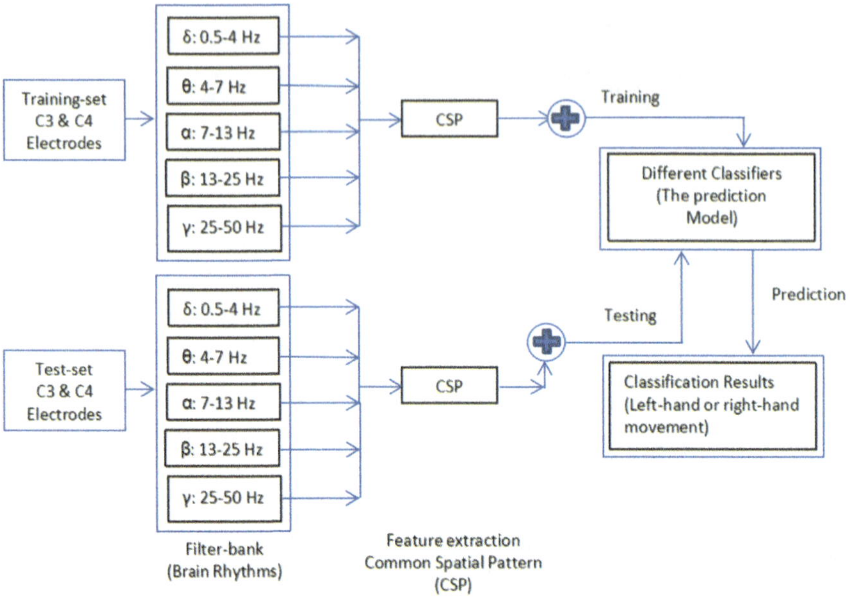

Fig. 11.7 The block representation of the filter-bank model-3

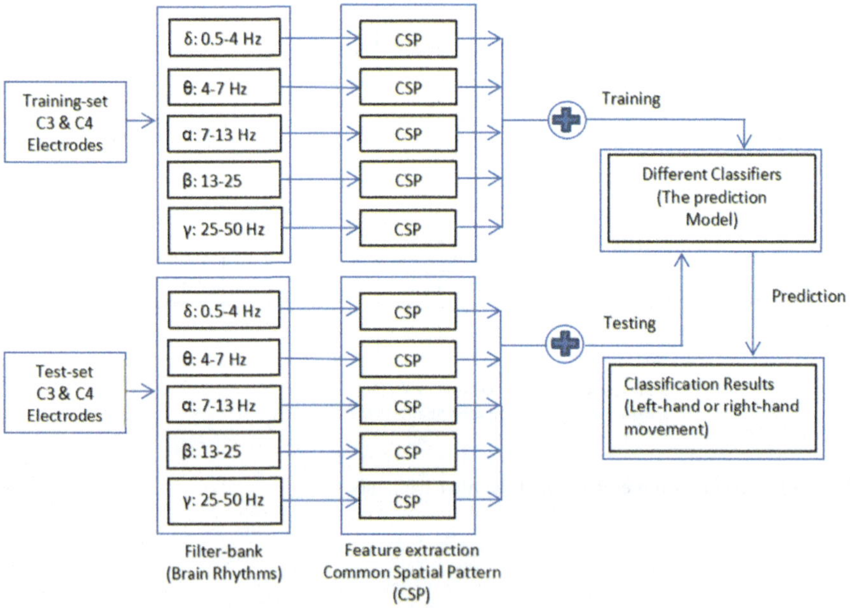

Fig. 11.8 The block representation of the filter-bank model-4

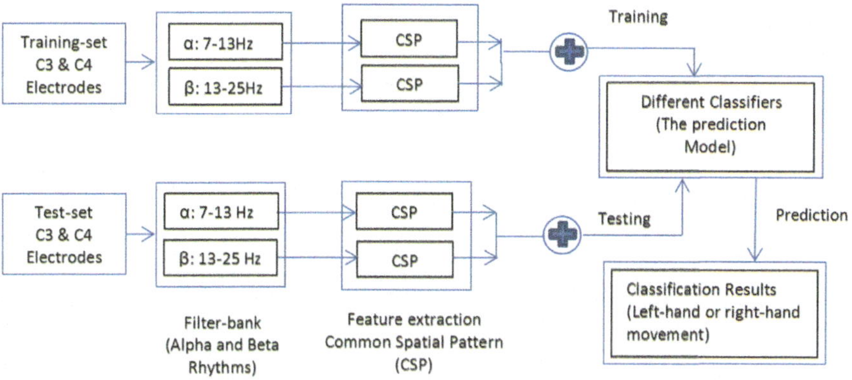

Fig. 11.9 The block representation of the filter-bank model-5

11.4 System Preparation

11.4.1 Dataset

The BCI competition II dataset III is used due to its long 6 s motor-imagery EEG binary signal [41]. The sampling rate of the dataset is 128 Hz. The EEG signal has been recorded from $C3$, Cz and $C4$ electrodes using the IEEE 10–20 electrode placement standard (Fig. 11.10). In our study, the observations from $C3$ and $C4$ electrodes are only taken for analysis due to their dominant role in acquiring human left and right hand movements EEG signal [42, 43]. The diagrammatic representation of a single trial for an electrode is shown in Fig. 11.11.

The total trials available in the dataset is 280 (that is, instances) containing equal number of left and right hand movements trials. The first 140 trials have been used for training and the remaining 140 trials are used for testing. An elliptic band-pass filter with cut-off frequencies of 0.5 and 50 Hz, is used to denoise the input EEG signal [6, 15, 43]. The brief description of the used dataset is also given Table 11.3 for easy understanding of the readers.

11.4.2 Resources

MATLAB 2016a installed on an Intel Core $i5-6200U$ CPU 2.40 GHz with 8 GB RAM and 64 bits Windows 10 Professional operating system has been used to carry out all the experiments of this chapter. The feature extractions and classifications of the used dataset has been done by separate MATLAB (`.m`) files. The code of differential evolution is taken from Rainer Storn Berkeley repository[1] [27]. However, the remaining techniques have been implemented using MATLAB scripts coded by us.

[1] http://www.icsi.berkeley.edu/~storn/code.html.

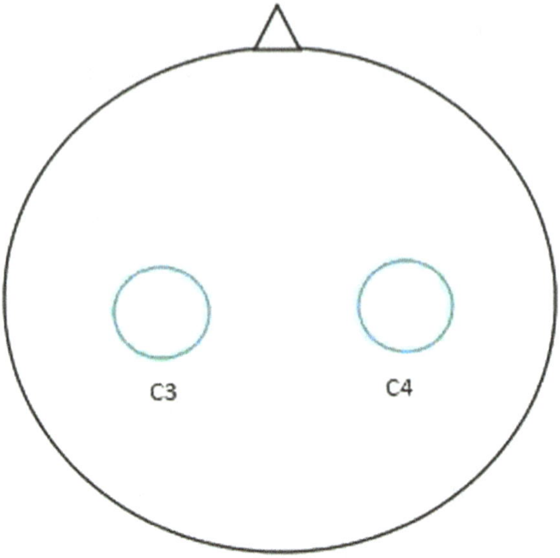

Fig. 11.10 IEEE 10–20 standard placement for $C3$ and $C4$ electrodes

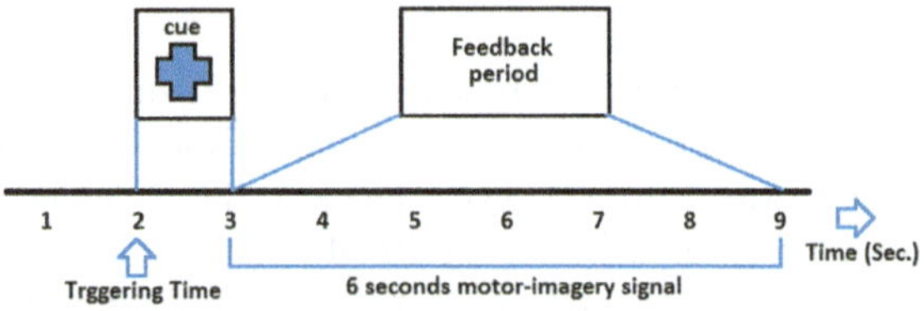

Fig. 11.11 Motor-imagery 6 seconds long EEG signal for an electrode

Table 11.3 Dataset description

Dataset	Electrodes	Sample size	Class label	Training/testing	Cut-off frequency
BCI competition II (dataset III)	C3 & C4	768 (6 s × 128 Hz)	1-left hand, 2-right hand movement	140/140	0.5–50 Hz

11.5 Experimental Discussion

This chapter includes different combinations of filter bank approaches subsequently with and without non-overlapping and overlapping temporal sliding window based feature extraction techniques (see Table 11.2). There are 10 variants of filter bank used with CSP to form the feature-sets. The smallest and largest obtained feature-set sizes are 4 and 30 respectively (available in last column of Table 11.2). Finally, mix-bagging, KNN, adaboost (Adab.) and logitboost (Logit.) have been implemented on the obtained datasets to examine the discriminating quality of the generated feature-sets given in Table 11.4. To get best possible result, K value is varied from 3 to 30 in

Table 11.4 Accuracies (%) obtained from different experiments

Experiment#	Mix-bag-DE	Mix-bag	K-NN	Adab.	Logit.	Mean-II (%)
Exp-1	85.71	85.00	83.57	82.86	82.86	84.00
Exp-2	81.43	80.71	79.29	77.14	76.43	79.00
Exp-3	84.29	83.57	82.14	81.43	82.14	82.71
Exp-4	82.14	80.00	79.29	78.57	79.29	79.86
Exp-5	79.29	79.29	65.71	61.48	60.00	69.15
Exp-6	78.57	77.85	70.71	77.14	78.29	76.51
Exp-7	82.14	82.14	79.29	68.57	72.86	77.00
Exp-8	86.43	84.29	82.14	77.86	77.86	81.72
Exp-9	82.14	79.29	72.86	69.29	69.29	74.57
Exp-10	82.86	82.14	72.14	69.29	68.57	75.00
Mean-I (%)	82.50	81.43	76.71	74.36	74.76	X

KNN and number of learners in both adaptive boosting and logit boosting are kept at 15 after a rigorous trials. In mix-bagging, the number of bag used is denoted by $m_{bag} = 5$ and the training-set bag sample size is indicated by m_{use} which is 65% of the actual training-set size (that is, 140 trials). The process has been executed $iter$ times and it checks whether the test-set accuracy obtained from the current iteration is better than the previous one, then store the current best ensemble configuration. This method is used so that the ensemble solution could not trapped in local optima trap. The set of samples chosen to form the each bag is done randomly with replacement technique (it means that some samples are repeatedly selected where remaining are discarded in formation of the next bag). This randomness brings exploration property to the system, however it lacks the mathematical guarantee to obtain the best result [in terms of classification accuracy (%)]. This issue has been addressed with a simple and popular optimization algorithm, that is, differential evolution. DE is used to minimize the classification error while building the training model. Literature says that if the classification error is reduced for the individual learner of an ensemble bagging model, then their combined prediction improves significantly. Here, mix-bagging introduces diversity in resultant decision boundary due to inheriting properties of different base classifiers (see Table 11.1). It uses the advantages of all its learners while reducing the disadvantages by combining the results using majority voting.

The mean accuracies are computed classifier-wise as well as experiment-wise from the results to understand and compare their individual performances (shown in Table 11.4). The **Mean-I** gives us clear view on classifier based mean accuracies obtained from all the 10 experiments. Our proposed DE-based mix-bagging provides best performances (that is, 82.50%) over other used classifiers including its traditional variant normal mix-bagging. Similarly, it is found that the experiment-1 (Exp-1) gives us good quality discriminating features which is validated by all the classifiers and can be realized through 84.00% **Mean-II** value. It needs to be noted that the feature-set size is ONLY 4 in the experiment-1 which is smallest among all the experimental feature-sets. However, the best classification accuracy is 86.43% which has been obtained from the experiment-8 using 30 features.

11.6 Conclusion

This chapter focuses on a comparative study of different filter bank approaches in terms of classification accuracy. Two fundamental types of filter banks have been used along with their non-overlapping and overlapping temporal sliding window based techniques. It is observed that the experiment 1 performs well irrespective of the classifier type. However, the highest classification accuracy obtained in our study is 86.43% from experiment 8. Again, a differential evolution based error minimized mix-bagging classifier has been introduced in this chapter. It is found that the proposed mix-bagging classifier which uses DE to minimize its overall training error, gives us 82.50% mean accuracy obtained using all the experiments and outperforms other used classifiers. This chapter can be concluded as: (i) traditional filter bank ranges from 4 to 24 Hz with a 4 Hz frequency band separation provides more discriminating features than others, (ii) The performance of proposed differential evolution based mix-bagging classifier improves over not only the traditional mix-bagging but also other used KNN and ensemble classifiers.

Here, the study is made using a binary classification BCI Competition II dataset III which has obtained EEG signals from a single subject. In future, we will extend the work in which more subjects are included and multiple decision classes based BCI datasets have been used.

References

1. Lotte, F.: Study of electroencephalographic signal processing and classification techniques towards the use of brain-computer interfaces in virtual reality applications. Ph.D. thesis. INSA de Rennes (2008)
2. Ilyas, M.Z., Saad, P., Ahmad, M.I.: A survey of analysis and classification of EEG signals for brain-computer interfaces. In: 2015 2nd International Conference on Biomedical Engineering (ICoBE)
3. Rao, R.P.N.: Brain-Computer Interfacing: An Introduction. Cambridge University Press (2013)
4. Nunez, P.L.: The brain wave equation: a model for the EEG. Math. Biosci. **21**(3–4), 279–297 (1974)
5. Kandel, E.R., Schwartz, J.H., Jessell, T.M., Siegelbaum, S.A., Hudspeth, A.J., et al.: Principles of Neural Science, vol. 4. McGraw-Hill, New York (2000)
6. Chatterjee, R., Bandyopadhyay, T.: EEG based motor imagery classification using SVM and MLP. In: 2016 2nd International Conference on Computational Intelligence and Networks (CINE), pp. 84–89. IEEE (2016)
7. Anderer, P., Roberts, S., Schlögl, A., Gruber, G., Klösch, G., Herrmann, W., Rappelsberger, P., Filz, O., Barbanoj, M.J., Dorffner, G., et al.: Artifact processing in computerized analysis of sleep EEG—a review. Neuropsychobiology **40**(3), 150–157 (1999)

8. Carretero, J., García, J.D.: The internet of things: connecting the world. Personal Ubiquitous Comput. **18**(2), 445–447 (2014)
9. Koskela, T., Väänänen-Vainio-Mattila, K.: Evolution towards smart home environments: empirical evaluation of three user interfaces. Personal Ubiquit. Comput. **8**(3–4), 234–240 (2004)
10. Varshney, U.: Pervasive healthcare: applications, challenges and wireless solutions. Commun Assoc Inf Syst **16**(1), 3 (2005)
11. Chatterjee, R., Maitra, T., Islam, S.K.H., Hassan, M.M., Alamri, A., Fortino, G.: A novel machine learning based feature selection for motor imagery EEG signal classification in internet of medical things environment. Future Gen. Comput. Syst. **98**, 419–434 (2019)
12. Bhaduri, S., Khasnobish, A., Bose, R., Tibarewala, D.N.: Classification of lower limb motor imagery using k nearest neighbor and naïve-bayesian classifier. In: 2016 3rd International Conference on Recent Advances in Information Technology (RAIT), pp. 499–504. IEEE (2016)
13. Chatterjee, R., Guha, D., Sanyal, D.K., Mohanty, S.N.: Discernibility matrix based dimensionality reduction for EEG signal. In: Region 10 Conference (TENCON), 2016 IEEE, pp. 2703–2706. IEEE (2016)
14. Chatterjee, R., Bandyopadhyay, T., Sanyal, D.K., Guha, D.: Dimensionality reduction of EEG signal using fuzzy discernibility matrix. In: 2017 10th International Conference on Human System Interactions (HSI), pp. 131–136. IEEE (2017)
15. Chatterjee, R., Bandyopadhyay, T., Sanyal, D.K., Guha, D.: Comparative analysis of feature extraction techniques in motor imagery EEG signal classification. In: Proceedings of First International Conference on Smart System, Innovations and Computing, pp. 73–83. Springer (2018)
16. Chatterjee, R., Bandyopadhyay, T., Sanyal, D.K.: Effects of wavelets on quality of features in motor-imagery EEG signal classification. In: International Conference on Wireless Communications, Signal Processing and Networking (WiSPNET), pp. 1346–1350. IEEE (2016)
17. Lemm, S., Schafer, C., Curio, G.: BCI competition 2003-dataset III: probabilistic modeling of sensorimotor/spl Mu/rhythms for classification of imaginary hand movements. IEEE Trans. Biomed. Eng. **51**(6), 1077–1080 (2004)
18. Bashar, S.K., Bhuiyan, M.I.H.: Classification of motor imagery movements using multivariate empirical mode decomposition and short time Fourier transform based hybrid method. Eng. Sci. Technol. Int. J. **19**(3), 1457–1464 (2016)
19. Chatterjee, R., Datta, A., Sanyal, D.K.: Ensemble learning approach to motor imagery EEG signal classification. In: Machine Learning in Bio-Signal Analysis and Diagnostic Imaging, pp. 183–208 (2018)
20. Han, J., Pei, J., Kamber, M.: Data Mining: Concepts and Techniques. Elsevier (2011)
21. Ang, K.K. , Chin, Z.Y., Zhang, H., Guan, C.: Filter bank common spatial pattern (FBCSP) in brain-computer interface. In: 2008 IEEE International Joint Conference on Neural Networks (IEEE World Congress on Computational Intelligence), pp. 2390–2397. IEEE (2008)
22. Ang, K.K., Chin, Z.Y., Wang, C., Guan, C., Zhang, H.: Filter bank common spatial pattern algorithm on BCI competition IV datasets 2a and 2b. Front. Neurosci. **6**, 39 (2012)
23. Zhang, H., Chin, Z.Y., Ang, K.K., Guan, C., Wang, C.: Optimum Spatio-spectral filtering network for brain-computer interface. IEEE Trans. Neural Netw. **22**(1), 52–63 (2010)
24. Rehman, N.U., Mandic, D.P.: Filter bank property of multivariate empirical mode decomposition. IEEE Trans. Sig. Process. **59**(5), 2421–2426 (2011)
25. Park, S.-H., Lee, D., Lee, S.-G.: Filter bank regularized common spatial pattern ensemble for small sample motor imagery classification. IEEE Trans. Neural Syst. Rehabil. Eng. **26**(2), 498–505 (2017)
26. Datta, A., Chatterjee, R.: Comparative study of different ensemble compositions in EEG signal classification problem. In: Emerging Technologies in Data Mining and Information Security, pp. 145–154. Springer (2019)
27. Storn, R., Price, K.: Differential evolution—a simple and efficient heuristic for global optimization over continuous spaces. J. Glob. Optim. **11**(4), 341–359 (1997)
28. Thomas, K.P., Guan, C., Lau, C.T., Vinod, A.P., Ang, K.K.: A new discriminative common spatial pattern method for motor imagery brain-computer interfaces. IEEE Trans. Biomed. Eng. **56**(11), 2730–2733 (2009)

29. DaSalla, C.S., Kambara, H., Sato, M., Koike, Y.: Single-trial classification of vowel speech imagery using common spatial patterns. Neural Netw. **22**(9), 1334–1339 (2009)
30. Wang, Y., Gao, S., Gao, X.: Common spatial pattern method for channel selection in motor imagery based brain-computer interface. In: 2005 IEEE Engineering in Medicine and Biology 27th Annual Conference, pp. 5392–5395. IEEE (2006)
31. Breiman, L.: Bagging predictors. Mach. Learn. **24**(2), 123–140 (1996)
32. Quinlan, J.R., et al.: Bagging, boosting, and C4. 5. In: AAAI/IAAI, vol. 1, pp. 725–730 (1996)
33. Datta, A., Chatterjee, R., Sanyal, D.K., Guha, D.: An ensemble classification approach to motor-imagery brain state discrimination problem. In: 2017 International Conference on Infocom Technologies and Unmanned Systems (Trends and Future Directions) (ICTUS), pp. 322–326. IEEE (2017)
34. Rahimi, M., Zarei, A., Nazerfard, E., Moradi, M.H.: Ensemble methods combination for motor imagery tasks in brain-computer interface. In: 2016 23rd Iranian Conference on Biomedical Engineering and 2016 1st International Iranian Conference on Biomedical Engineering (ICBME), pp. 336–340. IEEE (2016)
35. Rahman, A., Tasnim, S.: Ensemble Classifiers and Their Applications: A Review. arXiv preprint arXiv:1404.4088 (2014)
36. Alani, S.: Design of intelligent ensembled classifiers combination methods. Ph.D. thesis. Brunel University London (2015)
37. Nascimento, D.S.C., Canuto, A.M.P., Silva, L.M.M., Coelho, A.L.V.: Combining different ways to generate diversity in bagging models: an evolutionary approach. In: The 2011 International Joint Conference on Neural Networks (IJCNN), pp. 2235–2242. IEEE (2011)
38. Price, K., Storn, R.M., Lampinen, J.A.: Differential Evolution: A Practical Approach to Global Optimization. Springer Science & Business Media (2006)
39. Fleetwood, K.: An introduction to differential evolution. In: Proceedings of Mathematics and Statistics of Complex Systems (MASCOS) One Day Symposium, pp. 785–791. Brisbane, Australia, 26 Nov 2004
40. Price, K.V.: Differential evolution. In: Handbook of Optimization, pp. 187–214. Springer (2013)
41. BCI-Competition-II: Dataset III, Department of Medical Informatics, Institute for Biomedical Engineering, University of Technology Graz, Jan 2004 (accessed 6 June 2015)
42. Pfurtscheller, G., Neuper, C.: Motor imagery activates primary sensorimotor area in humans. Neurosci. Lett. **239**(2–3), 65–68 (1997)
43. Pfurtscheller, G., Neuper, C.: Motor imagery and direct brain-computer communication. Proc. IEEE **89**(7), 1123–1134 (2001)

Chapter 12
A Stacked Denoising Autoencoder Compression Sampling Method for Compressing Microscopic Images

P. A. Pattanaik

Abstract Standard stacked denoising autoencoder compression sampling (SDA-CS) approach improves compression sampling process by extracting features functional for disease detection from samples recorded using microscope. However, the clinical pre-processing and classification approach usually contains noise induced by camera illumination and lighting effects, resulting in the loss of information in the features that are essential for detecting disease. This chapter studied a novel strategy to design structured stacked denoising autoencoder (SDA) with binary high dimensional matrices of compressing sampling (HDM), which is a deep learning algorithm, based on promoting linear independence between rows by reducing the number of zero singular values. The design constraints establish a SDA-CS restoration method for simultaneous feature extraction, and compressive imaging by identifying global and invariant features and is robust against illumination noise. The simulation shows that the proposed method is faster and efficiently improves the quality of compression ratio by 49%, compared with the well known three traditional greedy pursuit methods.

Keywords Stacked denoising autoencoder compression sampling approach (SDA-CS) · Deep learning · Stacked denoising autoencoder · Compressing sampling

12.1 Introduction

During the past three decades, advances in artificial intelligence research and the significant efforts made in the medical field have allowed the acquisition of high-resolution images producing large amounts of data, which leads to high computational costs of data acquisition, storage, transmission, and processing [2]. This important yet difficult topic has gained more attention over recent years as researchers are engaged in finding the way in which disease detection and compression of huge database are possible using smart learning algorithms. The computational costs is a common issue in medical applications and can be tackled by using compressive

P. A. Pattanaik (✉)
Telecom SudParis, 9 Rue Charles Fourier, 91011 Evry Cedex, France

P. K. Pattnaik et al. (eds.), *Smart Healthcare Analytics in IoT Enabled Environment*, Intelligent Systems Reference Library 178,
https://doi.org/10.1007/978-3-030-37551-5_12

sampling and deep learning methods, allowing to reduce the amount of data and acquisition costs.

Compressing sensing (CS) has been considered for many real time applications such as MRI, medical imaging, remote sensing, signal processing, etc. SDA-CS method perform compression by summarizing useful features into single values, such as the mean and variance, ensue by feeding these encapsulated values into an SDA classifier [5] to determine disease fault status. Nevertheless, this approach often results in reducing the loss of using features that are vital for disease detection. Furthermore, this approach helps to concentrate on a specific feature which can detect the disease in one go rather considering all features leading to higher computational load and cost. The medical data usually contains noise inclusion induced by camera lightening and microscope adjustment disturbances. Stacked denoising autoencoder feedforward network [5] gives the excellent performance in reducing the noise as well as its removal.

The main task of this manuscript is as follows.

Firstly, we refine the compressing sampling procedure with compression delineation of stacked denoising autoencoder, and initiate the concept of error feedback in denoising autoencoder and combine the features of stacked denoising autoencoder into CS.

Secondly, this proposed approach is distinct from the traditional CS and brings the concept of recovery algorithm with stacked denoising autoencoder and compression sampling as a whole, increasing the efficiency of compression.

Thirdly, we propose an overhauled method to enhance the image quality of the noisy image, and simultaneously obliges the compression ratio with less computation time. This work assessed the effectiveness by evaluating the proposed method using three different medical based global disease datasets of filesize 864 MB.

The rest of the article is described as Sect. 12.2 describes the prior art, Sect. 12.3 describes the stacked denoising autoencoder compressing sampling (SDA-CS) based on stacked denoising autoencoder (SDA) with binary high dimensional matrices (HDM). The experimental detailed analysis performed for evaluation and benchmarking of the performance of our method vs three methods are described in Sect. 12.4. In Sect. 12.5, we conclude this chapter.

12.2 Review Work

In this section, we are dealing with information compression which is one of the main concerns in classifying images and grouped into lossy, irrespective of its kind [3]. A lot useful time is spend in the pre-processing step and clinical setups, demanding human expertise that severely limits the accuracy achievable by a clever learning algorithm. Deep learning (DL) known as stratified order learning, is a class of cascade multiple hidden layers of nodes for end to end feature extraction and classification. DL using auto encoders has gained research interest as it directs to grasp a compact depiction of the input while retaining the most crucial information [6]. Han et al. [4] proposed a sparse auto encoder compressing sampling method that helps in compressing the sampling process and chooses automatically appropriate sparsity by judging the error. The results show that the proposed methods help to find the concise measurement vector subject to obtained delusion. Majumdar [7] introduces a new auto encoder framework for image reconstruction using an adaptive approach and transform learning based methods. The framework gives better results than other broadly used methods in transform learning.

In sequence to explain our work in detail, the next subsection will expose particular examples related to compressing sampling and auto encoder.

12.3 Stacked Denoising Autoencoder Compression Sampling (SDA-CS) Approach

As mentioned above, the standard stacked denoising autoencoder compression sampling (SDA-CS) framework comprises of structured stacked denoising autoencoder (SDA) with compressing sampling (CS).

As shown in Fig. 12.1, we take three image datasets, namely intestine, malaria, leukemia datasets (DS), where the input data is feed into the encoder. If the information gained in the output section is similar to that of the input original data, then we conclude that the processing is reliable. In order to get minimum reconstruction error, the parameters of the encoder and decoder are adjusted and denoising limit is added to enable the reconstruct corrupted input data.

Hereby, we observe that the concept of stacked denoising autoencoder is homogeneous to the operation of compressive sampling. In SDA-CS framework, we have combined the idea of the stacked denoising autoencoder and CS and developed a compressing sampling process of CS.

In the method of CS measurement, we have considered two types of matrixes i.e. random projection matrix Ø = N × N and random measurement matrix β = M × N. For the value Ø, N is defines as number of rows as well as N as number of columns.

For the value β, M is defines as number of rows and N as number of columns.

Let ‘q’ is the measurement vector which can be defined as,

$$q = \beta a = \beta \phi_s \tag{12.1}$$

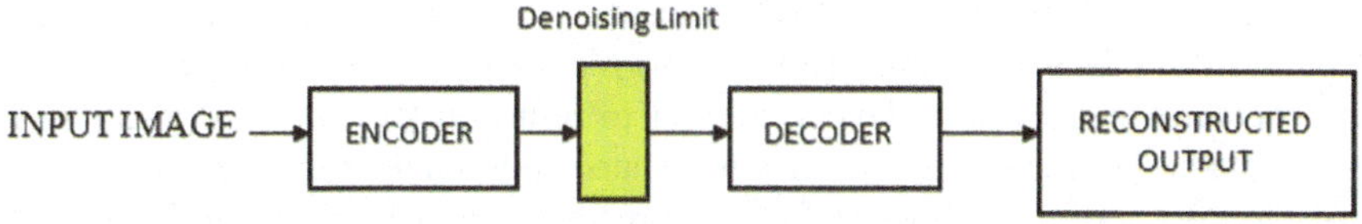

Fig. 12.1 The workflow of stacked denoising autoencoder (SDA)

where, 'a' is the space or time domain, and 's' is in the Ø domain. We define 's' as an N × 1 column vector.

Using Eq. (12.1), we can build a method and express function k,

$$k = \tilde{A}(\beta a) \tag{12.2}$$

We define $\tilde{A}(.)$ as the activation function of the given neural network, and '$\tilde{A}$' is given as follows:

$$\tilde{A}(t) = t \tag{12.3}$$

So,

$$k = \tilde{A}(\beta a) = \beta a \tag{12.4}$$

Hence, the measurement matrix β is random Gaussian matrix and elements $\beta_{i,j}$ are independent random variables.

$$\beta_{i,j} \sim N\left(0, \ldots, \frac{1}{n}\right) \tag{12.5}$$

In Fig. 12.1, the stacked denoising autoencoder has two operations i.e. namely encoding and decoding, which is almost similar to the compressing sampling and recovery process of CS, respectively. The whole SDA-CS method is updated by adjusting the measurement vector by calculating the error between the output reconstructive data and corrupted input data.

The minimal length of the measurement vector can be acceptable by considering the concept of Mean Square Error (MSE) [9]. In the input section, the original matrix can be replace by N × 1 matrix 'a'. The maximum compressing ratio 'p' is defined as,

$$p = \frac{Me}{N} \tag{12.6}$$

Equation (12.6), states that compact the length of the measurement vector the superior is the recovery. M_e is the expected length of the measurement vector 'q' and 'N' is the length of the projection matrix.

Figure 12.2, shows the entire SDA-CS approach where the input layer is x_i (i = 1, 2, …, n) is a N × 1 column vector and the recovery algorithm is used in between the encoding and decoding layers in order to refurbish the corrupted noisy input layer data x_i. The reconstruction error is updated between the recovery out-turn data and the in-turn data. In order to forge the recovery output data optimal, SDA-CS framework needs to adjust the extent of measurement vector and size of the error value.

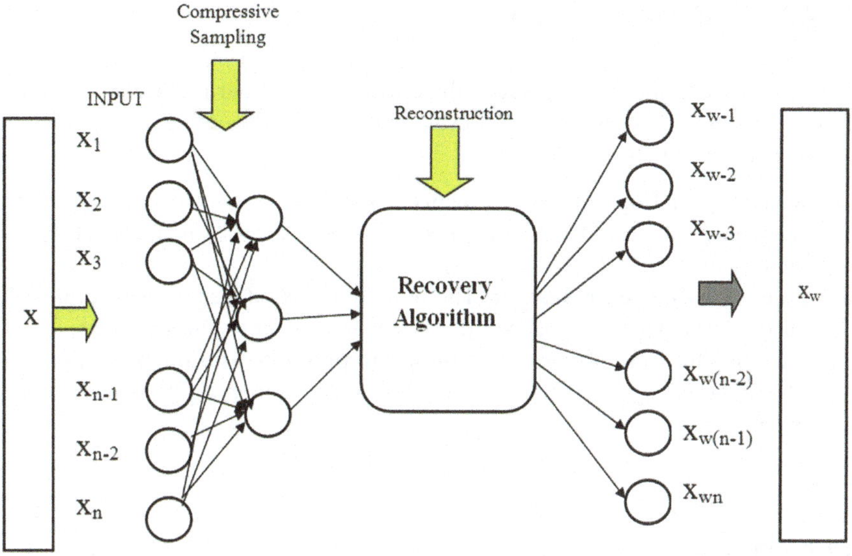

Fig. 12.2 The structure of SDA-CS approach

12.4 Experiments and Results

We demonstrate the applicability of our proposed method, all focussing on the aspect of identifying disease with improving the image quality, simultaneously improving the compression ratio and extensively compare it with benchmark CS methods.

12.4.1 Datasets

Intestine[1] (DS-I), Malaria[2] (DS-II) and Leukaemia[3] (DS-III) image datasets are the three publicly available databases obtained from the AI research group at Makerere University and University of Milan respectively. Our method uses the publicly available Field-stained malaria-infected blood smear microscopic images of 1182 count with 265 MB, 1217 count of the intestine parasite with 456 MB and 108 counts with 143 MB of Acute Lymphoblastic Leukemia (ALL) images obtained from Android smartphone to a Brunel SP150 microscope. Our method is performed using a server with an Intel Xeon E5 (Core TM i7-2600 k) processor, 32 GB RAM with software implementation with PyTorch 2.7, accelerated with CUDA 9.0. The entire framework was trained over 1000 epochs with a learning rate of 1×10^{-3} and decay rate of 0.1 per epoch. Average training time is ~45 s/epoch. The compressor has 365,234 learnable parameters and decompressor has 674,767.

12.4.2 Evaluation Metrics

Now, we analyze different aspects of the effectiveness of our proposed model and evaluate the procedure using various evaluation metrics. The observed quantitative measures are as follows:

i. **Baselines for Comparisons in terms of Running Time**: Effectiveness of the proposed model compared with other baseline popular CS methods in terms of running time.
ii. **Image Quality Improvement**: The proposed method incorporates to identify the disease in terms of image retrieval feature extractor representations.
iii. **Baselines for Comparisons in terms of compression ratio and noise analysis**: The proposed model performance is validated by comparing with the observed image.

12.5 Discussion

In prior to ratify the proposed design method, a lay of compressive measurements are considered. We compare the proposed SDA-CS method with existing traditional CS orthogonal matching pursuit (CS_OMP) method, traditional CS subspace pursuit (CS_SP) method and traditional CS regularized OMP (CS_ROMP) method [3, 11]. The three existing traditional methods receive significant attention due to their low complexity and are called greedy pursuit methods. These three greedy pursuit methods are deterministic in nature. The overall running time of the SDA-CS method is as shown in Table 12.1. Running time includes the encoding time for feature extraction and entropy coding. In the experiments, for the logarithm function is stated to the value of 2, with maximum MSE of 2.4 and maximum compressing ratio 'p' as 0.5 for SDA-CS, without having a dependency on these parameter values, the reconstruction results to be 2.4. We observed that the reconstruction MSE results of SDA-Cs referred to be 2.4, considering the different bases of logarithmic values, a variation of MSE and compression rate 'p'. By determining the size of the delusion value,

Table 12.1 Comparison results of running time between the SDA-CS method with three traditional greedy pursuits methods

MSE	Running time (in s)			
	SDA-CS	CS-ROMP	CS-OMP	CS-SP
2.4	240	880	910	940
2.5	180	800	820	860
2.6	150	780	790	800
2.7	130	700	720	780
2.8	90	650	660	700

the SDA-CS approach can continuously adjust the denoising limit and the extent of measurement vector to make the recovery out-term data to be the optimal.

Results demonstrate that proposed SDA-CS approach performs better in presence of noise. From Table 12.1, we can observe the recovery results with a significant increase in compression ratio with minimum running time. The proposed method improves the quality of compression ratio as much as 49% higher than those of the three compared traditional greedy pursuit methods. The compression ratio is being calculated using Huffman coding, which is an efficient entropy lossless algorithm used for data compression.

The use of entropy-based compression sampling method with stacked denoising autoencoder further boosts compression factor, and our SDA-CS helps to transfer the input code to a relatively flat image quality over a wide range of compression factors. In SDA-CS method, we can note that the running time is gradually reducing as contrast to the other three Greedy pursuit CS methods. With the SDA-CS, we improve the compressing sampling process to a very far extend with drastically reduction and are able to evaluate the delusion between the recovery data out-term and the corrupted in-term data.

As shown in Figs. 12.3 and 12.4, SDA-CS method is used for the purpose of enhancing the image quality and reducing the noise. As shown in Fig. 12.4, our proposed model SDA-CS automatically constructed observed image of good size,

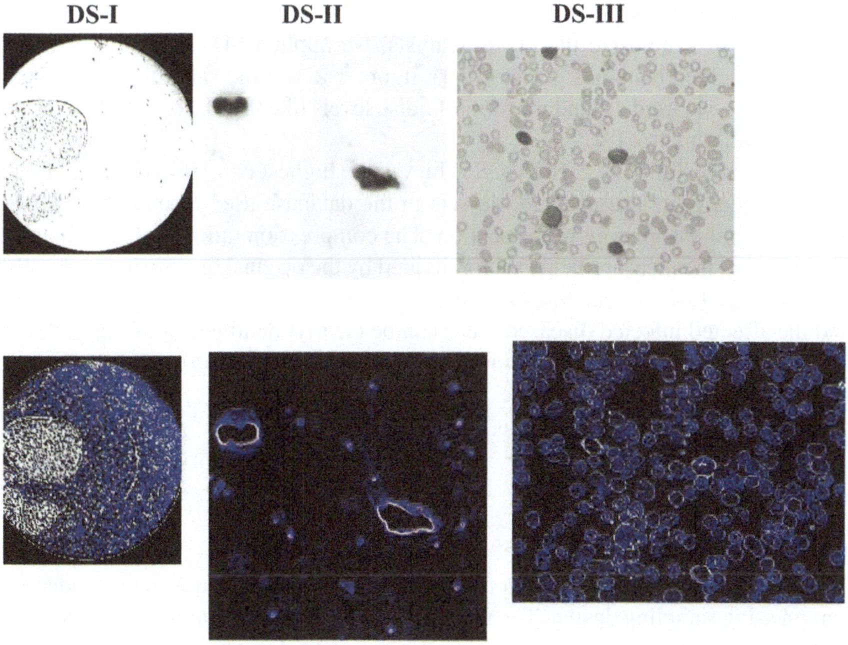

Fig. 12.3 Visualization of the overhauled image obtained by SDA-CS

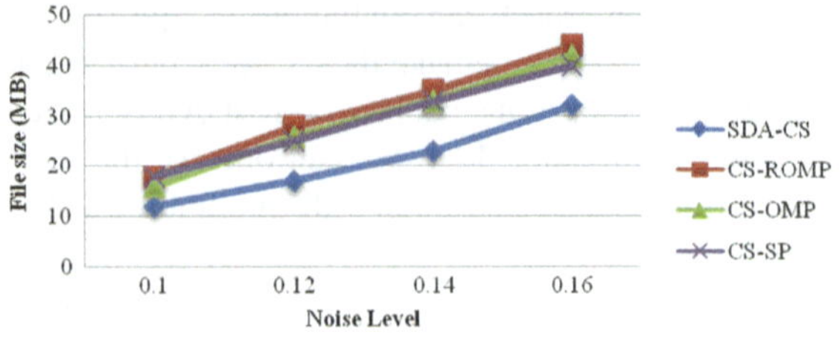

Fig. 12.4 The proposed method outperforms greedy pursuit methods in terms of compression ratio and noise analysis

Table 12.2 Comparison results of compression between the SDA-CS method with other three traditional greedy pursuits CS methods to scan medical images with real images

Methods	Compression ratio (%)
SDA-CS	49
CS-ROMP	29.16
CS-OMP	37.25
CS-SP	38.02

which provided good stability between providing enough data to encode the image while reducing the size of itself.

In order to synthesize the noise analysis, we applied SDA-CS to each of the images, which corresponds in Eq. (12.3). In order to test the validation of different blurry levels, we used a standard form of noise levels like 0.1, 0.12, 0.14, 0.16 as per Gaussian filter matrix [8].

In order to synthesize the noise analysis, we applied SDA-CS to each of the images, which corresponds in Eq. (12.3). In order to test the validation of different blurry levels, we used a standard form of noise levels like 0.1, 0.12, 0.14, 0.16 as per Gaussian filter matrix [8].

As shown in Table 12.2, SDA-CS achieves the highest compression ratio among all the challengers. The average file size in the database used is about 864 MB as described at the beginning of the section. The compression ratio is calculated as the dimension of the measurements vector divided by the original bit stream file size [8].

From Fig. 12.3, we can view that the image quality is visually improved by 5% and the affected infected diseased areas can be clearly identified from Fig. 12.3b as compared to original images shown in Fig. 12.3a. No substitution error was endowed in the SDA-CS compressed image.

12.6 Conclusion

This chapter states a new framework based on the denoising stack autoencoder and compressing sampling design. The method enables to solve an optimization problem without performing the product of large matrices, instead, it takes the advantage of the stacked and structure of compressing sampling providing a better performance than traditional greedy pursuit CS methods. The proposed approach is robust enough to obtain the minimal length of the measurement vector in the case of accepted reconstruction error. Experiments showed that the proposed SDA-CS method compared competitively with other three greedy pursuit CS methods, with the advantage of improving the reconstruction quality by 49%. It is concluded that SDA-CS has multiple benefits over noise reduction and compression methods in medical fields.

References

1. Bain, B.J.: Diagnosis from the blood smear. N. Engl. J. Med. **353**, 498–507 (2005)
2. Bench-Capon, T.J., Dunne, P.E.: Argumentation in artificial intelligence. Artif. Intell. **171**, 619–641 (2007)
3. Donoho, D.L.: Compressing sampling. IEEE Trans. Inf. Theory **52**, 1289–1306 (2006)
4. Han, T., Hao, K., Ding, Y., Tang, X.: A sparse autoencoder compressing sampling method for acquiring the pressure array information of clothing. Neurocomputing **275**, 1500–1510 (2018)
5. Jia, C., Shao, M., Li, S., Zhao, H., Fu, Y.: Stacked denoising tensor auto-encoder for action recognition with spatiotemporal corruptions. IEEE Trans. Image Process. **27**, 1878–1887 (2018)
6. LeCun, Y., Bengio, Y., Hinton, G.: Deep learning. Nature **521**(436) (2015)
7. Majumdar, A.: An autoencoder based formulation for compressing sampling reconstruction. Magn. Reson. Imaging (2018)
8. Qi, Y., Guo, Y.: Message passing with l1 penalized KL minimization. In: 2013 International Conference on Machine Learning, pp. 262–270 (2013)
9. Salari, S., Chan, F., Chan, Y.T., Read, W.: TDOA estimation with compressive sampling measurements and Hadamard matrix. IEEE Trans. Aerosp. Electron. Syst. (2018)
10. Singh, A., Kirar, K.G.: Review of image compression techniques. In: 2017 International Conference on Recent Innovations in Signal Processing and Embedded Systems (RISE), pp. 172–174 (2017)
11. Yao, S., Guan, Q., Wang, S., Xie, X.: Fast sparsity adaptive matching pursuit algorithm for large-scale image reconstruction. EURASIP J. Wirel. Commun. Netw. **1**(78) (2018)
12. Zhang, J., Ghanem, B.: ISTA-Net: interpretable optimization-inspired deep network for image compressive sensing. In: Proceedings of the IEEE Conference on Computer Vision and Pattern Recognition, pp. 1828–1837 (2018)

Chapter 13
IoT in Healthcare: A Big Data Perspective

Ritesh Jha, Vandana Bhattacharjee and Abhijit Mustafi

Abstract With the advent of Internet of Things, the entire world seems to be connected. Everything is connected to anything. It is natural that health care could not remain untouched, and smart health care systems are coming in practice. Wearable or implanted sensors form body area networks transmitting data at an enormous rate. This further brings in the huge amount of data, often called Big Data which needs to be stored and analyzed. In the era of Artificial intelligence, it is imperative that researchers look towards machine learning tools to handle this vast amount of medical data. This chapter presents a framework for data analytics using Random Forest classification technique. A comparison is done after applying feature selection. It is seen that the training time gets reduced substantially even though the accuracy does not suffer. This is the most important requirement of Big data handling. The algorithms are implemented on Apache Spark.

Keywords Apache spark · Big data · Random forest · Feature selection

13.1 Introduction

The internet connectivity of all the things and enhancement in telecommunication, is making the development and deployment of remote health monitoring systems feasible and serviceable. The dream of real time monitoring of users, analysis of medical data, diagnosis and automated communication with doctors or emergency personnel is now practically realizable. The figure shows how closely this ecosystem of things and people operating them is knit, where both are equal stakeholders and the decision making of both influence each other (Fig. 13.1).

R. Jha · V. Bhattacharjee (✉) · A. Mustafi
Department of Computer Science and Engineering, BIT Mesra, Ranchi, India
e-mail: vbhattacharya@bitmesra.ac.in

R. Jha
e-mail: riteshjha@bitmesra.ac.in

A. Mustafi
e-mail: abhijit@bitmesra.ac.in

P. K. Pattnaik et al. (eds.), *Smart Healthcare Analytics in IoT Enabled Environment*, Intelligent Systems Reference Library 178,
https://doi.org/10.1007/978-3-030-37551-5_13

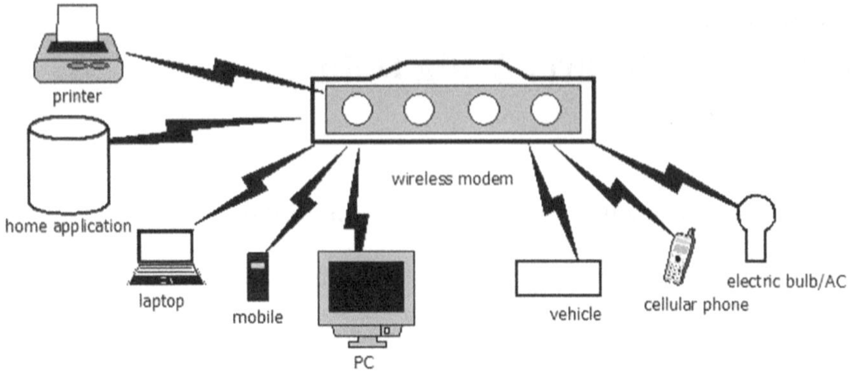

Fig. 13.1 IoT based interrelated communication between devices

The heterogeneous nature of Internet of Things (IoT) where various kinds of devices are interconnected over diverse protocols also opens up different application areas, medical systems being one of them. Smart transportation, electrical energy management systems, smart irrigation, sensor based disaster mitigation are several others [1–6].

The various types of sensors used in smart health care vary from pulse sensors to take a pulse reading [7], to respiratory rate sensors [10, 11], which utilize the fact that the air exhaled is warmer than the ambient air. This fact is also utilized in counting the number of breaths. There are also body temperature sensors [12–15] and blood pressure sensors [16–20]. Sensors are also used to measure the level of oxygen in the blood [26]. EEG sensors for monitoring brain activity and ECG sensors to detect heart strokes are very commonly used [21–25]. ECG sensors could be typically arm based, integrated into helmets or worn as chest straps. A very popular application of EEG sensors is to detect driver drowsiness and is being used by leading car manufacturers as an important safety feature. In this world of lone travelers, this could be a life saving boon!

Apart from sensors, there are examples of IoT systems that have been developed for detecting sleep disorders [27] and rehabilitation systems [41]. Gesture recognition systems have shown great potential of use for medical diagnosis of a person's state of mind [28–31, 37, 40].

Actually speaking, all this data being generated or collected requires to be stored and analyzed for any actionable insight [8, 9]. The rest of the chapter is organized as follows: in Sect. 13.2 we give an overview of the Big data framework. Section 13.3 presents the methodology explaining the Random forest classification technique which we aim to implement for classification of medical Big data. Section 13.4 presents the experimental set up. Section 13.5 presents the results and analysis, and Sect. 13.6 concludes the chapter.

13.2 Big Data Framework

Data handling of medical data to produce output in the current scenario is a four stage process, as shown in Fig. 13.2.

The data from medical or bio sensors is collected and subjected to transformation which could be preprocessing or cleaning, i.e., removal of erroneous data. This data is then transferred to the Big data framework such as Hadoop, Spark and analytics performed on it. Machine learning algorithms are applied to extract meaningful information. This then results in an output which could be specific recommendation to the user, or reference to a doctor or in extreme cases, emergency user assistance may be sought [32–36].

Data preparation is a very important step in data analytics [35, 38, 39]. The cleaning of data means handling NULL values, zeroes or special characters like "?", "NA" as examples. It is also important to find out the correlation among the attributes. Much of this exercise helps one in finding the correct set of features to be used in the machine learning model.

We now elaborate upon the SPARK framework, which is the system on which we have implemented our work. With the increase in the volume of data parallel data analysis is a compulsory requirement to be able to get real time solutions. As a result, practitioners in many fields have sought easier tools for this task. Apache Spark is a popular tool, extending and generalizing Map Reduce. There are several benefits. It is easy to use - the applications can be developed on a laptop, using a high-level API that lets one focus on the content of computation. Second, Spark is fast, enabling interactive use and complex algorithms. Figure 13.3 shows the Spark Flow Stack.

Apache Spark is a cluster computing platform which is fast and general purpose. The Map Reduce model has been extended to efficiently support more types of computations, including interactive queries and stream processing. Fast processing in large datasets means a lot between exploring data interactively and waiting minutes or hours. Spark has more speed due to its ability to run computations in memory, but the system is also more efficient than Map Reduce for complex applications running on disk. Spark is designed to be highly accessible, and it offers simple APIs in Python, Java, Scala, and SQL, and rich built-in libraries. Integration with other Big Data tools is also very easy. In particular, Spark can run in Hadoop clusters and access any Hadoop data source, including Cassandra. Spark can run over a variety of cluster managers, including Hadoop and YARN. Spark cluster consists of many machines, each of which is referred to as a node/slave. There are two main components of Spark: Master and Workers. There is only one master node which assigns jobs to

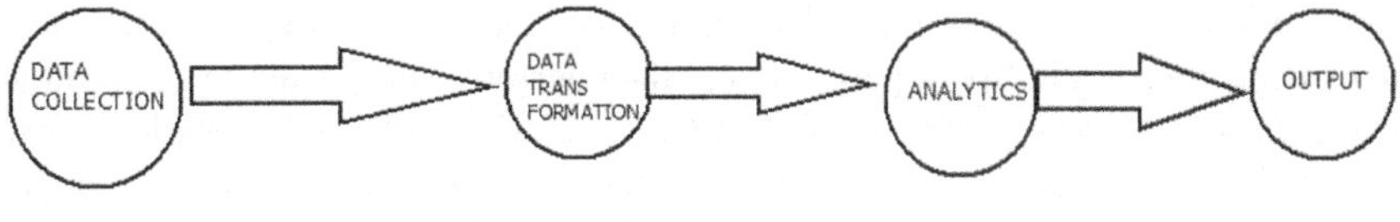

Fig. 13.2 Four stage data handling

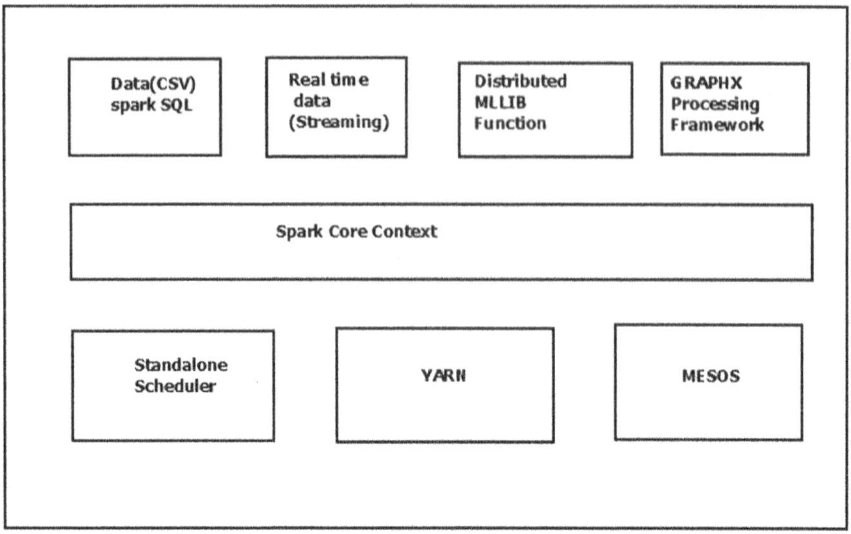

Fig. 13.3 Spark flow stack

the slave nodes. There can be any number of slave nodes. Data can be stored in HDFS or in local machine. A job reads data from the local machine/HDFS, performs computations on it and/or writes some output.

13.3 Methodology

The objective of Machine learning approach in big data is to identify the hidden patterns. This can be done either by classification or clustering techniques [33, 34]. Problem arises when the data is imbalanced and multi-class. In this chapter, random forest technique has been applied for classification. Further feature selection using PCA has been done and then classification results are compared with the previous results.

13.3.1 Random Forest Technique

Random forest is one kind of ensemble approach to boost the training phase. It forms many decision trees in Spark partition and then performs the voting mechanism to predict the class labels among the decision trees. However, the time complexity can be varied by tuning the parameters and varying the worker nodes, cores etc. In our case we applied this approach in EEG dataset. Two experiment have been conducted, (1) Random Forest without PCA, (2) Random Forest with PCA.

Algorithm 1: Random Forest

Input: Training data
Output: Class labels

1. Load the training data in dataframe of spark
2. Handle any missing values
3. Scale the dataset.
4. Split the dataset into 70% training, 30% testing
5. Apply randomForest() to train the model
6. Use testing data on trained model to predict the class label.

Algorithm 2: Random Forest with PCA

Input: Training data
Output: Class Label

1. Steps 1–3 are same as Algorithm 1
2. Apply PCA function(returns the increasing order of variance of each feature e.g., k = 2, k = 3…)
3. Apply RandomForest() with reduced features to train the model
4. Use trained model to predict the test data.

13.4 Experimental Setup and Dataset Description

The experimental setup used for this paper consisted of 5 Personal Computers: 1. Master Node and 4 Slave/Worker Nodes. Each system was identical with the following specifications: 8 GB DDR3 RAM, Intel Core i7 5th Gen Processors and a 1 Terabyte Hard disk drive. The Operating System used was Linux Ubuntu-18.04 with Apache Spark-2.4.3. Python Language has been used in Spark platform. Figure 13.4 shows the overall architecture of our Big medical data processing framework.

13.4.1 EEG DataSet

EEG (electroencephalography) data set is used to identify the electrical activity of human brain and disorders. The dataset has 15 features and 14,980 instances and also no missing value. The data is from one continuous EEG measurement with the Emotiv EEG Neuroheadset. The duration of the measurement was 117 s. In this dataset, the eye state was detected via a camera during the EEG measurement. Then, later on it was added to the file after analyzing the video frames. The eye-closed state is ‘1’ while ‘0’ indicates the eye-open state. All values are in chronological order with the first measured value at the top of the data.

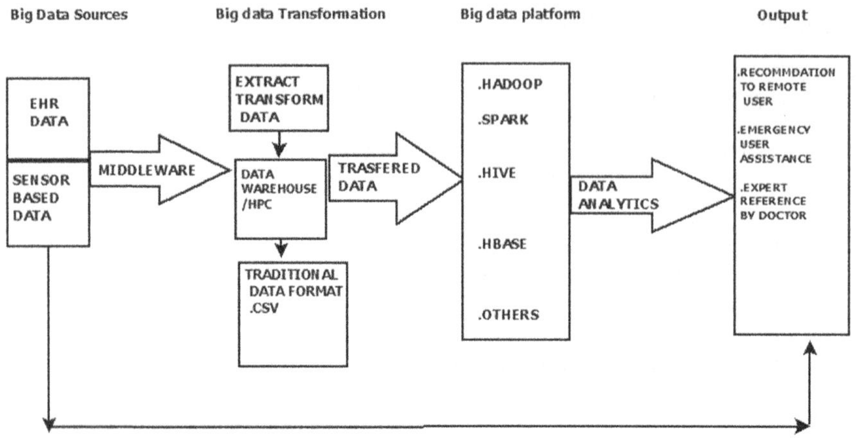

Fig. 13.4 Big data processing framework

Data is obtained from UCI and available at [41]. Pre-processing was performed to normalize it before applying random Forest algorithm. The dataset was divided into 30% testing and 70% training.

13.4.1.1 Classification Evaluation Parameters

To get the accuracy a confusion matrix is used which has the following entries.

From Fig. 13.5, the following entries are defined as follows:

1. TP: number of positive data correctly predicted by the model.
2. FN: number of positive data predicted as negative by the model.
3. FP: number of negative data predicted as positive by the model.
4. TN: number of negative data correctly predicted by the model.

Fig. 13.5 Confusion matrix for binary classification

		Predicted Class	
		TRUE	**FALSE**
Actual Class	**TRUE**	True Positive (TP)	False Negative (FN)
	FALSE	False Positive(FP)	True Negative (TN)

13.4.1.2 Classification Parameters

$$\textbf{Accuracy} = \text{TP} + \text{FN}/(\text{TP} + \text{FN} + \text{FP} + \text{TN}).$$

Sensitivity is called the true positive rate(TPR) as the fraction of positive data predicted correctly by the model:

$$\text{TPR} = \text{TP}/(\text{TP} + \text{FN})$$

Specificity is called the true negative rate(TNR) as the fraction of negative data predicted correctly by the model.

$$\text{TNR} = \text{TN}/(\text{TN} + \text{FP})$$

13.5 Results and Analysis

The Random forest technique was applied on the EEG Dataset, with and without PCA.

The Fig. 13.6 gives a plot of Accuracy versus number of features selected.

From Fig. 13.6 we can observe that accuracy increases as features are increasing and for feature value which are less than or equal to 6 the accuracy is less than 88%

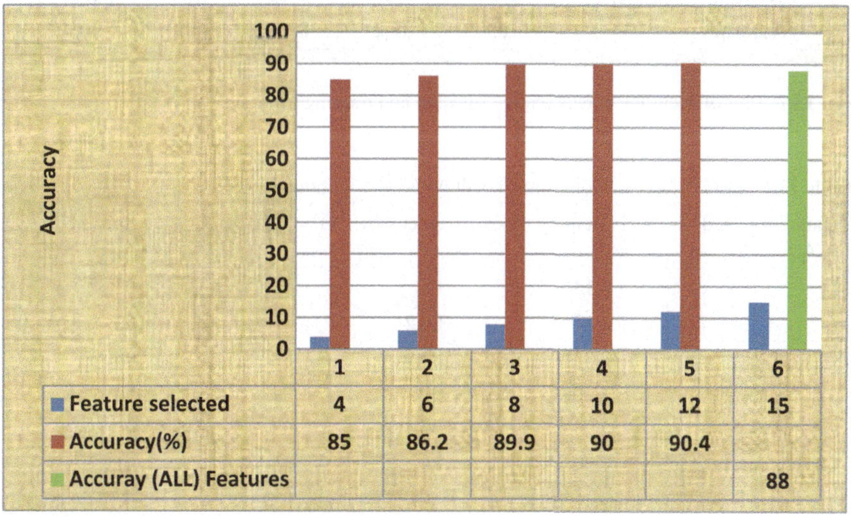

Fig. 13.6 Plot of accuracy versus feature selected, all features

then it starts increasing when feature value reached to 12. So for all cases when number of features is more than 6 accuracy is also greater than 88% (Fig. 13.7).

From Table 13.1 and Fig. 13.6 it can be seen that the increase in training time is correlated with increase in accuracy. For the a training time 2.25 s the accuracy has been found to be highest. So from Table 13.1 we find that accuracy has been increased from 88 to 90.4% when we selected 12 features and time also has been reduced from 2.90 to 2.25 s, which provides the ideal parameter selection in this dataset. This is an example of best dimensionality reduction for big data application in terms of reduced training time and accuracy.

From Fig. 13.8 we observe that specificity has increased up to 96% with 12 features while sensitivity has maximum value at 84.46 for 10 features.

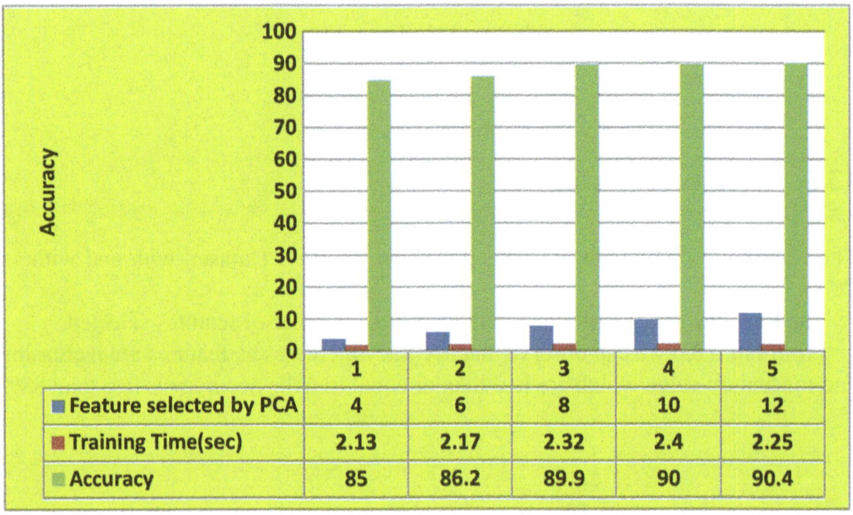

Fig. 13.7 Plot of accuracy versus feature selected and training time

Table 13.1 EEG dataset random forest result with PCA/without PCA

Feature selected by PCA	Training time(s)	Accuracy (%)	Sensitivity (%)	Specificity (%)
4	2.13	85	77	93
6	2.17	86.2	77	93
8	2.32	89.9	83	95
10	2.40	90	84.46	94
12	2.25	90.4	83	96
All (without PCA)	2.90	88	85	91.59

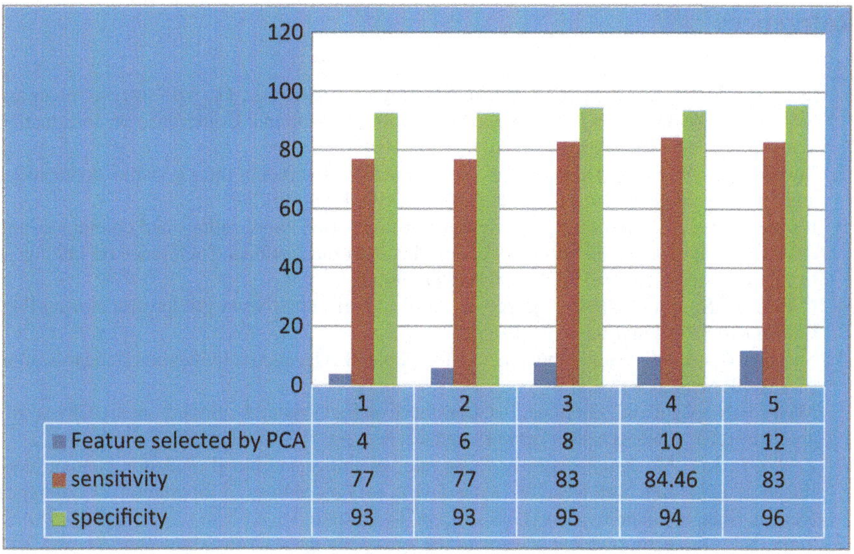

Fig. 13.8 Plot of feature selected, sensitivity and specificity

13.6 Conclusion

This chapter presented an overview of big data framework for analytics of medical data. The problems of huge dimensions and noisy data were also discussed. The large number of features lead to an increase in training time of the prediction models. This can be handled using feature selection approaches. The random forest classification technique is applied. It is shown that feature selection leads to an improvement in training time at the same time not compromising on accuracy. Having classified a disease related data, gathered from sensors, one can predict in real time regarding the present state of a patient through wearable or implanted sensors. This prediction can be used to generate one of the following outputs: 1. specific recommendation to the user; 2. reference to a doctor; or in extreme cases 3. emergency user assistance could be sought.

The discussion presented in this chapter brings out several important findings about data analytics of medical data. The first is that this facilitates making better health profiles of users, and due to which, better predictive models can be built. Secondly, analyzing the stored data from various sources with proper selection of features and application of machine learning techniques can lead to a better understanding of diseases. And finally, for the holistic development of all, it is necessary that patients be treated as partners in monitoring their own wellness and they be informed about any impending threat to their health. Our ongoing work aims at applying more classification techniques on real medical datasets, and to develop recommender systems based on the model. With big data analytics of medical data, we take a sure step in the direction of wellness for all!

References

1. Dohr, A., Modre-Opsrian, R., Drobics, M., Hayn, D., Schreier, G.: The internet of things for ambient assisted living. In: Proceedings of the International Conference on Information Technology: New Generations, pp. 804–809 (2010)
2. Miorandi, D., Sicari, S., De Pellegrini, F., Chlamtac, I.: Internet of things: vision, applications and research challenges. Ad Hoc Netw. **10**(7), 1497–1516 (2012)
3. Bhuvaneswari, V., Porkodi, R.: The internet of things (IoT) applications and communication enabling technology standards: an overview. In: 2014 International Conference on Intelligent Computing Applications. ISBN: 978-1-4799-3966-4
4. CASAGRAS: CASAGRAS Eu project final report. http://www.grifsproject.eu/data/File/CASAGRAS%20FinalReport%20(2).pdf
5. Smith, I.: Coordination and support action for global RFID related activities and standardization (CASAGRAS) (2008)
6. Murty, R.N., Mainland, G., Rose, I., Chowdhury, A.R., Gosain, A., Bers, J., et al.: City sense: an urban-scale wireless sensor network and test bed, pp. 583–588 (2008)
7. Ženko, J., Kos, M., Kramberger, I.: Pulse rate variability and blood oxidation content identification using miniature wearable wrist device. In: Proceedings of International Conference System, Signals Image Process (IWSSIP), pp. 1–4 (2016)
8. Terry, N.P.: Protecting patient privacy in the age of big data. UMKC Law Rev. **81**, 385–415 (2013)
9. Shrestha, R.B.: Big data and cloud computing. Appl. Radiol. (2014)
10. Milici, S., Lorenzo, J., Lázaro, A., Villarino, R., Girbau, D.: Wireless breathing sensor based on wearable modulated frequency selective surface. IEEE Sens. J. **17**(5), 1285–1292 (2017)
11. Varon, C., Caicedo, A., Testelmans, D., Buyse, B., van Huffel, S.: A novel algorithm for the automatic detection of sleep apnea from single-lead ECG. IEEE Trans. Biomed. Eng. **62**(9), 2269–2278 (2015)
12. Aqueveque, P., Gutiérrez, C., Rodríguez, F.S., Pino, E.J., Morales, A., Wiechmann, E.P.: Monitoring physiological variables of mining workers at high altitude. IEEE Trans. Ind. Appl. **53**(3), 2628–2634 (2017)
13. Narczyk, P., Siwiec, K., Pleskacz, W.A.: Precision human body temperature measurement based on thermistor sensor. In: 2016 IEEE 19th International Symposium on Design and Diagnostics of Electronic Circuits and Systems (DDECS), pp. 1–5 (2016)
14. Nakamura, T., et al.: Development of flexible and wide-range polymer based temperature sensor for human bodies. In: 2016 IEEE-EMBS International Conference on Biomedical and Health Informatics (BHI), pp. 485–488 (2016)
15. Eshkeiti, A., et al.: A novel self-supported printed flexible strain sensor for monitoring body movement and temperature. In: Proceedings of IEEE Sensors, pp. 1615–1618 (2014)
16. Heart Foundation. High blood pressure statistics (2017). Available: www.heartfoundation.org.au/about-us/what-we-do/heartdisease-in-australia/high-blood-pressure-statistics
17. Thomas, S.S., Nathan, V., Zong, C., Soundarapandian, K., Shi, X., Jafari, R.: Bio watch: a noninvasive wrist-based blood pressure monitor that incorporates training techniques for posture and subject variability. IEEE J. Biomed. Health Inform. **20**(5), 1291–1300 (2016)
18. Griggs, D., et al.: Design and development of continuous cuff-less blood pressure monitoring devices. In: Proceedings of IEEE Sensors, pp. 1–3 (2016)
19. Zhang, Y., Berthelot, M., Lo, B.P.: Wireless wearable photoplethysmography sensors for continuous blood pressure monitoring. In: Proceedings of IEEE Wireless Health (WH), pp. 1–8 (2016)
20. Wannenburg, J., Malekian, R.: Body sensor network for mobile health monitoring, a diagnosis and anticipating system. IEEE Sens. J. **15**(12), 6839–6852 (2015)
21. Rachim, V.P., Chung, W.-Y.: Wearable noncontact armband for mobile ECG monitoring system. IEEE Trans. Biomed. Circuits Syst. **10**(6), 1112–1118 (2016)

22. Von Rosenberg, W., Chanwimalueang, T., Goverdovsky, V., Looney, D., Sharp, D., Mandic, D.P.: Smart helmet: wearable multichannel ECG and EEG. IEEE J. Transl. Eng. Health Med. **4**, Art. no. 2700111 (2016)
23. Spanò, E., Pascoli, S.D., Iannaccone, G.: Low-power wearable ECG monitoring system for multiple-patient remote monitoring. IEEE Sens. J. **16**(13), 5452–5462 (2016)
24. Li, G., Lee, B.-L., Chung, W.-Y.: Smart watch-based wearable EEG system for driver drowsiness detection. IEEE Sens. J. **15**(12), 7169–7180 (2015)
25. Ha, U., et al.: A wearable EEG-HEG-HRV multimodal system with simultaneous monitoring of tES for mental health management. IEEE Trans. Biomed. Circuits Syst. **9**(6), 758–766 (2015)
26. Gubbi, S.V., Amrutur, B.: Adaptive pulse width control and sampling for low power pulse oximetry. IEEE Trans. Biomed. Circuits Syst. **9**(2), 272–283 (2015)
27. Amendola, S., Lodato, R., Manzari, S., Occhiuzzi, C., Marrocco, G.: RFID technology for IoT-based personal healthcare in smart spaces. IEEE Internet Things J. **1**(2) (2014)
28. Sahoo, P.K., Mohapatra, S.K., Wu, S.-L.: Analyzing healthcare big data with prediction for future health condition. IEEE Access **4**, 9786–9799 (2016)
29. Manzari, S., Occhiuzzi, C., Marrocco, G.: Feasibility of body-centric passive RFID systems by using textile tags. IEEE Antennas Propag. Mag. **54**(4), 49–62 (2012)
30. Krigslund, R., Dosen, S., Popovski, P., Dideriksen, J., Pedersen, G.F., Farina, D.: A novel technology for motion capture using passive UHF RFID Tags. IEEE Trans. Biomed. Eng. **60**(5), 1453–1457 (2013)
31. Amendola, S., Bianchi, L., Marrocco, G.: Combined passive radio-frequency identification and machine learning technique to recognize human motion. In: Proceedings of European Microwave Conference (2014)
32. Lin, K., Xia, F., Wang, W., Tian, D., Song, J.: System design for big data application in emotion-aware healthcare. IEEE Access **4**, 6901–6909 (2016)
33. Hung, C.-Y., Chen, W.-C., Lai, P.-T., Lin, C.-H., Lee, C.-C.: Comparing deep neural network and other machine learning algorithms for stroke prediction in a large-scale population-based electronic medical claims database. In: Proceeding in 39th Annual International Conference of the IEEE Engineering in Medicine and Biology Society (EMBC), pp. 3110–3113 (2017)
34. Park, J., Kim, K.Y., Kwon, O.: Comparison of machine learning algorithms to predict psychological wellness indices for ubiquitous healthcare system design. In: Proceedings of the 2014 International Conference on Innovative Design and Manufacturing (ICIDM), pp. 263–269 (2014)
35. Jagadish, H.V., Gehrke, J., Labrinidis, A., Papakonstantinou, Y., Patel, J.M., et al.: Big data and its technical challenges. Commun. ACM **57**, 86–94 (2014). https://doi.org/10.1145/2611567
36. Raghupathi, W., Raghupathi, V.: Big data analytics in healthcare: promise and potential Health Inform. Science Syst. **2**, 1–10 (2014). https://doi.org/10.1186/2047-2501-2-3
37. Lee, J.H., Lee, E.J.: Computer-aided diagnosis sensor and system of breast sonography: a clinical study. Sens. Transducers **180**, 1–10 (2014)
38. Schultz, T.: Turning healthcare challenges into big data opportunities: a use-case review across the pharmaceutical development lifecycle. Bull. Assoc. Inform. Sci. Technol. **39**, 34–40 (2013). https://doi.org/10.1002/bult.2013.1720390508
39. Olaronke, I., Oluwaseun, O.: Big data in healthcare: prospects, challenges and resolutions. In: Proceedings of 2016 Future Technologies Conference (FTC), pp. 1152–1157 (2006)
40. Fan, Y.J., Yin, Y.H., Xu, L.D., Zeng, Y., Wu, F.: IoT-based smart rehabilitation system. IEEE Trans. Ind. Inform. **10**(2), 1568–1577 (2014)
41. https://archive.ics.uci.edu/ml/datasets/eeg+database

Chapter 14
Stimuli Effect of the Human Brain Using EEG SPM Dataset

Arkajyoti Mukherjee, Ritik Srivastava, Vansh Bhatia, Utkarsh and Suneeta Mohanty

Abstract This chapter presents an Electroencephalography (EEG) based approach for brain activity analysis on the Multi-Modal face dataset to provide an understanding for the visual response invoked in the brain upon seeing images of faces (familiar, unfamiliar and scrambled faces) and applying computational modeling for classification along with the removal/reduction of noise in the given channels. Thus demonstrating the process of EEG analysis which may be used in various smart health care applications.

Keywords Electroencephalography (EEG) · Feature extraction · Multi-modal dataset · Visual stimuli

14.1 Introduction

The mechanism of thought generation or body movement is first carried out in the neurons. The brain accomplishes it by generating electrical pulses. The relay of messages from the human brain to the body is held in the form of the flow of ions from the brain to the specific muscles/nerves targeted. The movement of the limbs, the blinking of an eye and most of the voluntary, as well as the involuntary actions, start with the generation of said signals in the brain [1]. The idea that these signals may be harnessed for further analysis is the principal motive behind this chapter.

Using Electroencephalography (EEG) [2], brain activity may be visualized. It is a technique employed to map the synaptic potential fluctuations due to ion flow within the brain [3]. These fluctuations may be plotted in the form of quantifiable signals that would be utilized for running analytics and deriving insights as well as early diagnosis. In 1924, the first human electroencephalogram (EEG) recording, by German physiologist and psychiatrist Hans Berger (1873–1941) and the subsequent invention of the electroencephalogram has made EEG a standard non-invasive way of diagnosing coma, encephalopathies, sleep disorders, depth of anaesthesia and brain death. Despite the recent advancements in technology and the shift from EEG to

A. Mukherjee · R. Srivastava · V. Bhatia · Utkarsh · S. Mohanty (✉)
School of Computer Engineering, Kalinga Institute of Industrial Technology (KIIT) Deemed to be University, Bhubaneswar, Odisha, India

P. K. Pattnaik et al. (eds.), *Smart Healthcare Analytics in IoT Enabled Environment*, Intelligent Systems Reference Library 178,
https://doi.org/10.1007/978-3-030-37551-5_14

the high-resolution anatomical imaging techniques counterparts such as Magnetic resonance imaging, EEG still remains an inexpensive and highly accessible tool for researchers and diagnosis which offers temporal resolution in the millisecond range, something which is not possible with Positron emission tomography (PET) [4], Computed tomography (CT) [5] or Magnetic resonance imaging (MRI) [6].

Advancements in the field of Statistical Learning has helped researchers around the world in the classification of the EEG signals, facilitating them in understanding behavioral patterns, allowing for early diagnosis of diseases and detection of abnormal behaviour of the brain, which, in turn, has proved to be of much interest and merit for the early diagnosis of potential patients.

Using an EEG reading device, we may read these waves and run analytical algorithms on them in order to better understand the physical [7] and/or emotional behavioural [8] responses of a given wave corresponds to rendering and enable us to observe as well as predict the future behaviour a person is most likely to present and derive conclusions of interests from said predictions. This idea is novel and relevant as the use of said analytics has allowed us to predict seizures [9] and classify the emotional state a person is in [8] with higher accuracy than ever before.

14.2 Review of Related Works

Pfurtscheller et al. [10] classified the Electroencephalograph (EEG) signals of the 3 subjects imagining the movement of the left and right-hand movement. To classify the said movements a neural network provides the appropriate classification. Effect on the contralateral central area and the ipsilateral side was derived.

Vigario et al. [11] showed the results of using independent component analysis (ICA), proving it to be a useful method for artifact detection and extraction from MEG (Magnetoencephalographic) and EEG (electroencephalographic) recordings and also presented the findings of the application of this technique in their review.

Blankertz B et al. [12] BCIs (Brain Computer Interfaces) created a new transmission pathway between the brain and an output device by bypassing the general motor output relay of nerve and muscles. The system takes readings from the scalp (non-invasive), the surface of the cortex, or from inside the brain (invasive) and allowed the users to control a variety of different applications. The chapter briefly explores the six datasets and the outcomes with the workings of the best algorithms in the BCI competition 2003.

Barry et al. [13] conducted an analysis of EEG recordings of 28 university students during eye-closed and eye-opened states (resting) to determine the physiological response and behaviour. Later providing specific topographical representation and reflecting the region of generation of the signal while processing the EEG signal recorded. Detailed examination of the generation of alpha, beta, delta and theta bands is correlated from eye-closed to eye-opened condition.

Soleymani and Pantic [14] demonstrated the tagging of multimedia content without any direct input from the user. With the help of EEG signal, tagging and classification of the multimedia content is conducted on the basis of previous studies on emotional classification. This implicit method of classification provides a more suitable alternative approach for recognizing emotional tags overcoming the difficulties of self-reported sentiments by the person.

Liu et al. [15] Alcoholism causes severe damage to the functional neuro system. Consumption of alcohol over a long period of time may lead to blurred vision, lack of brain and muscle coordination and degradation of memory over time. The brain activity of alcoholic people and those in the normal state was examined. The study underlines the impact of alcoholism on the brain. The result of the study may be implemented for the rehabilitation of patients being affected by alcoholism.

Henson et al. [16] showed the study of multi-modal data through multiple steps involved along with neuroimaging data analysis of multiple human subjects. Performing the combined processing of EEG and MEG data for multiple subjects leading to forward modelling using structural MRI and finally mapping the data across all the subjects showing the increased power in the cortical source for faces versus scrambled face.

14.3 Relation Between Electroencephalography (EEG) and Magnetoencephalography (MEG)

While both EEG and MEG are used for mapping the brain signals, MEG is significantly better as it delivers an increased signal-to-noise ratio and also has more scalp based sensors in comparison to EEG, this allows MEG based reading to have greater spatial resolution and sensitivity [17].

In this study, the focus is on the EEG generated signals and their analysis due to its accessibility and inexpensive nature, which, while meaning that the scope of the analytical work may be reduced, at the same time allows for mobile as well as flexible deployment of the technique in lesser developed areas.

14.4 Applications of EEG

Understanding of the EEG signal provides insights into brain activity to formulate methods for physiological and psychological recovery to brain stimuli. Conversion of the brain signals to a digital format that may be construed by researchers has opened the gates for the use of all conventional techniques over EEG data. With the advancement in machine learning the recorded electrical activity of the brain may be interpreted using state-of-the-art algorithms to find patterns in the signal recorded. Classification and anomaly detection have paved the way for numerous healthcare applications. EEG data may assist in providing aid to the challenged persons and act as assistance in their specific needs.

14.4.1 Depth of Anaesthesia

Depth of anaesthesia provides a breakdown of the impact of the drug on the nervous system under clinical supervision [18]. The EEG signal of the brain electrical activity gives a descriptive view of the features of the drugs and their effect on the human body. The reading is taken at a scale of milliseconds. EEG provided an accurate report about body stimuli. Blood pressure and heart rate cannot be trusted completely during a surgical operation with regard to intraoperative consciousness as it may differ from person to person as per their medical condition. The neurophysiological parameters involved during the changeover from awake to deep anaesthesia must be carefully governed. EEG provides a comprehensive real-time analysis to facilitate this purpose.

14.4.2 Biometric Systems

Biometric systems are designed on individual physiological, physical characteristics such as fingerprint, iris, etc. [19]. In the current scenario the fingerprint-based biometric systems are prevalent however the EEG signals based on the mental task performed by an individual are reliable for the recognition system. Combining EEG signals with the existing security systems for recognition may further strengthen it and reduce the high dependence on a unique biological feature. The benefit biometric system based on EEG is that the brain signal may not be acquired at a distance. Thus being a challenge for replicating the signal artificially [20].

14.4.3 Physically Challenged

Physically challenged people who are incapable to use a joystick or keyboard required to operate the wheelchair may be provided assistance to walk through other means as witnessed in the past. So a much-sophisticated technique was developed using EEG [21]. The electrical activity of the brain is precisely sent as the command for controlling the wheelchair and reinforcing their movement.

14.4.4 Epilepsy

Epilepsy is a well known neurological disorder, affecting about 1% of the population. The sporadic nature of the onset of an epileptic episode may lead to serious implications due to the nature of these fits affecting the daily life of a patient. The prediction of the occurrence of such an episode is extremely useful for patients suffering from the said disorder as it allows us to prevent the seizures (ictal events) with the clinical methods like electric treatment or pharmacological [22, 23]. This is extremely beneficial for patients who have become resilient to drug-based treatments. Multiple methods for seizure prediction using EEG exist such as using hybrid feature selection [24] and using spatiotemporal correlation structure of intracranial EEG [25].

14.4.5 Alzheimer

Alzheimer's is a brain disease which diminishes reasoning and loss of memory over time. As Alzheimer's disease progresses, the brain tissues shrink. The clinical methods for the treatment are available in the form of drugs. However, the effectiveness of these drugs decreases with an increase in the severity of the disease. That is why early diagnosis helps in early recovery which might not be possible at later stages. Techniques like MRI and PET imaging are effective, though still developing and remain costly. On the contrary, EEG provides inexpensive means to the clinical community for an accurate diagnosis [26].

14.4.6 Brain Death

Brain-death analysis may be performed with EEG confirmatory test [27]. This clinical practice is relatively safe as recording and monitoring of EEG signals do not cause stress on other organs. The permanent loss of all brain and brainstem functions is referred to as brain death. As human life ends with brain death the clinical practices for the examination of brain death are also done using apnea test, brainstem reflexes test, pupil test and many others. EEG signals are registered continuously for a time and the positive response of the EEG test concludes that the brain is functioning.

14.4.7 Coma

Coma is a brain-state in which a person will have some brain activity whereas the brain-dead person does not show any response [27, 28].

Understanding the difference between the states of coma and brain death is crucial. Thus requiring an accurate and fast diagnosis. This diagnosis does not require unplugging the ventilator. Therefore it's safe.

EEG is helpful in providing us with valuable information with regard to the thalamocortical function in comatose patients when it is clinically inaccessible [29]. Continuous EEG observations on such patients may allow us to observe any potentially treatable conditions as well as analyze the effects of therapy. It may play a role in the establishment of a prognosis of possibly neuronal death-causing diseases.

14.5 Challenges

EEG signals in the brain are recorded in three major ways—non-invasive, invasive, intracortical. These represent the position of the electrodes in the brain and each of these methods must go through a tough risk evaluation before it is used for a particular purpose. Each of these has its own advantages and corresponding disadvantages.

The action potentials produced by neurons of the brain, decay exponentially with distance from its source of production. This implies that the EEG signals are dominated by the collective sum readings from major dominant neuron clusters whose fields add up and reach the electrodes on the scalp where the readings are collected via electrodes [30].

As tissues act as a natural low pass filter, The Non-invasive EEG signals are comprised of low-frequency Electrical signals (<=90 Hz) ignoring high-frequency Signal Fields [31].

EEG signals recorded via Non-Invasive EEG Caps are non-resistive to artifacts such as distortion of our collected EEG signal due to eye blinks and other frequent common human activities that depend on a person to person basis [32].

The invasive methodology is a more accurate and detailed data Collection Technique. Here the electrodes are placed directly on the brain of the subject. This is only possible by removing a part of the skull and then place the sophisticated electrodes on the top of the exposed brain with the help of surgeries. It becomes an Expensive as well as a tedious task [33].

As these electrodes are placed on the brain via surgery there is a chance of infections that may lead to potentially permanent damage to the brain [34]. Due to these reasons, there is a considerably low acceptance rate of invasive over the Non-Invasive technique [35].

The Intracortical Technique takes a step further than the invasive technique. Here the Electrodes are placed deep in the grey matter of the subject's brain and are used to record Electricals signals produced by Electrodes. These adds on both the benefits and challenges. As these electrodes are placed deep inside the Grey Matter, this destroys all obstructing neurons that come in the way of implementation [36].

Neurodegeneration is also a great risk in intracortical implantation which may lead from damage to complete death of neurons in the brain of the subject. Also, we face a Time-dependent degradation in the recording quality. This technique is prone to most clinical risks and should be implemented with great care and responsibility [31].

As the EEG data is highly non-stationary and non-linear and that too is prone to artifacts, one has to choose the most effective technique for feature extraction and selection that is itself a tedious task [37–39].

Brain-computer interface for a particular subject requires a lot of training for that particular subject which becomes unacceptably time-consuming for a practical system, hence not only the collection of data but also the training procedure must be planned and designed carefully.

EEG signals may be affected by the posture and mood of the subject. An upright posture tends to prove the focus of the subject and improve the quality of the EEG signals collected [40].

There is a difference between EEG signals of a healthy subject as compared to an unhealthy subject that has undergone some health issues hence while designing BCI's this factor should be taken care of [41, 42].

Overall the invasive technique is far more accurate in comparison with the non-invasive techniques as we have a far more accurate data as compared to the non-invasive techniques. But The non-invasive technique has an unignorable benefit of less complexity, cost-effectiveness and is also risk-free as compared to invasive Techniques.

Furthermore, a very crucial aspect that can't be neglected is the Social-Ethical Issues like privacy, mind reading and remote control, especially, this is much more vulnerable in invasive techniques as the Electrodes are embedded in the subject and collect data for an extended period of time.

14.6 Visual Stimuli Analysis

Python [43] alongside the third-party libraries such as "MNE" [44] have been used In order to read the data and process it as necessary.

Experiments were run on a computer with an Intel i5 processor running at 2.5 GHz using 8192 MB of RAM, running Windows version 10.0. The experiment is to analyze as well as visualize the brain responses to visual stimuli presented to them in the form of faces (familiar, unfamiliar and scrambled) (Multi-modal Face Dataset (SPM) [33].

The EEG signal recorded is cleaned by removing artifacts and unnecessary noise in the recording and studied with the help of various visualisation techniques. The cleaned EEG data may be fed into a machine learning for further exploration and classification. The processes are explained in detail in later sections.

The brain produces responses in certain areas upon receiving different forms of stimulus. Knowing which part of the brain is being activated during known stimuli is a very important form of diagnosis in the medical community, as it helps detect abnormalities and defects if the proper response is not initiated in the brain.

14.6.1 EEG Data Preprocessing

Preparing the data is necessary by filtering the raw data using a low and a high pass filter of 40 Hz and 1 Hz respectively.

In Fig. 14.1, the plotting of frequency (Hz) versus decibel (dB) shows the power spectral density of the data which helps us visualize all the channels in waveform with any abnormal power fluctuations caused by external factors.

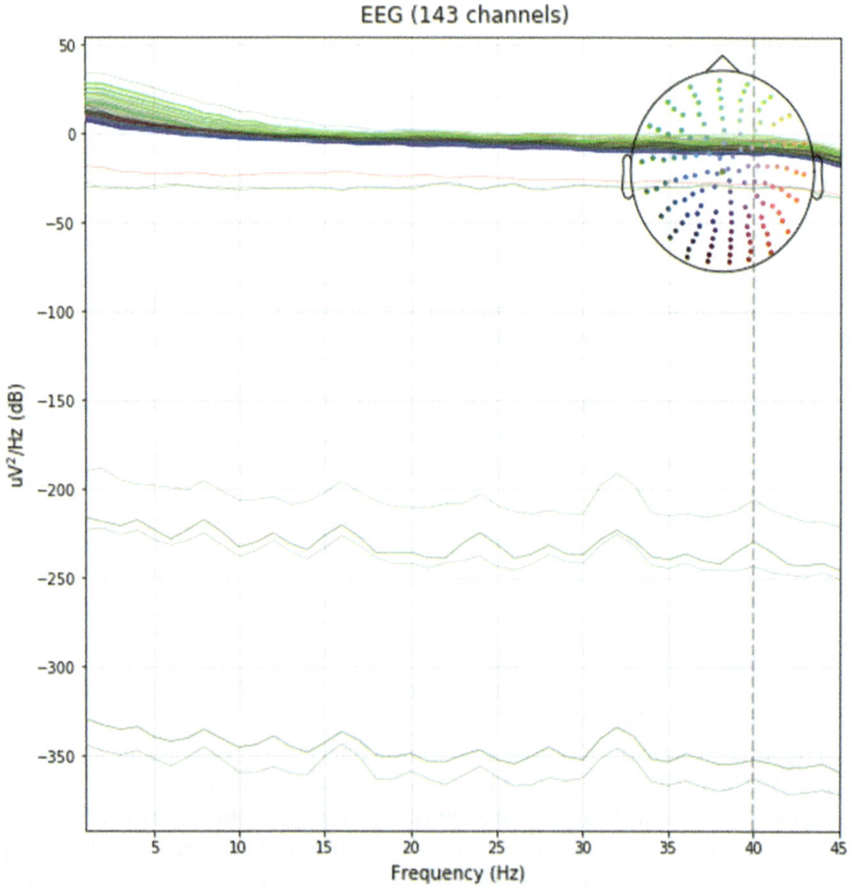

Fig. 14.1 Power spectrum density graph

14.6.2 Visualising the Data

Visualization is a key step to making the data human-understandable and hence analysable by medical professionals. The basic step of visualizing the data is to plot the raw signal data in a single EEG epoch.

In Fig. 14.2, the raw signals are plotted for the respective channels to understand the nature of the EEG recording. Although modern techniques like automatic classification using machine learning are useful, these data visualization techniques are useful for all medical practitioners.

In Fig. 14.3 equips to investigate the region of the brain active during the presence of the stimuli. Topological maps aid in finding the regions of activation during various time frames. The average evoked-response of the brain along with the topological maps helps in identifying the peaked response magnitude along with the time of occurrence and the position of activation as detected by the electrode sensor locations.

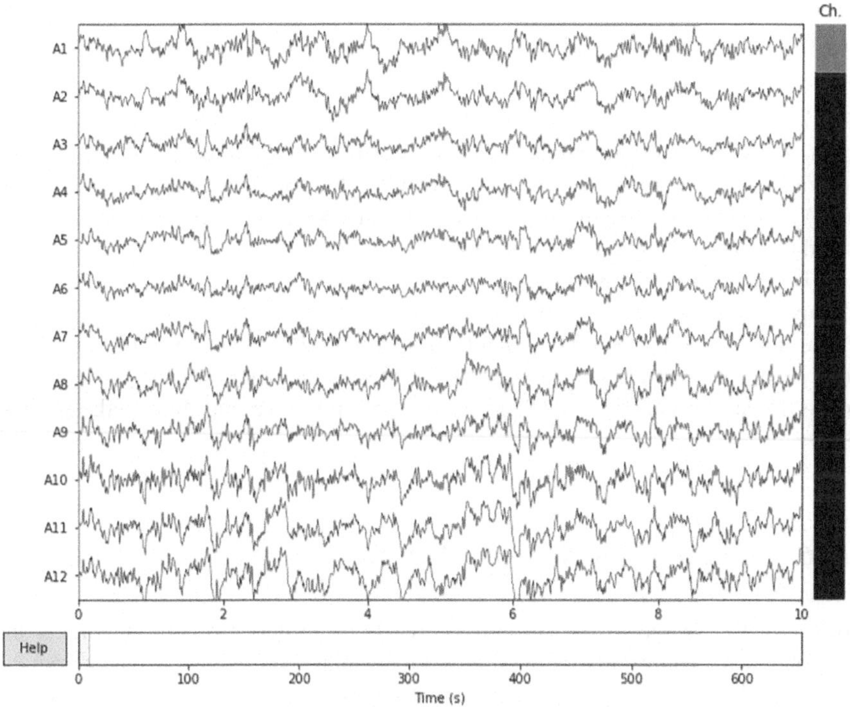

Fig. 14.2 Raw signals from the EEG channels

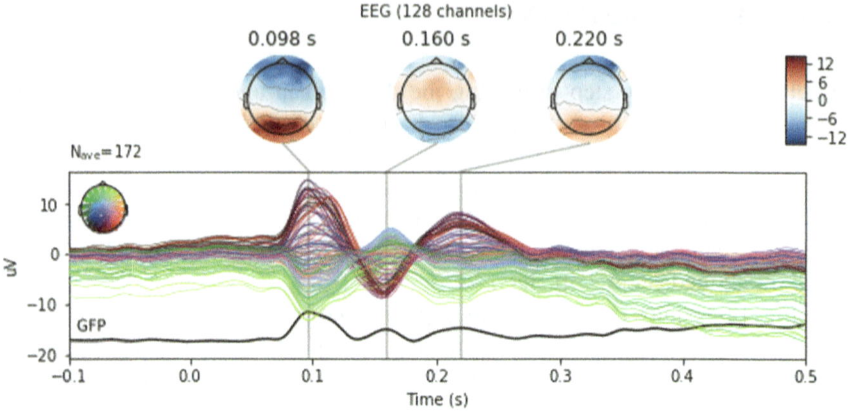

Fig. 14.3 Topological maps of the region of brain activity during the presence of the stimuli

14.6.3 Artifact Removal

EEG data, especially non-invasive EEG recordings pick up unwanted noise in the data. These noise in the data are known as artifacts, which are to be removed by various statistical methods. One such method is Independent Component Analysis (ICA). Through ICA we may remove various muscles and eye artifacts and clean up the data thus avoiding misclassification.

Using ICA, the multivariate (EEG) time series is split into separate additive subcomponents. The way ICA works is that it finds directions in the feature space corresponding to high non-Gaussianity projections. This decomposes the signal into independent components thus localizing the effect of the artifacts within these components. Detecting and removing these components minimizes the effect of the artifacts [45].

14.6.4 Locating the Response Source

Investing the source of the stimulus in the brain is performed by averaging the response across time and plotting it on a T1MR image, thus showing the anatomical region of the brain where the response is strongest.

In Fig. 14.4 the red area depicts that the occipital region (lower back) of the brain which is the most activated during the conduction of the experimental paradigm. The green area denotes the white matter of the brain. More such derivations and insights about the experiment and EEG signal may be obtained upon using the derived data to generate more visually explanatory plots.

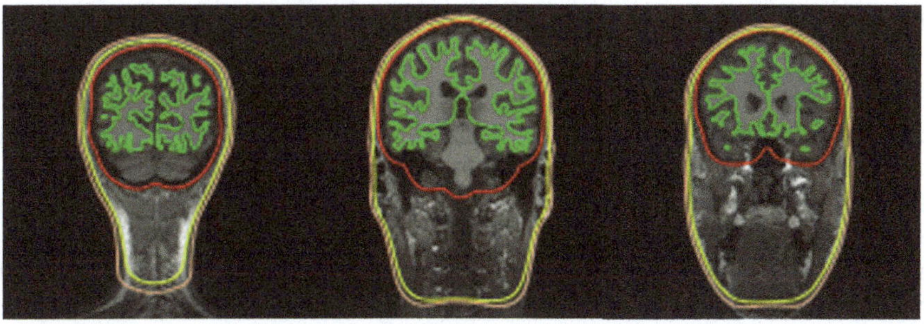

Fig. 14.4 T1MRI images of the brain with highlights on the regions of activation

In Fig. 14.5, breaking the responses into categories may show that familiar and unfamiliar faces do not produce responses in different parts of the brain but scrambled faces show a clear distinction in terms of activation in the brain that we may further segregate using multiple statistical techniques and gain better insight into the working of the visual cortex.

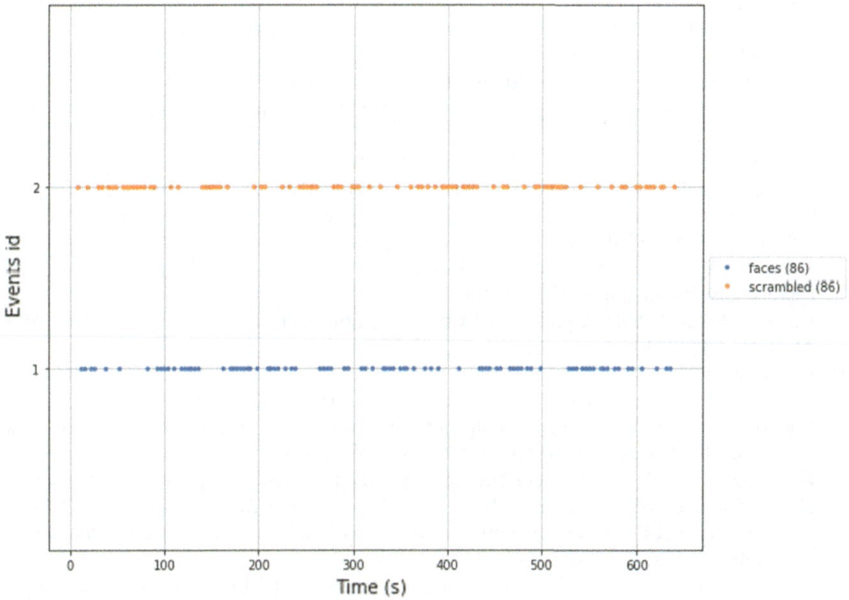

Fig. 14.5 The classification of scrambled versus unscrambled faces

14.7 Conclusion

In the contemporary era, the EEG based diagnosis contributes to the smart health care systems by offering a dynamic analysis of the data of a person. The realisation of the brain responses for the visual image stimuli provides a diagnosis of brain activity to be employed in clinical and therapeutic study. This work demonstrates that the EEG can be used as an efficient technique for brain signal analysis as it provides a flexible and variable usage. The future scope of this work shall entail the use of real-time data to gain a better understanding of the mental state of a patient and use it as a means for forming a prognosis for the given subject.

References

1. William, N., et al.: Cyclic variations in EEG during sleep and their relation to eye movements, body motility, and dreaming. Electroencephalogr. Clin. Neurophysiol. **9**(4), 673–690 (1957)
2. Niedermeyer, E., da Silva, F.L.: Electroencephalography: Basic Principles, Clinical Applications, and Related Fields. Lippincott Williams & Wilkins (2004)
3. Anderson, C.W., et al.: EEG signal classification with different signal representations. In: Proceedings of the 1995 IEEE Workshop on Neural Networks for Signal Processing, 31 Aug–2 Sept 1995
4. "PET Imaging". GE Healthcare. Archived from the original on 2012-05-04
5. "CT Scan (CAT Scan, Computerized Tomography) Imaging Procedure". MedicineNet. Retrieved 2018-11-29
6. Chou, I.: Milestone 19: (1990) Functional MRI. Nature. Retrieved 9 Aug 2013
7. Jana, G.C., et al.: Enhancing the performance of motor imagery classification to design a robust brain computer interface using feed forward back-propagation neural network. Ain Shams Eng. J. **9**(4), 2871–2878 (2018)
8. Wang, X.-W., et al.: Emotional state classification from EEG data using machine learning approach. Neurocomputing **129**, 94–106 (2014)
9. Lehnertz, K., et al.: Seizure prediction by nonlinear EEG analysis. IEEE Eng. Med. Biol. Mag. **22**(1), 57–63 (2003)
10. Pfurtscheller, G., et al.: EEG-based discrimination between imagination of right and left hand movement. Electroencephalogr. Clin. Neurophysiol. **103**(6), 642–651 (1997)
11. Vigario, R., et al.: Independent component approach to the analysis of EEG and MEG recordings. IEEE Trans. Biomed. Eng. **47**(5), 589–593 (2000)
12. Blankertz, B., et al.: The BCI competition 2003: progress and perspectives in detection and discrimination of EEG single trials. IEEE Trans. Biomed. Eng. **51**(6), 1044–1051 (2004)
13. Barry, R.J., et al.: EEG differences between eyes-closed and eyes-open resting conditions. Clin. Neurophysiol. **118**(12), 2765–2773 (2007)
14. Soleymani, M., Pantic, M.: Multimedia implicit tagging using EEG signals. In: 2013 IEEE International Conference on Multimedia and Expo (ICME) (2013)
15. Liu, J., et al.: Clinical decision support system for alcoholism detection using the analysis of EEG signals
16. Henson, R.N., et al.: Multimodal integration of M/EEG and f/MRI Data in SPM12. Front. Neurosci. **13** (2019)
17. Hall, E.L., et al.: The relationship between MEG and FMRI. NeuroImage **102**, 80–91 (2014)
18. Shalbaf, A., et al.: Monitoring the depth of anesthesia using a new adaptive neurofuzzy system. IEEE J. Biomed. Health Inf. **22**(3), 671–677 (2018)

19. Maiorana, E., et al.: On the permanence of EEG signals for biometric recognition. IEEE Trans. Inf. Forensics Secur. **11**(1), 163–175 (2016)
20. Das, R., et al.: EEG biometrics for user recognition using visually evoked potentials. In: 2015 International Conference of the Biometrics Special Interest Group (BIOSIG) (2015)
21. Turnip, A., et al.: Brain-controlled wheelchair based EEG-SSVEP signals classified by nonlinear adaptive filter. In: 2015 IEEE International Conference on Rehabilitation Robotics (ICORR) (2015)
22. Güttinger, M., et al.: Seizure suppression and lack of adenosine A1 receptor desensitization after focal long-term delivery of adenosine by encapsulated myoblasts. Exp. Neurol. **193**(1), 53–64 (2005)
23. Esteller, R., et al.: Comparison of line length feature before and after brain electrical stimulation in epileptic patients. The 26th Annual International Conference of the IEEE Engineering in Medicine and Biology Society
24. D'alessandro, M., et al.: Epileptic seizure prediction using hybrid feature selection over multiple intracranial eeg electrode contacts: a report of four patients. IEEE Trans. Biomed. Eng. **50**(8), 1041–1041 (2003)
25. Williamson, J.R., et al.: Epileptic seizure prediction using the spatiotemporal correlation structure of intracranial EEG. 2011 IEEE International Conference on Acoustics, Speech and Signal Processing (ICASSP) (2011)
26. Staudinger, T., Polikar, R.: Analysis of complexity based EEG features for the diagnosis of alzheimer's disease. 2011 Annual International Conference of the IEEE Engineering in Medicine and Biology Society (2011)
27. Chen, Z., et al.: An empirical EEG analysis in brain death diagnosis for adults. Cognitive Neurodyn. **2**(3), 257–271 (2008)
28. Cui, G., et al.: EEG analysis for differentiating between brain death and coma in humans. Int. J. Comput. Technol. **15**(11), 7189–7201 (2016)
29. Young, G.B.: The EEG in coma. J. Clin. Neurophysiol. **17**(5), 473–485 (2000)
30. Waldert, S. Invasive vs. non-invasive neuronal signals for brain-machine interfaces: will one prevail? Front. Neurosci. **10** (2016)
31. Waterstraat, G., et al.: Non-invasive single-trial EEG detection of evoked human neocortical population spikes. NeuroImage **105**, 13–20 (2015)
32. Ball, T., et al.: Signal quality of simultaneously recorded invasive and non-invasive EEG. NeuroImage **46**(3), 708–716 (2009)
33. Neuroimaging, Welcome Centre for Human. Multi-Modal Face Dataset. UCL. www.fil.ion.ucl.ac.uk/spm/data/mmfaces/
34. Ahmadian, P., et al.: How capable is non-invasive EEG data of predicting the next movement? A mini review. Front. Hum. Neurosci. **7** (2013)
35. Blabe, C.H., et al.: Assessment of brain-machine interfaces from the perspective of people with paralysis. J. Neural Eng. **12**(4), 043002 (2015)
36. Riera, A.: Invasive vs non-invasive EEG ready to become a cyborg? Blog Neuroelectrics (2015). www.neuroelectrics.com/blog/invasive-vs-non-invasive-eeg-ready-to-become-a-cyborg/
37. Ang, K.K., et al.: Filter bank common spatial pattern (FBCSP) in brain-computer interface. In: 2008 IEEE International Joint Conference on Neural Networks (IEEE World Congress on Computational Intelligence) (2008)
38. Tabar, Y.R., Halici, U.: A novel deep learning approach for classification of EEG motor imagery signals. J. Neural Eng. 14(1), 016003 (2016)
39. Yang, H., et al.: On the use of convolutional neural networks and augmented CSP features for multi-class motor imagery of EEG signals classification. In: 2015 37th Annual International Conference of the IEEE Engineering in Medicine and Biology Society (EMBC) (2015)
40. Caldwell, J.A., et al.: Body posture affects electroencephalographic activity and psychomotor vigilance task performance in sleep-deprived subjects. Clin. Neurophysiol. **114**(1), 23–31 (2003)
41. Cheng, D., et al.: Exploring motor imagery EEG patterns for stroke patients with deep neural networks. In: 2018 IEEE International Conference on Acoustics, Speech and Signal Processing (ICASSP) (2018)

42. Hara, Y.: Brain plasticity and rehabilitation in stroke patients. J. Nippon Med. Sch. **82**(1), 4–13 (2015)
43. Welcome to Python.org. Python.org. www.python.org/
44. MNE–MNE 0.19.dev0 Documentation. www.nmr.mgh.harvard.edu/mne/dev/
45. "Artifact Correction with ICA." Artifact correction with ICA—MNE 0.18.2 documentation. www.nmr.mgh.harvard.edu/mne/stable/auto_tutorials/preprocessing/plot_artifacts_correction_ica.html#sphx-glr-auto-tutorials-preprocessing-plot-artifacts-correction-ica-py

Chapter 15
Securing the Internet of Things: Current and Future State of the Art

Sharmistha Roy, Prashant Pranav and Vandana Bhattacharjee

Abstract Internet of Things (IoT) is an emerging area of research and has attracted many researchers because of its potential use in diversified fields of social life viz. healthcare, agriculture, home and industrial automation, etc. Internet of Things is a connection of devices having sensors for collection of data from physical world, sharing information through reliable communication channel for making devices act smartly in real life system. With the increase in the number of IoT devices there is a proportional growth of data which leads to numerous security and privacy risks. Thus, assuring security features and protection mechanism is of high concern and talk of the scientific world. This paper aims to present state-of-the-art research relating to various IoT features, its architecture, security features and mechanisms, the security threats that have emerged from IoT, different mechanisms to provide a secure working environment to an IoT system, the research work in progress in the domains of security and challenges that are faced in IoT systems. Since, healthcare system is a very sensitive field, thus failure of IoT applications in medical field is of utmost importance and highly significant. Thus, this paper aims to address security issues, requirements and various secure mechanisms that can be adopted to provide a secure healthcare system.

Keywords Internet of Things (IoT) · Security · IoT features · Smart healthcare system · Security requirements · Security mechanism · RFID · Attacks · Security issues

15.1 Introduction

We are living in the new era of digital communication and technology where Internet of Things (IoT) is a buzzword and is considered as an emerging area of research. Presently the use of Internet is increasing exponentially thus making significant

S. Roy (✉) · P. Pranav
Faculty of Computing and Information Technology, Usha Martin University, Ranchi, India

V. Bhattacharjee
Department of Computer Science and Engineering, BIT Mesra, Ranchi, India
e-mail: vbhattacharya@bitmesra.ac.in

P. K. Pattnaik et al. (eds.), *Smart Healthcare Analytics in IoT Enabled Environment*, Intelligent Systems Reference Library 178,
https://doi.org/10.1007/978-3-030-37551-5_15

changes in the daily life of people. Earlier days people used to communicate among each other by sending letters which took up to several days to reach. However, the Internet has reduced the communication time by sending emails, WhatsApp and Facebook posts, various tweets which get delivered to the recipients anywhere in this world within a fraction of seconds. Internet of Things is one such invention in this digital world which not only reduces time but also make daily life of people much more efficient and convenient. Internet of Things is a revolution to this world which connects any physical objects or devices to the Internet, having the capability to capture information from the physical world, sharing those captured information between other terminals, computing power which results in designing devices to perform intelligently. As per the statistical record of Statista [1], the number of devices connected to the Internet will gradually increase from 26.66 billion in 2019 to 75.44 billion in 2025. Internet of Things has a wide range of applications starting from smart home, smart city, smart agriculture and perhaps the most important smart healthcare. Internet of Things enabled medical applications is an essential requirement for providing better and up-to-date medical facilities for the patients, with the ability to also be provided remotely [2]. Keeping in view the increasing population rate, rise in chronic diseases and constraint in the medical facilities, IoT is a boon for the healthcare system which provides high quality medical care to the patients [3]. Figure 15.1 shows IoT devices present in real world.

Internet of Things technology comprises of several components which includes RFID readers, sensors for capturing data from the physical world, wireless technologies for communication and sharing of data among the devices, storage facility, computing and processing power to provide various applications and services. Apart from these, with the fast growth of IoT devices and applications, there is also a need for privacy and security mechanisms to enable a secure IoT system [4]. With the increasing number of threats and vulnerabilities, there is a basic need for designing systems to provide basic security features, allow data to flow securely between

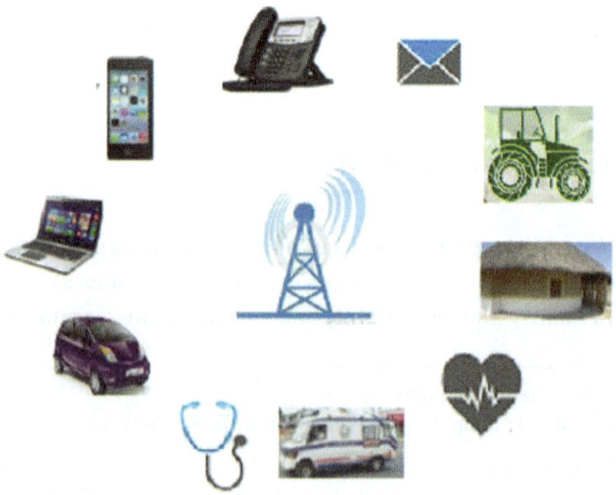

Fig. 15.1 Internet of Things in real world

devices and also have the capability to detect new threats. Since, healthcare is a crucial system, thus it is very essential to share patients data confidentially among the devices and designing vulnerability-proof smart healthcare system [5].

This paper mainly focuses on the privacy and security concerns of the smart healthcare system. The paper is organized as follows. Section 2 gives the concept and basic characteristic features of IoT system. Section 3 discusses the different layers of IoT architecture. Section 4 focuses on the various security features and requirements. Section 6 highlights on the known security threats and vulnerabilities that can affect healthcare system. Section 7 discusses the various security mechanisms and algorithms that can detect threats. Several researchers are working on the security issues of IoT enabled system which are discussed in Sect. 8. Section 9 describes the security challenges and issues for IoT enabled system. Finally, conclusions and future scope of work is presented in Sect. 10.

15.2 Concepts and Basic Characteristics of Internet of Things

The marvelous benefits provided by IoT system have made it highly popular and in demand in every field. The potential use of Internet of Things in healthcare system is in very early stage, but it is still being explored and several initiatives have been undertaken towards developing smart healthcare systems.

Internet of Things is the interconnection of devices that has the capability to collect information from real world, share among the devices, perform computation and act intelligently. IoT is having basic four components such as [6]:

Comprehensive perception. IoT enabled devices includes physical equipments such as RFID readers, sensors which can gather information from physical world. Moreover, IoT devices also support Machine-to-Machine (M2M) communications.

Heterogeneous network access. IoT devices support connection among diversified computing devices having wired/wireless networks using different access technologies.

Reliable communication. The main objective of IoT enabled devices is to provide reliable and trustworthy transmission of data among the devices. Various encryption algorithms and security protocols are available to provide reliable transmission of data with high accuracy.

Smart processing. IoT devices have the capability to compute intelligently using soft computing techniques and cloud computing technology, thus can analyze collected information to meet demands of users.

To understand the concept of IoT and their need for privacy and security requirements, we have discussed several features of IoT which are categorized in Fig. 15.2 [7]:

Interdependence. Internet of Things is a collection of multiple devices, thus Interdependence among various devices is there. Controlling of one device or environment

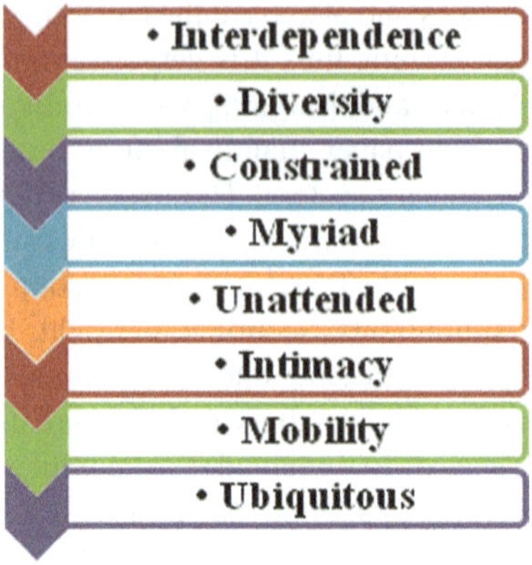

Fig. 15.2 Feature of Internet of Things

behavior using several other devices is known as interdependence. Security mechanism is very much essential for enabling dependencies among various devices so as to avoid any malicious activities.

Diversity. Internet of Things is spread across diversified applications having different physical environment, different networking protocols. Thus, many applications are dependent on the cloud platforms which provide physical resources and software applications on demand basis to manage different IoT devices. At the same time, due to diversified applications, they are also vulnerable to different security threats. Thus, there is requirement of Intrusion Detection System (IDS) and Intrusion Prevention System (IPS) to protect variety of attacks.

Constrained. Shortage of memory area, less computational ability, limited power supply and delay in transmission of data on real time processes are the constraints of the IoT enabled devices. Due to these constraints there is huge probability of security attacks and vulnerabilities to IoT enabled systems. Hence, security mechanisms are undertaken for providing security to those devices with such limited resources.

Myriad. The number of IoT enabled devices is increasing gradually which also lead to generation of enormous amount of data which is described as myriad. IoT devices are built in such a manner that they do not have safety test mechanism to detect vulnerabilities and malware. Thus, various researchers have carried out research work to develop secure algorithms that can distinguish malicious activities from the legitimate ones in the communication network.

Unattended. Many IoT devices in the field of healthcare system, agricultural fields, and military regions remain disconnected from the external interface for a longer time period i.e. the devices remain unattended. However, the devices have to perform effectively even in that unattended situation. Hence, it requires certain security mechanisms to detect whether the devices have been attacked remotely or not.

Intimacy. Intimacy is one of the necessary feature of IoT devices which helps to establish relationship between users and IoT devices by collecting information from the environment and users which are nearby the IoT devices. However, intimacy can be misutilized by the attackers which may compromise security and privacy issues of the devices.

Mobility. Mobility is one of the beneficial features of IoT devices which enable them to move around and communicate with neighboring devices. At the same time, this feature also helps the attackers to inject malicious program into the IoT devices which may release sensitive information to the hackers. Enabling the IoT devices to change configuration dynamically by following the security conditions and measures may help the mobility feature from being compromised.

Ubiquitous. Day-to-day life of all human being in near future is surely to be ruled by many IoT devices, which describes the ubiquitous nature of IoT devices. The increasing number of IoT devices owned by a human being may create security management problem. Users may not be aware of the security issues and configuration of every device. Thus, manufacturers have to minutely focus on the security measures of the IoT devices during its configuration.

Here we have summarized some of the features of IoT and necessary security mechanisms which may be undertaken for ensuring secure IoT devices.

15.3 IoT Architecture

The fundamental idea behind Internet of Things is to behave as an intelligent system that has the basic three characteristics namely information gathering, reliable data transmission and intelligent computation. These three characteristics are categorized in three different layers as shown in Fig. 15.3 and discussed [8]:

Perception Layer. It is the lowest level layer of IoT architecture which consists of RFID reader, sensors, barcode readers as objects for collecting necessary information from the physical world and converts this information into digital signal and then transfer to network layer through M2M terminal.

Network Layer. This is the middle level layer of IoT architecture which is ubiquitous in nature, and consists of networking infrastructure and communications protocols

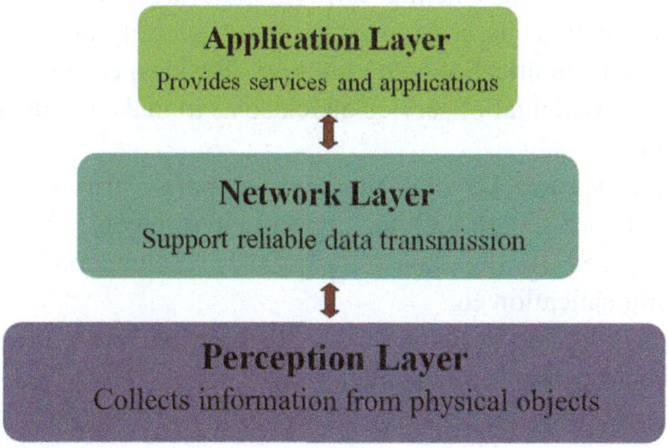

Fig. 15.3 Various layers of IoT architecture

for reliable data transmission. Various types of networks can be used such as Internet, wireless network, mobile networks for essential transfer of information between the devices.

Application Layer. This is the top most layer of IoT architecture which provides social, technical, professional services according to users need. This layer consists of various computing platforms for performing intelligent computing. This layer acts as the interface between users and IoT devices through various applications.

Providing security in each layer of IoT architecture is a challenging task and thus requires lots of effort for real-time implementation.

15.4 Security Features and Security Requirements of an IoT System

An IoT system is vulnerable to various types of security threats and requires incorporating numerous security features [9]. This section is going to describe various security features and necessary requirements for providing security and privacy in different layers of IoT architecture [10].

Perception Layer. This layer consists of various sensors and RFID devices having less power supply and restricted memory space. Thus, it is difficult to apply encryption algorithm and other secure protocols. In absence of such secure algorithms the devices lack necessary security principles like confidentiality, integrity, authentication etc.

Perception layer requires physical security for the objects present and for secure data collection. Thus, necessary security mechanisms are required such as authentication mechanism for avoiding illegal access.

Network Layer. This layer is susceptible to viral attack, illegal access, denial of service attack, man-in-the-middle attack and various security issues while transmitting data from one terminal to another. IoT devices require transmission of bulk of information through M2M terminal which creates network congestion, preventing timely data transmission.

Integrating existing cryptographic algorithm in communication layer is still a research. Thus, it requires necessary security algorithms to provide confidentiality, user authentication, data integrity. Besides, cryptographic protocols are required to remove denial of service attack so as to make the data available to intended devices and users.

Application Layer. This layer supports various kinds of services which require different secure architecture and environment. Different security mechanisms are required in this layer for privacy protection, access control, key agreement, authentication etc.

Providing necessary authentication protocols and key agreement algorithms for heterogeneous IoT applications is one of the security requirements for application layer. Moreover, privacy preservation and data protection are also necessary security requirements [11].

15.5 Security Threats in an IoT System: Current and Future Scenario

The importance of the Internet of Things (IoT) is growing rapidly with the reliance of one and all on the use of the internet and smart devices for day to day use. However, the malicious activists keep on trying their luck on every growing technology for fulfilling their unprecedented acts. So, the race to keep up with the security challenges of strongly and smartly connected devices is rapidly gaining momentum. The connected devices share mutual bonding and they exhaustively send and receive data to each other upon recognition. This sharing of data is done without the use of any protection and identification protocol. Breaching into the security channels of the IoT devices may result in physical harm to the communicating devices and human and in the worst case, the loss of life. In recent years, the security issues of IoT have sparked controversy and the use of IoT for a smart living has embroiled debates across the globe. The most common security threats include but are not limited to: hijacks, leaks, home intrusion and unsecured devices.

Routers, printers, thermostats, refrigerators, webcams are some of the devices connected to the IoT. Smart locks, smart watches and many more such gadgets also use in one way or the other, the power of the IoT. These are the devices we carry with us or wear. Amazon Alexa and Google Assistant which uses Artificial Intelligence are some home automation hubs using IoT. In the coming ages, there will be more and more devices connected to the IoT. With this growing wave of devices and gadgets deploying IoT, the need of security mechanism to protect these devices is even greater than what we can think of. Some of the most common security threats as of now which have or will gain momentum in the coming ages are listed below:

IoT Botnet Attacks. In the year 2016, the internet was brought down due to one of the severe attacks on the IoT. Most prominent of the IoT devices viz. routers and IP cameras were breached by Mirai Botnet. A botnet is a collection of internet connected computers that are controlled remotely by some outside party. The data of some IoT devices were hacked and the devices were transferred to the botnet. The centrally controlled IoT botnets flooded the traffic of a DNS provider, Dyn, which eventually deprived millions of users worldwide, the access of the internet.

IoT Devices sending Spams. Smart devices used in home automation such as smart locks and smart refrigerators have the computing power and functionality of a modern tablet. This led the attackers to use the smart devices as email servers and further utilize the power of these appliances to send thousands of spam emails without the owners of the devices being aware of the mischief.

The Shodan IoT Search Engine. The Shodan search engine has been revealing quite a few security flaws with the main focus on Australia. John Matherly, the developer of Shodon, wrote a few years back, how Telstra media, configured networking devices such as wireless routers running a popular IoT suite, OpenSSH with a same shared key on more than 50,000 devices. A hacker equipped with remote management of routers can easily break into the automation system by taking the advantage of same key.

Privacy Leaks. Trained hackers can utilize the leakage of IP addresses from unsecured IoT devices and can cause considerable amount of damage by accurately locating the residential address of the users. The use of VPN on the router for encrypting all the traffic through a specific ISP has been proposed by experts to counter these types of threats.

Unsecured Devices. These threats are most harmful which are proceeding in a gradual and subtle way. The device manufactures are partly involved in such threats as when the smart devices are shipped with a default username and password, the consumers cannot be solely expected to change the password to a reasonably strong one without a proper documented referenced materials.

Home Intrusions. This is the scariest threat. As discussed above, the unsecured devices broadcast IP addresses, which may be known through the Shodan searches and hackers can make use of this drawback, to locate proper addresses and sell the gathered information to outside criminal outfits.

Remote Vehicle Hijacking. Imagine the consequences of a remote hacker getting full access to a moving vehicle. So, the threat remains on how to prevent these smartly monitored cars from being hijacked. Automobile market is paying close attention to fix this vulnerability.

Experts and IT professionals are continuously examining security threats and measures to thwart the vulnerabilities. They have advised managers, engineers and developers to first follow a risk assessment of the devices in order to determine and prioritize their security issues. The Fig. 15.4 [12] depicts the risk assessment

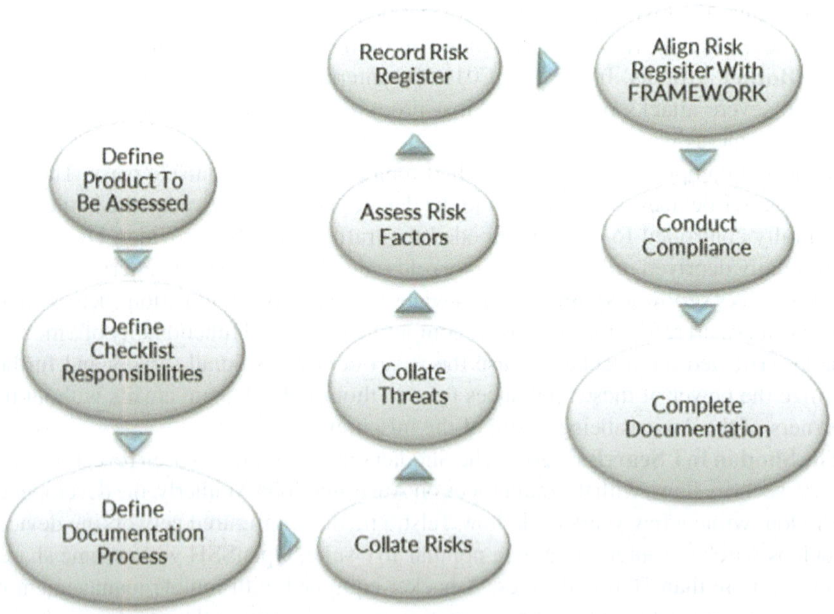

Fig. 15.4 Risk assessment process [12]

framework. The process endorses a proper supervision of device lifecycle starting from the manufacturing phase to its end of service. In order to deny any security issue of the device, it will be beneficial to insert a security checkpoint at each step of the device development life cycle.

15.6 Security of IoT Enabled Healthcare System

IoT enabled Healthcare system has the potential to reduce the cost, improve health quality, has the ability to monitor remotely, and enable smooth and continuous functioning of the medical devices. Providing effective, secure and trust worthy architecture and communication channel is still an area of research. In an healthcare system, data required are collected from patients which needs to be sent through secure communication channel that supports confidentiality, authentication and prevents any security attacks. Secure smart healthcare system is basically client-server architecture. Patients are the clients who are responsible for data acquisition and the server is stored in the cloud which stores the data acquired from the clients. Client system consists of sensor nodes which collects data from patients such as blood pressure, sugar level, heart rate, pulse rate etc. Since the sensor nodes are mobile in nature and have limited storage capacity and computing facility, thus the acquired data are transmitted through secure channel to the server. Transmission can be done through wired or wireless mode. However, this transmission channel should have basic security principles like confidentiality, integrity, authentication and availability. The server machine should have the storage facility, provides data management and security. Data can be stored in audio, video, structured, semi-structured, un-structured data and many more. Data management is required for efficient searching, analysis and predictions. And data security is essential for encryption of data, assigning security rights and roles, prevents different types of attacks, enables access control mechanism and backup recovery. Since, IoT devices are vulnerable to security threats and attacks, thus secure IoT based smart healthcare system is a mandatory one.

15.7 Security Mechanisms in an IoT System: Current State of the Art

Because of varied devices working as a unit and many a communication protocols in an IoT system, implementation of traditional security measures for an IoT system is not sufficient and possible. The Open Web Application Security Projects (OWASP), suggests three different layers of an IoT system namely hardware, communication links and interfaces/services. Hence, the implementation of IoT security mechanism at all the three levels as shown in Fig. 15.5, is deemed fit for the overall security of an IoT system.

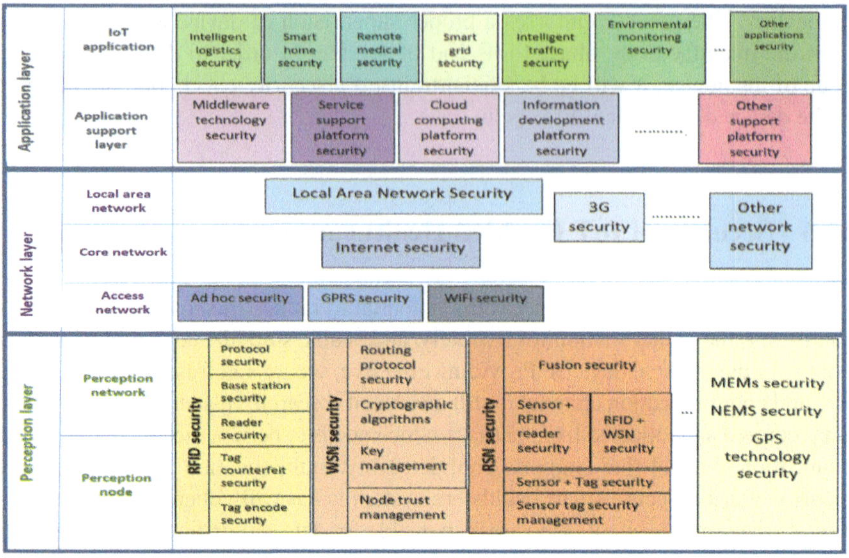

Fig. 15.5 Security mechanism at different layers of an IoT system [13]

The main objectives of a security mechanism in an IoT system are to:

- Provide privacy
- Confidentiality of data
- Provide security to the end users
- Provide security to the devices
- Guarantee the availability of the services offered by the system.

Current research trends suggest that authentication is still the most popular technology for ensuring security in an IoT system. Trust management is also gaining popularity followed by low cost encryption for a lightweight device.

Authentication. Authentication is the way by which users and devices are identified and monitored over an insecure communication channel and the required access is granted to authorized users and devices only. Some of the well known attacks in an IoT system such as Man-in-the middle attack, impersonating attack and reply attack can be overcome through the deployment of a proper authentication mechanism. Authentication is still the most popular technology for granting access to users at application layer and also to devices. Recently, the demand for lightweight authentication is gaining momentum to be used in low-cost and low-power devices such as RFID.

Encryption. It is the mechanism by which the transmitted data is converted into an unreadable format-cipher text at the sender device. In case of an IoT system, the transmitting nodes are encrypted. Conventional cryptographic protocols are not suitable for achieving encryption in an IoT system. Due to the requirement of an IoT system to be constrained in terms of power and resources, the traditional used cryptographic protocols such as AES, RSA, Blowfish are not suitable for encrypting the nodes of an IoT system. So, the demand for a lightweight encryption protocol is on increase. PRESENT is one such protocol most widely used for the purpose of encryption of smart devices. Other notable lightweight encryption protocols include AESL (where 'l' stands for lightweight), HEIGHT, and TEA.

Trust Management. Trust management's aim is to identify and remove vulnerable nodes and to provide access control securely. Current trends of research in this field include trust calculation where the trust values of participating nodes in an IoT system is verified and validated in an automatic and dynamic way. Most of the researches till date have covered only identifying the malicious nodes and only a few trust based access control mechanism have been proposed. Trust evaluation is very less used as of now as a security mechanism, but is a very powerful security mechanism for an IoT system due to its ability to calculate a node's trust score dynamically and henceforth ensure a secure communication.

Secure Routing. The most important elements in an IoT network are sensors and actuators, which are prone to security issue due to the possibility of IP leak. Most of the sensors and routers used in an IoT system are low-power, resource constrained and besides sharing information they can also store the data and perform some computations. IoT network uses IPv6 due to the large connections of devices in the system. Due to the lack of authentication at IPv6 layer, there is a possibility of security breach. Some of the mechanism for securing routers and sensors focuses on building protocols for establishing point to pint and multipoint communication in the network of connected devices. One such protocol is RPL (low power and lossy network protocol), which is specifically designed for devices having constrained in power and resource.

Besides the above discussed mechanism two new technologies namely Blockchain and SDN (Software Defined Network) are prominently researched in the field of security solutions to an IoT system. SDN deals with problem of resource alloca tion in an IoT device by formulating the idea of separate network control and data control which ensures both centralized control and dynamic management of the network. Blockchains, the backbone of cryptocurrency will allow the IoT system to take advantage of its secure transactions and its decentralization of communication and processes.

15.8 Current Research Trends Related to IoT Security

A survey of literatures in the area of IoT security shows an upward increment in developing mechanism for authentication and encryption. The survey is presented below in Tables 15.1 and 15.2. Table 15.1 shows the trends of the literatures with respect to the methodology used and results achieved. Table 15.2 shows the benefits, limitations and future scope of the existing methodologies.

Table 15.1 Literature survey: introduction, methodology and result analysis

Title	Introduction	Methodology	Result
THE CONSUMER SECURITY INDEX FOR INTERNET OF THINGS (Lot): A PROTOCOL FOR DEVELOPING AND IMPROVING CONSUMER DECISION MAKING AND TO INCENTIVIZE GREATER SECURITY PROVISION IN Lot DEVICES [14]	Consumer Security Index is used for secure decision making in IoT devices. The index is developed in coordination with consumers and security experts. With the use of focus groups handled by IoT security experts, many studies were conducted. Security features required by consumers were identified by one study and other uses an online hiring formulated consumer preferences	Seven participants with the expertise on IoT security were selected and a Nominal Group Technique (NGT) is used for formal consensus development	Findings suggest that- data collection from security experts as well as consumers helps in formulating valuable information in terms of labeling the security requirement of these groups. The first label is systematically developed many groups such as retailers, government and others. An analytical inclusion with regards to communicating information to users about crime prevention in the manuals
ON DEMAND SECURITY CONFIGUIRATION FOR IoT DEVICES [15]	An on demand configuration of security features is proposed in the paper which can include security features as and when required without hampering the device image	Configuring security functions and generating device image Generation of device image is done by collecting many sets of Security profiles (SPs) for the device in question through the help of other devices having same hardware features same as the incorporating device. Once the analysis of SPs are done, functional modules was identified after analyzing security functional modules of these profiles while keeping in check the function dependencies among different profiles. Once these two are collected, a configuration map of the whole SFM was calculated	The technique proposed guarantees the creation and configuration of a device image for the configuration of real time security. The proposed security profiles can be used to collect information and reassess the reliability of the modules

(continued)

Table 15.1 (continued)

Title	Introduction	Methodology	Result
SOLVING THE SECURITY CHALLENGES OF loT WITH PUBLIC KEY CRYPTOGRAPHY [16]	The advancement in the computational powers of cyber criminals make them even more innovative in finding ways to break into devices for their own uses. The paper shows the role of PKC to solve security issues in n IoT system	An identity-based public key cryptography viz MIKEY-SAKKE is used as a cryptographic tool. The used protocol enables organizations to manage their own independent key management server (KMS) platform	The result shows that the devices can work with each others as well as the system with the use of MIKEY-SAKKE technology. The developed products employing these technologies can be used across sectors providing a better degree of security
DATA SECURITY OF SMART CITIES [17]	The flow of data exchange between the connected devices of a smart city and users is described in order to identify the rule behind these exchanges	The methodologies used include many cases such development of technologies bricks to secure data by label products and their services	The data given by device are reliable and authentic once it is identified. The device cannot perform any action without proper notification
INTERNET-OF-THINGS SECURITY AND VULNERABILITIES:TAXONOMY,CHALLENGES AND PRACTICE [18]	Some security attacks in the devices connected through the IoT system are discussed and rules formulating and classifying are developed based on the application domain and defining architecture of the system. architecture	The used methods include providing authentication and encryption at all the 4 layers of the IoT security architecture	Security threats and concerns of privacy were developed and identified at each layer of an IoT system
REMOTE SECURITY MANAGEMENT SERVER FOR loT DEVICES [19]	The paper seeks to propose a mechanism to improve safety of connected devices by deploying a functional architecture for security management remotedly	The securing of IPs of the devices is suggested by securing remote servers. The main method is to secure the overall communication channel in the IoT distributed environment	Devices connected through the IoT network provide enhanced security and breaching into devices is shown to be formidable

(continued)

Table 15.1 (continued)

Title	Introduction	Methodology	Result
A SECURE MULTI –HOP ROUTING FOR IoT COMMUNICATION [20]	The paper instigates a multi-hop routing protocol which in turn validates the communication in secured devices in an IoT system. The routing protocol authenticates devices before joining any other device in the network	Network security of IoT devices are tested by two sets of experiments namely Field test1 (indoor) Computer Data Center and Field test 2 (outdoor) Water Filtration Plant on three security parameters. UCID scheme was developed for time sensitivity on IoT device. Synchronization of IoT devices is done using NTP (network time protocol) server	Analysis of the test results suggest that the SMRP produces a secured multi-hop IoT communication and that too without the cost of degradation in the system performances
BLOCKCHAIN MECHANISM FOR IoT SECURITY [21]	This paper underlines IoT environments where Block Chain Mechanisms (BCMs) plays a vital role with an emphasis that blockchains are only part of security solutions of an IoT network	The transmission of the data and transaction over an IoT network can be done by using the methodology deployed by a blockchain. The blockchains are in themselves unbreakable and the use of the mechanism in an IoT system further solidifies the network	Results suggests that block chains can be used at the lower layer of the communications model to provide cohesion for information carry over a chained links
A FULL STACK FOR QUICK PROTOTYPING FOR IoT SOLUTIONS [22]	The paper seeks to represents a novel approach for prototyping devices connected strongly in an IoT network	The methods used include developing a specific prototype for connected devices which allows the developers focus on the product functionality instead of security issues	The propound solution permits to speed up the prototyping and allows more strain on coding the devices functionality
THREE DIMENSIONAL VORONOI DIAGRAM-BASED SELF DEPLOYMENT ALGORITHM IN IoT SENSOR NETWORKS [23]	Authors deployed an algorithm for 3D WSNs on the basis of Voronoi diagram. The features of adjacency as well as rapid partitioning are employed	The algorithm utilizes the benefits of Voronoi diagram to become aware of the facts of a 3D division and monitoring is carried out in a faster way	Analysis shows that performance of the algorithm can be achieved by using similar nodes by increasing the coverage ratio of the algorithm

Table 15.2 Literature survey: advantages, disadvantages and future scope

Title	Advantages	Disadvantages	Future scope
THE CONSUMER SECURITY INDEX FOR INTERNET OF THINGS (IoT): A PROTOCOL FOR DEVELOPING AND IMPROVING CONSUMER DECISION MAKING AND TO INCENTIVIZE GREATER SECURITY PROVISION IN IoT DEVICES [14]	Coordination of research can be done with the collaboration of customers and experts Integration of consumers into the design process provides a better degree of self realization to a consumer in the terms of product usage	The proposed approach is having the drawbacks as it relies on the consumer's hypothetical engagement with the label The study outline represents the initial development of the CSI but a proper understanding must be carried on solidify the consumers purchase behavior	Further research can be done on the findings of the research to disseminate on the public and wider community through IoT UK
ON DEMAND SECURITY CONFIGUIRATION FOR IoT DEVICES [15]	The feature allows consumers to be realistic about the security functionalities of the device they use. The on time monitoring of security issues further enhances their reliability on the device	Lack of experience in challenges related to IoT security may speed up as proper security features are not prepared in robust way	Research on efforts to identify problems on OS for security and configuration management in an IoT system
SOLVING THE SECURITY CHALLENGES OF IoT WITH PUBLIC KEY CRYPTOGRAPHY [16]	The proposal of network-agnostic mode to secure data in an IoT system may address some of the security challenges in an IoT system	The growth of IoT into a complex eco-system, the main procedure is just limited to securing the networks managing the operated IoT devices	Requirement of a security solution beyond PKC, which can be simple, less costly and effective
DATA SECURITY OF SMART CITIES [17]	The paper suggests that accessing and responding to threats in a smart city must be accompanied through a proper risk management process. A proper restoration plan must be carried out in order to reduce the chances of damage	The paper introduces a formulation of a risk assessment and management protocol for avoiding the damages in the connected devices	The result shows that the formulation of the procedure for risk management and assessment cat each step of the device development can enhance the security of the device and henceforth ensure the users that the devices connected are free from any bugs

(continued)

Table 15.2 (continued)

Title	Advantages	Disadvantages	Future scope
INTERNET-OF-THINGS SECURITY AND VULNERABILITIES:TAXONOMY,CHALLENGES AND PRACTICE [18]	The paper studies in depth the security issues and vulnerabilities in an IoT system	Some of the special challenges of an IoT such as communication through a channel, data protection are discussed in depth and protocols for handling such issues have been proposed	Further research is deemed for developing an architecture that best fits into the security mechanism of an IoT network
REMOTE SECURITY MANAGEMENT SERVER FOR IoT DEVICES [19]	In remote security management server various security functions are integrated, comprehensive and systematically provided. This eliminates security threats and vulnerabilities of IoT devices enhancing the securities and safety of IoT devices	Security management functions for existing IoT devices are rarely provided or only a few functions such as device authentication are still vulnerable to week levels	Research on to obstruct and prevent various infringements incidents that may occur in the IoT environment by using systematic remote management function in advance
A SECURE MULTI –HOP ROUTING FOR IoT COMMUNICATION [20]	A proposal of multi hop routing protocol secures the IPs provide by the service provider which ensures the users that same IPs for many devices connected through the network can be avoided	All the IoT devices cannot provide a service because of resource limitations within each device. Further, it only focuses on securing the channel through which the devices communicate	Further focus can be done on securing the devices and network used for IoT system
BLOCKCHAIN MECHANISM FOR IoT SECURITY [21]	The feature of the blockchains that it cannot be broken as of now can be employed to the IoT security which ensures providing security at lower level of the layered architecture of the IoT systems	Due to the complexity with which a blockchain works, it may be very tough to implement a full blockchain security mechanism to the IoT infrastructure	Further research may be done on developing a secured blockchain based architecture which may be suitable for lightweight applications

(continued)

Table 15.2 (continued)

Title	Advantages	Disadvantages	Future scope
A FULL STACK FOR QUICK PROTOTYPING FOR loT SOLUTIONS [22]	Advantages of programming with the approach include a very lightweight approach which includes (i) coding in Python or Hybrid C/Python which captures very less memory of the network	It is significant noting that a lot of operational load is encountered due the connection in both the directions through the Zerynth ADM in scenarios when the algorithm is to deal with hundreds and thousands of devices	Future work will be directed towards (1) Extension in the number of supported RTOS, MCU architectures, and boards (2) Extension of the device and cloud network facilities (3) Improvement in the stack with a native connection to decentralized security (4) Development of new sensors, actuator, and industrial protocol interfacing libraries
THREE DIMENSIONAL VORONOI DIAGRAM-BASED SELF DEPLOYMENT ALGORITHM IN loT SENSOR NETWORKS [23]	The proposed algorithm guarantees uses device authorization and data encryption for securing data in the network	The algorithm is quite focused and global information is deprived of it	As a future scope of work Optimization of the algorithm can be done in order to adapt heterogeneous IoT networks

15.9 Security Issues and Challenges

Security is still the key for an IoT network with the concern of paramount data security. With more IoT applications becoming a trend via cloud providers, adding devices connected to each other will become a matter of a click, which will eventually create tremendous security issues in an IoT network. In the coming time, security issues will dominate as opposed to development and innovations. Some of the key security issues which are getting attention are:

More Dangerous Attacks: In recent botnets have used the drawbacks of IoT devices and used them to send much traffic to unsuspected websites. With the involution of computation power of the hijacker, attacks against IoT devices targeting critical infrastructure such as the power critical infrastructure may evolve. Most of the critical infrastructures which bridge the gap between our digital and physical world are outdated and not well equipped to handle attacks on them. Recent studies have shown that much of such system run on outdated software leaving them open to destructive malware and other such targeted attacks.

Increase in IoT Based Financial Crime: Electronic payment is getting popular and convenient now a days. Companies involved in electronic payment may witness a rise in financial crime and identity fraud. Fraud detection using deep learning can be utilized for early detection of unwanted signals.

Machine Phishing: Hackers may infiltrate into IoT devices and communication channel to send false signal which may force owners to take precautionary measures which can be damaging.

With a day by day increment in number of IoT device operating in uncontrolled, complex and insecure environment, securing the overall IoT system presents a number of unique challenges.

Secure Constrained Devices: IoT devices in general have limited amount of resources, storage and low computing power. Traditional encryption protocols are not suitable for these devices as real time transmission of data using the traditional and complex encryption mechanism is much time consuming. IoT devices are as such prone to many side channel attacks. To make up for these device limitations, IoT devices must be secured through multiple layers of protection.

Authorization and Authentication of Devices: Device authorization and authentication is a critical challenge, with many a device showing signs of failures within an IoT system. Identity matching mechanism must be used in order to establish a secure connection between devices and allow them to propagate through gateway of services and apps. The manufacturer must ensure that the end user copes up well with the prescribed limit of device authentication password.

Manage Device Updates: This is the most of challenges to update regularly the security patches and apply to the software running on IoT devices. A proper monitoring of different available updates and consequently applying them to the distributed environment should be done.

Secure Communication: Once the devices are secured, the next important challenge is to secure the communicating links between the IoT devices and cloud services or applications. The recommended practice is to encrypt the messages apriori and adapt standards like TSL.

Ensure Data Privacy and Integrity: The storage and protection of data once it is done with transmission must be done securely. Data privacy includes information hiding of the data before it is stored or using data separation to break up the data into two and extract the personally identifiable information from the payload.

15.10 Conclusion

Adapting a multi-layered architecture to ensure data and device protection is very essential with the growing threat of security breach in an IoT network. The vulnerabilities of an IoT system can be utilized with ease to break into the security channel as well as the connected devices of the distributed network.

Incorporating security mechanisms such as authentication and encryption can partly secure the devices and data, but cannot solely secure the whole system. There are a number of security issues and challenges which must be addresses with proper risk assessment process in order to make the hackers incompetent breaking into the IoT system.

Current security research trends suggest the focus on developing a trust model and blockchain based techniques to secure the devices and transmission of data. Further, securing the communication channel is also a way to provide confidentiality and integrity of data in an IoT network.

References

1. The Statistics Portal: Internet of Things (IoT) connected devices installed base worldwide from 2015 to 2025 (in billions) (2019). [Online]. Available: https://www.statista.com/statistics/471264/iot-number-of-connected-devices-worldwide/
2. Baker, S., Xiang, W., Atkinson, I.: Internet of Things for smart healthcare: technologies, challenges, and opportunities. IEEE Access **5**, 26521–26544 (2017)
3. Banka, S., Madan, I., Saranya: Smart Healthcare monitoring using IoT. Int. J. Appl. Eng. Res. **13**(15), 11984–11989 (2018)
4. Joshitta, R.S.M., Arockiam, L.: Security in IoT environment: a survey. Int. J. Inf. Technol. Mech. Eng. IJITME **2**(7), 1–8 (2016)
5. Madhugundu, D.K., Ahmed, F., Roy, B.: A survey on security issues and challenges in IoT based smart home. In: Proceedings of 3rd International Conference on Internet of Things and Connected Technologies (ICIoTCT), pp. 423–427 (2018)
6. Gou, Q., Yan, L., Liu, Y., Li, Y.: Construction and strategies in IoT security system. In: IEEE International Conference on Green Computing and Communications and IEEE Internet of Things and IEEE Cyber, Physical and Social Computing, pp. 1129–1132 (2013)
7. Zhou, W., Zhang, Y., Liu, P.: The effect of IoT new features on security and privacy: new threats, existing solutions, and challenges yet to be solved. IEEE Internet of Things J. 1–11 (2018)

8. Nandhini, R., Aparna, R., Srilakshmi, P.: Study on security issues in Internet of Things. In: Proceedings of International Conference on Social Impact of Internet of Things (IoT)- Boon or Bane, pp. 130–134 (2018)
9. Suo, H., Wan, J., Zou, C., Liu, J.: Security in the Internet of Things: a review. In: Proceedings of International Conference on Computer Science and Electronics Engineering, pp. 648–651 (2012)
10. Suchitra, C., Vandana, C.P.: Internet of Things and security issues. Int. J. Comput. Sci. Mob. Comput. **5**(1), 133–139 (2016)
11. Vippalapalli, V., Ananthula, S.: Internet of things (IoT) based smart health care system. In: International Conference on Signal Processing, Communication, Power and Embedded System (SCOPES), pp. 1229–1233 (2016)
12. IoT Security Foundations. https://www.iotsecurityfoundation.org/. Accessed 3 May 2019
13. Noor, M., Hasan, W.H.: Current research on Internet of Things (IoT) security: a survey. Comput. Netw. **148**, 283–294 (2019)
14. Blythe, J.M., Johnson S.D.: The consumer security index for loT: a protocol for developing an index to improve- customer decision making and to incentivize greater security in loT devices. In: Proceedings of the conference on Living in the Internet of Things: Cybersecurity of the IoT, pp. 1–7 (2018)
15. Chung, B., Kim, J., Jeon, Y.: On-demand security configuration for loT devices. In: Proceedings of International Conference on Information and Communication Technology Convergence (ICTC), IEEE, vol. 8, no. 16, pp. 1082–1084 (2016)
16. Roderick, H., Secure, C.: Solving the security challenges of loT with public key cryptography. Netw. Secur. **2019**(1), 17–19 (2019)
17. Ainane, N., Ouzzif, M., Bouragba, K.: Data security of smart cities. In: Proceedings of the 3rd International Conference on Smart City Applications (2018)
18. Chen, K., Zhang, S., Li, Z., Yi, Z., Deng, Q., Ray, S., Jin, Y.: Internet-of-Things securities and vulnerabilities: taxonomy, challenges and practice. J. Hardw. Syst. Secur. **2**(2), 97–110 (2018)
19. Yoon, S., Kim, J.: Remote security management server for loT devices. In: International Conference on Information and Communication Technology Convergence (ICTC), IEEE, pp. 1162–1164 (2017)
20. Chze, P.L.R., Leong, K.S.: A secure multi-hop routing for loT communications. In: IEEE World Forum on Internet of Things (WF-IoT), pp. 428–432 (2014)
21. Minoli, D., Occhiogrosso, B.: Blockchain mechanisms for loT security. Internet of Things **1**(2), 1–13 (2018)
22. Mazzei, D., Balldi, G., Montelisciani, G., Fantoni, G.: A full stack for quick prototyping of loT Solutions. In: 2018, Cloudification of the Internet of Things (CIoT), IEEE, pp. 1–5 (2016)
23. Tang, X., Anbar, H., Minji, W.: Three–dimensional Vorinoi diagram-based self-deployment algorithm in loT sensor networks. Ann Telecommun. 1–13 (2018)

The manufacturer's authorised representative in the EU is Springer Nature Customer Service Centre GmbH, Europaplatz 3, 69115 Heidelberg, Germany. If you have any concerns regarding our products, please contact ProductSafety@springernature.com

Printed and bound by CPI Group (UK) Ltd, Croydon, CR0 4YY
30/09/2026
02225693-0004